BRADY

Essentials
of Prehospital
Maternity Care

Bonnie Urquhart Gruenberg
CNM, MSN, RN, EMT-P

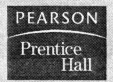

PEARSON
Prentice
Hall

Upper Saddle River, New Jersey 07458

Publisher: Julie Levin Alexander
Publisher's Assistant: Regina Bruno
Executive Editor: Marlene McHugh Pratt
Senior Acquisitions Editor: Stephen Smith
Senior Managing Editor
  for Development: Lois Berlowitz
Associate Editor: Monica Moosang
Editorial Assistant: Diane Edwards
Executive Marketing Manager: Katrin Beacom
Director of Marketing: Karen Allman
Marketing Coordinator: Michael Sirinides
Director of Production and
  Manufacturing: Bruce Johnson
Managing Production Editor: Patrick Walsh
Production Liaison: Julie Li
Production Editor: Lisa S. Garboski, bookworks
Media Product Manager: John Jordan
Manager of Media Production: Amy Peltier
New Media Project Manager: Tina Rudowski
Manufacturing Manager: Ilene Sanford

Manufacturing Buyer: Pat Brown
Senior Design Coordinator: Cheryl Asherman
Interior Designer: Amy Rosen
Cover Designer: Michael Ginsberg
Cover Image: Custom Medical Stock
Photo Director, Image Resource Center: Melinda Reo
Manager, Rights and Permissions: Zina Arabia
Manager, Visual Research: Beth Brenzel
Manager, Cover Visual Research
  and Permissions: Karen Sanatar
Image Permission Coordinator: Jennifer Puma
Composition: The GTS Companies/York, PA Campus
Printing and Binding: R.R. Donnelley & Sons,
  Harrisonburg
Cover Printer: Phoenix Color Corporation

Pearson Education LTD
Pearson Education Singapore, Pte. Ltd
Pearson Education Canada, Ltd
Pearson Education—Japan
Pearson Education Australia PTY, Limited

Pearson Education North Asia Ltd
Pearson Educación de Mexico, S.A. de C.V.
Pearson Education Malaysia, Pte. Ltd
Pearson Education, Upper Saddle River, New Jersey

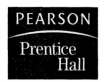

10 9 8 7 6 5 4 3 2 1
ISBN 0-13-119990-0

Contents

Chapter 6   Normal Delivery Management   149

Chapter 7   Maternal and Fetal Complications of Labor and Delivery   177

Chapter 8   Postpartum Adaptation   209

Chapter 9   The Neonate   225

Chapter 10   The High-Risk Neonate   247

Chapter 11   Gynecology   289

Preface

Working as an urban paramedic, I became keenly aware of the need for improved education in emergency obstetrics, gynecology, and neonatology. Many ambulance calls involved situations never covered in textbooks or formal training. When I looked for books on these topics specifically written for EMS personnel, I was astonished to find that none existed. After earning an MSN from the University of Pennsylvania and becoming a certified nurse-midwife and OB-GYN nurse practitioner, I embarked upon filling this gap.

Essentials of Prehospital Maternity Care seeks to explain current principles and practices in obstetrics, gynecology, and neonatology with all the thoroughness expected in the classroom while maintaining strict applicability to emergencies in the field. It also emphasizes the holistic, patient-empowering approach that is finally commanding a central role in many disciplines of health care.

Pregnancy brings about a complete redefinition of a woman's concept of self and a reordering of her life. Childbirth is a pivotal moment, a rite of passage that transforms a woman into a mother. The health care provider who shepherds her through these transitions connects with her at a level at which social artifice is suspended and physical boundaries disappear.

Within these pages, underlying all the clinical information, medical facts, and careful research, burns my abiding passion for the subject. Working with pregnant women is a joy and a challenge, one that forges a vital connection between provider and patient. It is ameliorating the pain of the woman in labor and welcoming newborn infants with gentle hands. It is the rapid, rhythmic whoosh of fetal hearts and the undulations of maternal bellies. It is steadying the woman on her emotional roller coaster. It requires investment of time and energy, mind and heart, and its crises demand skill and expertise. Its reward is life itself.

This is what I hope to transmit to the EMS professional above all else—the love, the wonder, the realization of privilege. This book will prepare you to facilitate the natural process of birth and stand ready to intervene should complications arise. But I hope that it will also nurture an abiding sense of awe.

Note: In this text, the fetus and newborn are referred to as male to avoid pronoun confusion with the mother.

Acknowledgments

Because every writer is shaped by the people in his or her life, every book is a product not only of individual effort but also of countless influences, connections, and interactions. Many people in my life made this book possible by supporting, helping, and encouraging me.

Alex Gruenberg has been a blessing through the creation of this book. Most of the text was written while I worked 45 to 116 hours per week as a midwife. Often I put in a frenetic day seeing patients in the office, came home, and wrote for hours before bed. As deadlines approached, Alex supported my creative endeavors by tending to mundane chores so that I might immerse myself in the project. He is a constant, loving presence, listening to my concerns when I come home exhausted from a long delivery, augmenting my productivity, and providing a revitalizing counterbalance to the stresses of life.

Alex's participation marks prodigious growth for him. When we first met, he professed exceptional squeamishness. But within several months, he could tolerate graphic birthing tales without flinching. Recently I recounted a dramatic hemorrhage over dinner, and he never put down his fork. To my abundant joy, he even saw fit to commit irrevocably to this lifestyle—we were married the summer of 2004.

John Bryans has been indescribably helpful in helping me to negotiate the complicated world of book publishing. His schedule is hectic, but he has always made time to help me and allay my concerns. I value his expertise, his generosity, his unceasing willingness to assist me, and his friendship.

Stephen Smith and Monica Moosang, my main contacts at Prentice Hall, have performed admirably despite joining this project halfway through—a feat similar to building an airplane in flight.

The Plymouth Volunteer Ambulance Corps of Plymouth, Connecticut, kindly posed for some of the illustrations in this book. Special thanks to Diane Croce, Rebecca Achilli, Ryan Rigon, Lisa McCoy (and her son, Noah), Lindsay Smith, Chris Smith, Becky Rancourt, and my dear friend Skip Mudge. Skip and Becky coordinated the photo shoot and have been supportive and enthusiastic about this project. Longtime friend Michael Levesque, who delivered many babies in the field despite being totally unnerved by laboring women, always offers me a place to stay on my many ventures back to Connecticut.

My deepest appreciation goes to my colleagues at Lake Erie Women's Center in Erie, Pennsylvania: my midwife partners Peggy Boyd, Jennifer Bozza, and Kelli Gevas; obstetricians Greg Ballengee, Peter Levinson, Mark Townsend, Lakshmi Vemulapalli, and Elizabeth Wise; nurse practitioners Rosemarie Malek, Lynn McGrath, and Lyn Straub; Diana Zenewicz, who keeps the practice in balance and helps us in countless ways, always with an optimistic smile; and nurses, medical assistants, and other staff. All are knowledgeable resources and support-ive friends.

The nurses at Hamot Medical Center in Erie are a godsend. As I de-veloped professionally, they supported, nurtured, and advised me. As I worked on the manuscript during odd hours between births, they shared ideas, ferreted out reference material, and encouraged me. Their company is one reason I look forward to my days on call.

My instructors at University of Pennsylvania helped lay the founda-tions of this book, and I wish to thank them, especially Wendy Grube, Kate McHugh, Barbara Reale, Marilyn Stringer, Bill McCool, and Dawn Durain. Phyllis Block oversaw most of my clinical training, and under her wise, patient tutelage I developed confidence and proficiency. Kathleen Raffleur and Ruth Schlegel were also instrumental in my clinical education.

My own mother, Joyce Urquhart, deserves special thanks for more than the obvious reason. She loves babies and birth almost as much as I do, appreciates my work, and applauds all that I undertake.

And of course my deep appreciation goes to the women whom I am privileged to serve. With every birth, office visit, and significant interac-tion, they help me learn, grow, and become a better provider.

Reviewers

MARY E. MAKRIS, EMT-P, MPH
Associate Professor
Texas Tech University Health Sciences Center
Lubbock, TX

KATHERINE P. RICKEY, NREMT-P; EMS I/C
Barnstead, NH

MARK A. SIMPSON, CCEMT-P; NREMT-P; RN
Muscle Shoals, AL

RHONDA M. WATSON, PARAMEDIC
Troy, NC

About the Author

Bonnie Urquhart Gruenberg is a native of Southington, Connecticut. She entered EMS in 1987 and worked full-time for more than a dozen years, first as an EMT, then as a paramedic in various Connecticut localities. She obtained her BSN at Southern Vermont College in Bennington, Vermont, graduating as valedictorian. She then attended graduate school at the University of Pennsylvania, where she earned a double master's degree as a certified nurse-midwife and an obstetrics and gynecology nurse practitioner. Her training included high-risk obsterics in a Harrisburg hospital and delivering Amish babies at home by gas lamp in Lancaster County. She currently practices as a certified nurse-midwife in Erie, Pennsylvania. Her first book, *Hoofprints in the Sand: Wild Horses of the Atlantic Coast,* was published by Eclipse Press in 2002.

She is a self-taught artist whose paintings and photography express a reverence for life, the vitality reflected in the flash of galloping hooves or the eyes of a newborn child. She also enjoys Web design and has written articles for publications as different as *Equus* and the *American Journal of Nursing.* Long years as an urban paramedic have taught Bonnie that nobody is promised a tomorrow, so she tries to milk every bit of living out of each day. She also enjoys horseback riding and cherishes her time on the trail with her horse, Fancy (The Pone). She is the mother to grown sons Mark Bryan Scianna and Keith Scianna and wife to Alex Gruenberg.

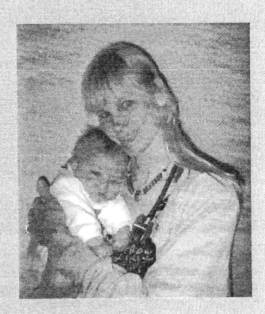

CHAPTER 1

The Woman
and the Fetus

Objectives

By the end of this chapter you should be able to

- Describe the basic structure and function of the female reproductive system

- Describe the common malformations of the female reproductive tract

- Explain the major points of fetal development through each of the three trimesters

- Explain how common complaints of pregnancy relate to physiological changes

CASE
Study

Just after sunrise, Yolanda and Victor parked the ambulance behind the apartment building and climbed the stairs to apartment 306. The woman who answered the door introduced herself as Julia. She was 24 weeks' pregnant, and she had called for an ambulance after finding pink stains on the toilet paper after urinating. She was reasonably sure that the blood had come from her vagina, and she was very worried although she was not experiencing any pain. Her obstetrician had cautioned her to have any bleeding evaluated right away. Her husband was at work with the car, and she had no other way to reach the hospital.

Victor took a rapid history and discovered that this was Julia's seventh pregnancy and that this was the longest she had carried any of them. The other six had spontaneously aborted without warning, often in the second trimester. "I have a unicornuate uterus," Julia explained. "I probably will never make it to full term, but my doctor thinks that I can carry this one until it is mature enough to survive outside the womb. We have been doing weekly ultrasound scans. The baby is growing, and my cervix has stayed long and closed."

Victor learned that she had undergone a digital cervical examination in the office the day before. He knew that the bleeding could have been related to the exam and did not necessarily herald another pregnancy loss. Examination of Julia's abdomen revealed palpable fetal movement and no obvious contractions. "I might have been having some painless tightenings and pelvic pressure last night," Julia said. "I'm not sure. It didn't really affect my sleep." She offered to walk down the stairs, but the EMTs cautioned her that it was inadvisable to let her walk, and she was carried down in a stair chair. They positioned her in a left lateral position on the stretcher and checked her perineum for additional bleeding and signs of imminent delivery. There were none. Her vital signs were 108/60, 88, and 20. The ambulance did not carry a Doppler, and fetal heart tones were inaudible with a stethoscope, but fetal movement was both palpated by the crew and reported by the mother.

Questions

1. What is a unicornuate uterus? What risks does it pose to mother and fetus?
2. Yolanda and Victor guessed the positioning of the fetus upon hearing Julia's history. What fetal presentation is likely and why?
3. If Julia is about to deliver, what can Yolanda and Victor expect of a 24-week fetus. Is it viable? How large should it be?
4. Julia denies pain, and there are no obvious contractions. Could Julia be in labor?

Introduction

Of all the wondrous workings of the human body, reproduction may be the most awe inspiring. It is amazing that the union of two microscopic cells from two individuals can produce a new unique person in a matter of months. The embryo develops according to ancient blueprints with no external direction and grows into an infant with organ systems and a complex metabolism that sustains life outside the protection of the uterus. It is a process that encompasses profound changes in not only the fetus but also the mother who sustains it to viability.

Women and girls make up roughly half the population, substantially more in some locations and age groups. Prehospital health care providers often encounter pregnancy, birth, spontaneous abortion, sexual assault, and numerous other obstetrical and gynecological issues. In order to recognize deviations from normal, it is essential for the EMS professional to understand the structure and function of female anatomy and the basics of fetal development.

Female Internal Reproductive Anatomy and Physiology

Ovaries

The female gonads, known as ovaries, lie on either side of the pelvis and are attached by a fold of tissue to the posterior broad ligament of the uterus. See Figures 1-1 and 1-2. They are also connected to the uterus by the ovarian ligament and to the pelvic wall by the suspensory ligament. Mature ovaries are oval shaped and range from 2 to 5 cm long and 1.3 to 3.0 cm wide. A full bladder can significantly displace the ovaries anteriorly and superiorly.

A woman's ovaries produce ova and hormones crucial to sexual development and function—chiefly estrogen, progesterone, and testosterone. Estrogen is primarily responsible for female secondary sex characteristics and cyclic changes in the vaginal epithelium and the endometrium of the uterus. Progesterone is responsible for changes in the uterine lining to prepare for the implantation of the conceptus, development of the placenta after implantation, and breast development. Testosterone in females influences sex drive and is necessary for other bodily functions.

Each ovary consists of several important structures. The hilus is the entry point for blood vessels and nerves. The cortex contains ova, primordial and developing follicles, the corpus luteum, and a connective

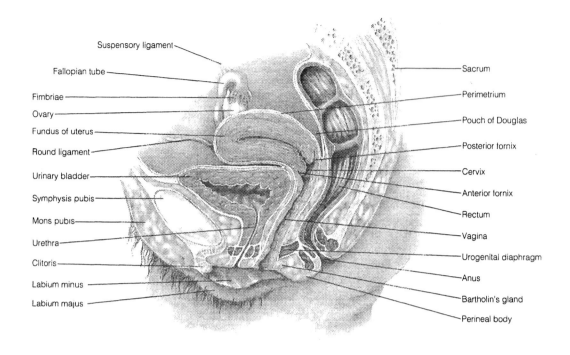

FIGURE 1-1

Female Internal Reproductive Organs.

A nonpregnant woman, side view in cross section. In most women, the uterus is anteverted or anteflexed; that is, it leans forward over the bladder. A retroverted or retroflexed uterus tilts toward the sacrum. The nonpregnant uterus is normally not palpable above the pubic bone.

tissue, the theca. The cortex surrounds the medulla, which contains nerves, blood vessels, lymphatic tissue, and smooth muscles.

Ovaries are homologous to the testes; the tissue that develops into the ovaries in a female embryo becomes the testes in the male, and both testes and ovaries have the same function: producing gametes (sex cells) and hormones.

The ovaries of a female fetus at 20 weeks' gestation contain more ova than she will ever have again in her life—about 5 million–7 million. From then through menopause, many of these ova die. By the time of her birth, she will have about 2 million ova. By puberty, only 300,000–400,000 will remain. Thereafter, with each menstrual cycle about 18–20 oocytes will begin to ripen within follicles—of which only one per cycle will ripen and release. Over her lifetime she will ovulate an average of 400 times. By menopause, about age 50, her ovaries will contain few, if any, ova.

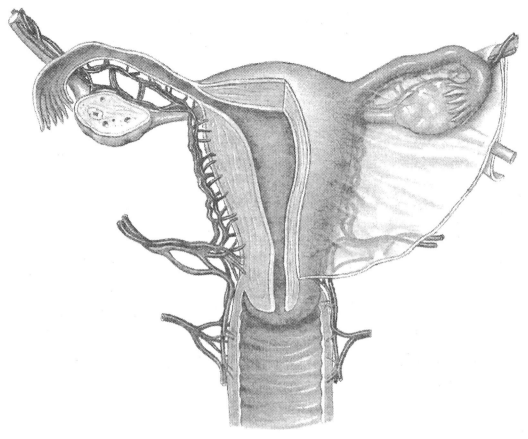

FIGURE 1-2
The Uterus.
Blood supply to female reproductive organs have a rich blood supply that increases greatly during pregnancy.

Fallopian Tubes

The fallopian tubes, or oviducts, are hollow structures about 10 cm (4 in.) long connecting the ovaries to the uterus. The interstitial portion, the passage from the proximal end of the tube into the uterus, is only 1 mm in diameter—the width of a pencil lead. The distal end is larger, funnel-shaped, and fringed with projections called fimbriae that intercept the ova upon ovulation. The ampulla comprises the outer two-thirds of the tube and is the site of fertilization. The lining of the fallopian tubes produces a protein-rich fluid that transports and nourishes the ovum, and ciliated cells and peristaltic contractions propel the ovum toward the uterus. Any delay or malfunction of this mechanism or obstruction from scarring or malformation can result in the conceptus implanting in the tube instead of the uterus (ectopic pregnancy).

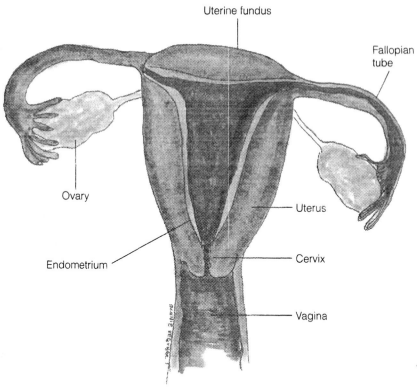

Uterine fundus

Fallopian tube

Ovary

Uterus

Endometrium

Cervix

Vagina

FIGURE 1-3
Female Reproductive Organs.
In the nonpregnant state, a woman's internal reproductive organs reside within the pelvis. Major organs and structures include ovaries, fallopian tubes, uterus, and vagina.
Illustration by Bonnie U. Gruenberg

Uterus

The nonpregnant uterus (womb), which sustains the fetus to viability, is located deep within the female pelvis. See Figure 1-3. (By the end of pregnancy, the uterus expands until it reaches the xyphoid process.) In the adult it is about the size and shape of a small, flattened pear, but it has an unparalleled facility for growth and expansion. Before pregnancy, its capacity is about 10 ml, but in a full-term pregnancy its capacity increases to 5,000 ml or more. Enlargement of existing muscle cells produces most uterine growth in pregnancy; but these cells also increase in number, and connective tissues become more elastic.

The uterus is secured by three groups of supports. The broad and round ligaments stabilize the upper parts. The cardinal pubocervical and uterosacral ligaments support the central part. The muscles of the pelvic floor provide a secure base for the uterus and lower reproductive tract. Only the cervix is stabilized laterally, allowing the body of the uterus mobility.

The uterus often inclines anteriorly, over the bladder (anteverted); but it may tilt backward or lie on the midline instead. The position of the uterus is influenced by parity (number of children she has birthed), bladder and rectal distention, posture, and muscle tone.

The uppermost part of the uterus, above the attachment of the fallopian tubes, is the **fundus.** The main body of the uterus is the corpus. The narrow, elastic neck of the uterus is the cervix. In a nonpregnant woman, its os (opening) barely admits a cotton swab, but in childbirth it must stretch to 10 cm wide. With pregnancy it becomes the lower uterine segment. During labor the lower uterine segment and cervix do not actively contract, but are stretched thin by the action of the upper uterine musculature. Most cesarean births involve incision through the lower uterine segment.

The cervical canal is lined with columnar ciliated epithelium that contains mucus-secreting glands. At ovulation, these glands secrete copious clear, alkaline mucus to facilitate the passage of sperm to the upper reproductive tract. At other stages of the menstrual cycle, cervical mucus becomes thick, sticky, and acidic, inhibiting the passage of sperm. Cervical mucus also lubricates the vagina and retards bacterial growth.

The uterus consists of three layers of involuntary (smooth) muscle. The muscle fibers of the outer layer run longitudinally, mostly over the fundus. During labor, every rhythmic contraction of this layer shortens the muscle fibers in the fundus, causing the muscle to thicken in the upper part of the uterus and become thinner in the lower uterine segment, expelling the fetus. In the middle layer, muscle fibers interlace in a figure-eight pattern. Large blood vessels pass through this mesh, and contraction of the uterus after delivery serves to compress these vessels to reduce bleeding, like crimping a hose to stop the flow. The innermost layer of musculature is composed of circular fibers that form sphincters at openings of the fallopian tubes and cervix. This layer helps to keep the cervix closed in pregnancy and prevents menstrual blood from flowing into the fallopian tubes.

fundus
The uppermost part of the uterus, between and above the openings of the fallopian tubes.

PEARLS Most uterine bleeding after childbirth is controlled by uterine compression and loops of muscle tightening around blood vessels, not by clotting mechanisms. Women with low platelets and other clotting deficiencies often lose no more blood than do other women during delivery.

endometrium
The mucous membrane lining the uterus.

The uterus is lined with a mucosal layer, the **endometrium,** which proliferates and degenerates in response to the monthly cycle of hormonal stimulation. The endometrium is composed of columnar epithelium laden with branching coiled glands and blood vessels that respond to estrogen and progesterone stimulation. The upper layers of the endometrium are shed in the menses every month if conception does not occur. The uterus is richly supplied with blood and lymphatic vessels, and perfusion increases in pregnancy.

The uterus is innervated by the autonomic nervous system. Even without an intact nerve supply, it can contract effectively, which is why a paraplegic woman will start labor normally, though she may be unable to bear down in the second stage. The pain of contractions is transmitted though the 11th and 12th thoracic nerve roots, but the pudendal and ilioinguinal nerves carry vaginal and cervical pain sensations. The motor fibers for pushing originate within the 7th and 8th thoracic vertebrae.

Vagina

The vagina, from a Latin word meaning "sheath," is a muscular tube, lined with mucous membrane, extending from the external genitals to the uterus. It accepts a penis during coitus and stretches to accommodate an infant head during childbirth. It is also the conduit for menstrual flow to leave the body.

The walls of the vagina are ridged with folds of tissue (rugae) that allow it to stretch during parturition (childbirth). Whereas the lower third of the vagina is richly innervated and sensitive to stimulation and pain, the upper vagina is relatively insensitive to either, though it can perceive pressure. After childbirth, lacerations to the upper vagina are usually painless and often do not require local anesthetic for repair. Injuries to the vaginal introitus, however, are extremely sensitive. The upper part of the vagina is termed the vaginal vault, and the area around the cervix is the fornix.

The hymen is a thin ring or partial ring of tissue surrounding or partly occluding the vaginal opening. An intact hymen is not a reliable indicator of virginity. The hymen can be torn by strenuous physical activity, trauma as from a bicycle accident, riding horses bareback, tampon use, or certain masturbation practices. Some women are born with hymens that never cover the vaginal opening. In childbirth, the hymen often ruptures into numerous hymenal tags that remain for life.

The vagina keeps bacteria away from the upper reproductive tract through several mechanisms. A continuous flow of moist secretions washes bacteria away, especially at the end of pregnancy. Many species of microorganisms live in the warm, dark, moist environment of the vagina, and they generally remain in balance. Beneficial bacteria such as *Lactobacilli* break down the glycogen secreted by the vaginal epithelial cells and produce lactic acid, which retards the growth of more harmful microorganisms. During the reproductive years, a healthy vagina has a pH of about 4.0–5.0. Use of systemic antibiotics, douches, and scented feminine products can upset the microbial balance and allow other organisms to dominate and cause infection.

Pregnancy and childbirth effect permanent changes in a woman's anatomy. After pregnancy the uterus, for example, will be larger, and after vaginal delivery the cervical os will change from round to slit like.

Bony Pelvis

The pelvis serves to protect several vital organs and support upright posture and ambulation. In girls and women, it is constructed to allow passage of an infant through its bony hollow. The pelvis comprises four bones held together by ligaments. The lateral margins are the innominate (hip) bones. Each innominate bone consists of a pubis, an ischium, and an ilium. These join anteriorly at the symphysis pubis and articulate with the sacrum in the back, at the sacroiliac joints. The coccyx, which loosely joins the lower edge of the sacrum, performs no clear function, but it can fracture during childbirth. In most quadrupedal (four-legged) mammals, offspring pass easily through a simple pelvic ring at birth. When humans became bipeds, the pelvis changed to accommodate upright posture, pushing the pubic bone forward and the sacrum down. Human infants must pass the sacrum and pubis simultaneously, making birth more difficult. To compensate, the previously rigid pelvic joints loosen in pregnancy, becoming hinges that shift and separate during birth. One cannot determine pelvic adequacy from the appearance of a woman's hips. A woman with a broad hips may have a narrow pelvic passage and vice versa. See Figure 1-4.

The doctor or midwife assesses the maternal pelvis early in pregnancy and again at term, measuring the distances between bony landmarks and determining the shape of the pelvic passage to anticipate possible problems during delivery.

There are four basic female pelvic shapes that are not specific to race or population. The internal configuration of pelvic bones is important during childbirth because it strongly influences what position and mechanism of birth the fetus will adopt.

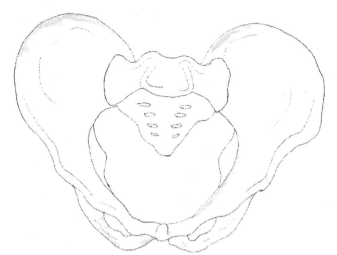

FIGURE 1-4
The Pelvis.
The shape of the female pelvis is influenced by racial heritage and individual variations. A pelvis optimal for birthing has a roomy central passage and few bony obstructions, but the true test is how well it accommodates the fetus in question. Pelvises of all shapes have the capacity to expand in childbirth. A woman with a narrow pelvic opening may have no difficulty delivering small, well-positioned babies.
Illustration by Bonnie U. Gruenberg

The gynecoid pelvis is ideal for childbearing—roomy in all dimensions with minimal bony projections obstructing the passage. The anthropoid pelvis is most common among non-Caucasian women (40.5%, but only 23.5% of Caucasian women) and is deeper than it is wide. The android pelvis (occurring in 32.5% of Caucasian women and 15.7% of others) is similar in many ways to the male pelvis, with a heart-shaped pelvic inlet, narrow pubic arch, and encroaching ischial spines, all of which can obstruct birth. The platypelloid pelvis (occurring in 3% of all women) is wider than it is deep and is not well suited to vaginal delivery.

deflexed
Not flexed, partially or completely extended. In a deflexed fetus, the chin is not pressed against the chest, potentially making birth more difficult by presenting a wider portion of the head to the pelvic inlet.

The EMS provider does not evaluate pelvic architecture in the field, but awareness of the different pelvic shapes can lend insights during labor and delivery. Babies often negotiate the pelvis however they fit it best. If a baby unexpectedly emerges with his shoulders in transverse position, you may conclude that the woman's pelvis probably has platypelloid tendencies. If a woman has been pushing for a long time and the fetus is not visible, one reason for her lack of progress may be a bony obstruction. If this is so, no amount of pushing will produce a vaginal delivery.

It is also important to remember that maternal pelvic shape is only one part of the bony equation. The other is the fetal skull. A small baby in a good position may have no difficulty negotiating a small pelvis. A large baby who holds his head tilted and **deflexed** may have trouble coming through a roomy pelvis.

External Reproductive Anatomy

The external female genitals are termed the vulva, including the mons pubis, labia, clitoris, vaginal vestibule, and associated structures. The appearance of female genitals varies greatly between individuals.

In a woman, the front of the symphysis pubis is covered by a rounded mound of soft, fatty tissue called the mons pubis. It serves to cushion this sensitive area during sexual intercourse. The adult woman's mons pubis is covered with pubic hair, usually in a triangular pattern, but almost diamond-shaped in some women.

Labia majora are the fleshy, hairy outer lips of the vulvar cleft that merge at the perineum. They are homologous to the scrotum in males and arise from the same tissue in the embryo. They serve to protect the more delicate structures that lie beneath them. Labial varicosities are not uncommon during pregnancy, especially in the third trimester, when the weight of the fetus and uterus restricts venous return from the vulva.

PEARLS Labial varicosities can rupture, especially in childbirth, causing a hemorrhage that may be difficult to control. Firm, direct pressure and application of ice will often stop the bleeding.

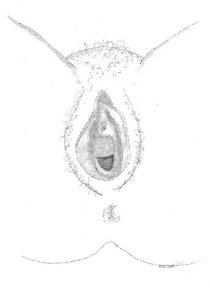

FIGURE 1-5
External Female Genitalia.
A woman's genitals show great individual variation. Labia minora may be small and hidden, long and exposed, or asymmetrical. The clitoris may be covered by a large, fleshy hood, or it may be small and inconspicuous. The urethral meatus may be distinctive or difficult to identify.
Illustration by Bonnie U. Gruenberg

Labia minora, or inner lips, are soft, moist, sensitive structures bordered laterally by the labia majora and merging below the vaginal opening. The surfaces of the labia are mucous membrane, and their interior contains erectile tissue, connective tissue, and abundant blood vessels and nerves. They are very sensitive to touch and pain, and they engorge with blood during sexual arousal. Sebaceous glands on the inner labia lubricate and waterproof the vulva and resist bacteria. Size, shape, and symmetry vary widely among women.

The clitoris is analogous to the penis and is as rich with blood vessels and nerve endings. The clitoris is the only organ in the body of either sex that exists purely to deliver pleasurable sensations. The glans of the clitoris is partially sheltered by a tent of labial tissue called the prepuce or clitoral hood. This is analogous to the male foreskin. Much of the clitoral body is buried in the vulvar flesh—only the tip is exposed. See Figure 1-5.

The vaginal vestibule is bordered by the labia minora and contains the introitus (vaginal opening), the urethral meatus, paired Skene's glands that lubricate during arousal, and two Bartholin's glands, also for secreting mucus.

 PEARLS Bartholin's glands sometimes become infected and form abscesses. This condition presents as painful swelling at the 5 or 7 o'clock position of the vaginal vestibule.

perineum
The area between the vaginal opening and the anus.

The **perineum** is the area between the vaginal opening and the anus. Beneath the perineal skin lie important muscles that support the pelvic floor, which thin and stretch in the second stage of labor to allow the birth of the infant. Most childbirth lacerations involve the perineum. An episiotomy is an incision of the perineum to enlarge the vaginal opening and is not a field procedure.

The mammary glands (breasts) are specialized sebaceous glands capable of producing the milk that can sustain one or more infants through early life. Breast size is determined by the amount of fatty tissue present—most women have similar amounts of glandular tissue and therefore similar capacity for lactation. Breasts, especially nipples, are richly innervated and sensitive to touch, so they are often involved in sexual arousal. See Figure 1-6.

The nipple is composed of erectile tissue and surrounded by the heavily pigmented areola. Fifteen to 20 milk ducts open onto the surface of the nipple, so milk emerges in a shower-spray fashion. The ducts widen into lactiferous sinuses behind the areola, fed by lactiferous ducts that

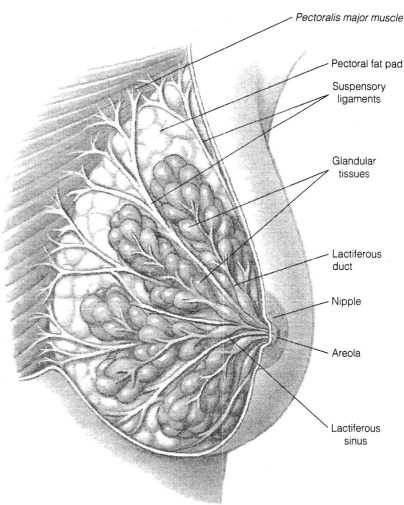

FIGURE 1-6
The Breast.
A woman's breasts function to produce the milk that will sustain her infant for at least the first year of life. The milk is produced by alveoli deep within the breast. The letdown reflex propels milk into the lactiferous sinuses, and the suckling of the infant presses on the sinuses and sends the milk through the nipple.

Pectoralis major muscle

Pectoral fat pad

Suspensory ligaments

Glandular tissues

Lactiferous duct

Nipple

Areola

Lactiferous sinus

drain lobes and lobules deeper in the breast. Tiny alveoli within the lobes produce the milk, and a letdown reflex triggered by the hormone oxytocin propels the milk into the lactiferous sinuses, where the baby can extract it.

Human milk confers incalculable advantages to the infant, many of which science is just beginning to recognize. Breast milk meets the needs of the individual infant. It varies in composition with the time of day, maternal nutrition, gestational age of the infant at birth, and stage of lactation; and it is richer in calories and fat toward the end of the feeding. The breastfed infant receives immunity against many diseases and is less susceptible to many common infections. The chemical composition of breast milk is optimal for neurological development. Consequently, breastfed infants tend to score higher on intelligence tests. Further, the intimacy of breastfeeding can enhance the bond between mother and child. The American Academy of Pediatrics supports breastfeeding for at least the first year of life, though longer breastfeeding confers greater health benefits. In some cultures it is customary to nurse infants to age 3 or 4 years—or even longer.

PEARLS Breastfeeding causes endogenous release of the hormone oxytocin, which both releases milk and contracts the uterus. By putting the baby to breast after delivery, the EMS professional can encourage a boggy (flaccid and toneless) uterus to stay contracted, reducing postpartum blood loss.

Women with Müllerian abnormalities often have problems with infertility, spontaneous abortion, ectopic pregnancy, preterm delivery, fetal growth restriction, uterine rupture, and fetal malpresentations.

Müllerian ducts
A pair of embryonic structures that gives rise to the reproductive organs in the female, but disappears in the male.

In contrast, studies have shown that formula-fed infants in developed countries have higher rates of diarrhea, respiratory infection, otitis media, bacteriemia, bacterial meningitis, urinary tract infection, sudden infant death syndrome, diabetes, adolescent obesity, Crohn's disease, ulcerative colitis (and other chronic digestive diseases), lymphoma, and allergic diseases over a lifetime than do breastfed infants. As a manufactured, bottled, and marketed product, infant formula is also more expensive than breast milk, and its associated packaging and energy consumption have a negative impact on the environment.

Uterine Abnormalities

The uterus is formed by the 10th week of fetal development by the fusion of two structures called **Müllerian ducts.** Fusion begins in the center and proceeds toward the upper and lower segments. A cavity forms in the lower portion, beneath a septum of tissue. This tissue gradually retracts and forms the uterine cavity by the 20th week of gestation. Disruption of this process results in deformities involving a uterus divided entirely or partially by a septum, or separate uterine horns. Other Müllerian abnormalities include absence of the vagina or a vagina partially or completely divided by a septum.

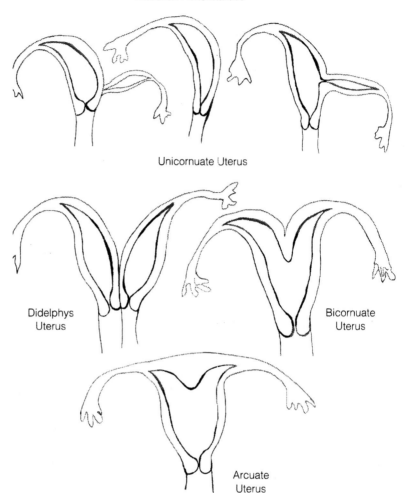

Mullerian Abnormalities

Unicornuate Uterus

Didelphys
Uterus

Bicornuate
Uterus

Arcuate
Uterus

FIGURE 1-7

Müllerian Abnormalities.

Müllerian abnormalities may involve a uterus divided entirely or partially by a septum, separate uterine horns, absence of the vagina, or a vagina divided by a septum.

Illustration by Bonnie U. Gruenberg

There is a wide range of Müllerian abnormalities spanning from subtle to severe, and there may be associated renal and ureteral problems in some patients. It is estimated that 2–3% of women have some type of Müllerian defect, though it appears that only about 1 in 400 of pregnant women will present with this condition at delivery. These statistics probably reflect the high rate of infertility and spontaneous abortion associated with these anomalies. See Figure 1-7.

A woman with a Müllerian defect may have been born with complete or partial agenesis (lack of development) or hypoplasia (underdevelopment) of the vagina, cervix, fundus, fallopian tubes, or any combination of these structures. Women born with these anomalies may be unable to bear children, though a vagina can be surgically created if one is absent.

A unicornuate uterus is a malformation involving a banana-shaped half uterus that may have a rudimentary uterine horn attached. About 51% of pregnancies involving a unicornuate uterus result in spontaneous abortion, and an additional 15% of fetuses are born prematurely, often before or on the cusp of viability. Women with a unicornuate uterus also have a higher rate of ectopic pregnancy, malpresentation, fetal growth restriction, and uterine rupture. The fetus will usually adopt a breech position as he attempts to conform to the narrow confines of the uterine cavity.

The woman with uterine didelphys has two uteri, two cervixes, and usually two vaginas. Each uterus has an associated fallopian tube and ovary. The condition confers the same risks to pregnancy as a unicornuate uterus (as mentioned), but with a slightly higher rate of successful outcome. Didelphys uterus carries a miscarriage rate of 30–40% and a 20% likelihood of preterm delivery, and fully 43% of the fetuses are breech presentation at delivery.

Most Müllerian abnormalities involve either a bicornuate or a septate uterus. With a bicornuate uterus, the woman has a single-chamber cervix and vagina that divides into two separate, but connected uterine cavities. The uterus is divided completely or partially by a muscular septum extending from the fundal region, sometimes as far as the cervical os. When examining the woman with a bicornuate uterus in pregnancy, the provider may feel a notch on the uterine fundus. A similar defect is the septate uterus, which involves a single uterus with a partial or complete midline septum. The rate of pregnancy loss before 20 weeks is 66–70% for complete bicornuate uterus and as high as 88% for septate uterus. The preterm delivery rate is 20% for women with partial bicornuate uterus and higher for complete. Breech presentation is likely.

Surgical correction of Müllerian abnormalities often improves reproductive outcomes. A cerclage procedure is sometimes performed on women with uterine didelphys, unicornuate, or bicornuate uteri and on women with a poorly formed cervix. This involves inserting a suture looped like a drawstring around the cervix to encourage it to stay closed. If a cerclage is still in place while the woman is in active labor, the risk of uterine rupture is increased.

Puberty

At puberty, a girl's secondary sexual characteristics begin to develop, and she gains the ability to reproduce. The timing of puberty is largely genetic, but better nutrition, greater body fat percentage, better general health, and psychological state all speed the onset of puberty. Girls who live close to the equator, in urban settings, and at lower altitudes also experience earlier puberty, as do the blind. Athletic and anorexic girls often have delayed puberty due to low weight and lower body fat percentage. African American girls tend to develop pubertal changes earlier than Caucasian girls. In Western Europe the average age of puberty for girls declined 4 months each decade between 1850 and 1960. This trend, now halted, has been attributed to better nutrition and healthier living conditions. In North America, the average girl attains puberty at about 12 years of age.

The mechanisms that trigger puberty are poorly understood, but maturation clearly involves an interplay of hormones secreted by the hypothalamus, pituitary, and ovaries. Female pubertal changes occur in an orderly sequence over a predictable span, usually about 4.5 years. The first signs are accelerated growth, usually occurring between the ages of 8 and 14, and breast budding, usually between ages 8 and 13, followed by the appearance of pubic hair, another growth spurt, and **menarche** (first menses) between 11 and 14 years. Initial menstrual periods are often irregular and anovulatory (lacking ovulation).

menarche
The beginning of menstruation.

For about the first 8 years of a girl's life, gonadotropin-releasing hormone (GnRH) is secreted in small, infrequent pulsations by the hypothalamus while she sleeps. Pubertal changes begin when the hypothalamus increases these nocturnal GnRH pulses in both amplitude and frequency, causing the pituitary to increase release of follicle-stimulating hormone (FSH) and luteinizing hormone (LH), which had preciously been restricted to very low levels. The ovaries are thus stimulated to produce estrogen, which triggers breast development, vaginal and uterine maturation, skeletal growth, and the female fat distribution that rounds hips and buttocks. Adrenal glands secrete androgens that cause the growth of pubic and axillary hair. Midway through the pubertal process, estrogen has caused the endometrial lining to thicken, and menarche occurs. Girls usually do not begin to ovulate until late in the pubertal process, often a year or more after menarche.

PEDIATRIC
NOTES

Pubescent girls are often embarrassed by and reticent about reproductive issues. Use tact and sensitivity when evaluating obstetric and gynecologic conditions in these patients.

The Menstrual Cycle

Throughout her childbearing years, a woman's fertility occurs in monthly cycles. See Figure 1-8. Although a man produces his gametes, spermatozoa, continuously and in vast quantities, a woman ripens and releases a single ovum per menstrual cycle. The intricacies of the menstrual cycle are complex, and it is beyond the scope of this book to present more than an overview.

Every cycle commences with the goal of initiating a pregnancy. If conception does not occur, the body abandons preparations and begins another attempt. Normal menstrual cycles are generally regarded as averaging 28 days; but only 15% of women have regular 28-day cycles, and normal range is 23–35 days. Age, stress, illness, vigorous exercise, and excessive weight loss can affect the length, regularity, and duration of menstrual cycles.

The reproductive life of the typical American woman is drastically different from that of her forebears. Compared to women who lived dozens, hundreds, or thousands of years ago, she reaches puberty sooner, has fewer children and bears them later in life, breastfeeds for a shorter interval if at all, and lives a significant percentage of her years after the age of menopause. Most women who live in industrialized nations ovulate about 450 times through their reproductive years. Before industrialization women were pregnant or lactating much of their reproductive lives and experienced at least one-third fewer lifetime ovulations. (Present-day women in nonindustrialized nations also tend to ovulate less than their counterparts in America and Western Europe.) In America women of certain subcultures such as the Amish have very large families and have few menstrual periods during the childbearing years. It appears that a prehistoric woman might have ovulated only about 50 times during her shorter life span.

follicular phase
The first part of the ovarian cycle, during which an ovum matures and is released.

The **follicular phase** is the first part of the ovarian cycle, during which an ovum matures and is released. It corresponds with the proliferative phase of the uterine cycle, during which the endometrial glands enlarge, lengthen, and wind in response to rising estrogen levels. The endometrium becomes six to eight times thicker, and cervical mucus becomes thin, clear, elastic, and alkaline to promote the passage of spermatozoa. In most women the follicular/proliferative stage lasts 10–17 days.

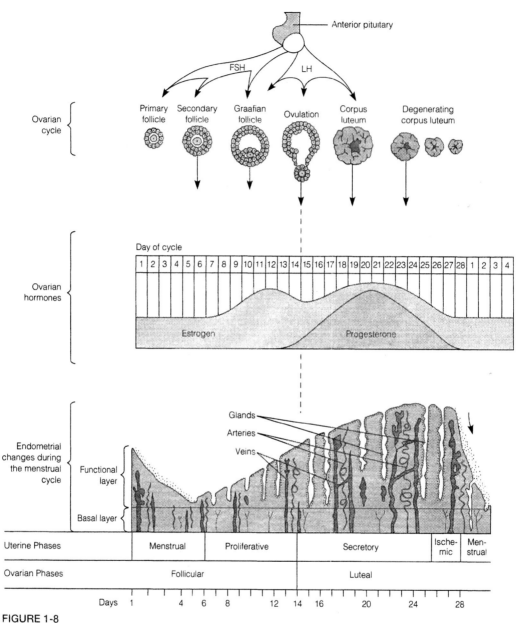

FIGURE 1-8

Female Reproductive Cycle.

Hormonal stimulation causes cyclic changes in the ovaries and the uterine endometrium.

The **luteal phase,** from ovulation to the onset of menses, corresponds with the secretory phase of the uterine cycle, during which estrogen continues to thicken the lining. But progesterone causes the uterine surface to ripple and endometrial glands to coil, dilate, and secrete fluid that can help implantation of a fertilized ovum. The uterus and endometrium become highly vascular, a process that continues if implantation occurs.

The menstrual cycle begins with the hypothalamus, which sends gonadotropin-releasing hormone (GnRH) to the anterior pituitary and prompts it to send follicle-stimulating hormone (FSH) and luteinizing hormone (LH) into the bloodstream. The ovary responds to FSH by producing many follicles at once, beginning the maturation process for an average of 18–20 ova. These follicles secrete increasing levels of estrogen as they grow. This estrogen stimulates the endometrium to proliferate and become thick and vascular to provide a potential implantation site for an embryo.

Rising estrogen levels, through a negative feedback mechanism, tell the pituitary that FSH is no longer needed. This mechanism is similar to a household thermostat: When the room reaches the desired temperature, the thermostat sends a message to the furnace to produce less heat. When the room cools, the thermostat tells the furnace to produce more heat. Many other hormonal processes are regulated by positive and negative feedback mechanisms.

The recruited follicles develop rapidly until one follicle surges ahead of the rest. This dominant follicle produces more estrogen than the others and develops more FSH receptors to capture most of the declining quantities of FSH in the bloodstream. Unable to secure adequate quantities of FSH, the competing follicles degenerate.

The dominant follicle continues to produce high levels of estrogen. When estrogen levels have exceeded a critical threshold for 2–3 days, positive pituitary feedback causes a surge of LH and FSH. (Commercial ovulation prediction kits detect rising LH levels.)

The ovum completes its maturation and prepares itself for fertilization. Twenty-four to 36 hours after the LH surge, ovulation occurs. The follicle ruptures, and the mature ovum is extruded into the abdominal cavity, to be quickly shepherded into the fallopian tube by the action of the fimbriae. This is the critical time for initiating a pregnancy; the ovum is capable of fertilization for a maximum of 24 hours. The woman may feel ovulation as sharp pain (**Mittelschmerz**) on one side or the other. Vaginal discharge changes, becoming slippery, abundant, and very hospitable to sperm.

After the follicle ruptures, the hormone-producing follicular cells shift gears metabolically, forming the corpus luteum and commencing to produce progesterone. Progesterone suppresses the growth of new follicles and causes secretory changes in the endometrium, priming it to allow embryonic implantation should conception occur. The luteal phase typically lasts 14 days unless the woman becomes pregnant. If she does not ovulate, she will not produce progesterone. Progesterone causes a slight elevation in basal body temperature, so a woman can keep a temperature chart to determine whether ovulation has occurred.

If no embryo implants in the uterus, the corpus luteum atrophies, and progesterone and estrogen levels drop. Without hormonal support, the uterine lining degenerates and begins to slough. Menstrual bleeding begins. Menstrual discharge includes blood, fluid, mucus, bacteria, vaginal and cervical secretions, and cellular debris. It amounts to an average total of 30–40 cc over 4–6 days. Meanwhile, the hypothalamus sends a releasing hormone to the pituitary and prompts it to release FSH and LH, beginning the process again.

 Inadequate follicular development can lead to low levels of progesterone, which may result in an inadequately developed endometrium and an increased risk of spontaneous abortion. This is called a luteal phase defect. Some pregnant women with low progesterone levels are prescribed progesterone (oral or vaginal suppositories), which maintains adequate maternal progesterone levels until the placenta is mature enough to take over the task, at 8–12 weeks. The EMS provider should realize that a woman on progesterone can still miscarry because progesterone will not prevent loss of a nonviable pregnancy.

Menopause

Menopause, also known as the climacteric or change of life, marks the end of a woman's reproductive years. The average age of menopause in the United States is 51.4 years (range 45–52 years). Thus an American woman who reaches the average life expectancy of a girl born in 2000, 79.5 years, will live more than one-third of her life after menopause. About 1 % of women enter menopause before age 40, usually in families with a history of early menopause. **Perimenopause**, the transitional period surrounding the climacteric, may begin while a woman is in her 30s and continue for 5–6 years, but sometimes as many as 10–15 years. Menopause, by commonly accepted definition, begins one year after the final menstrual period, but symptoms such as hot flashes can continue for 5–10 years after the last menses.

Menopause is a shift from a cyclic to a noncyclic hormone pattern, its onset marked by the cessation of ovulation and monthly menses. Fewer of a woman's ovarian follicles are responsive to pituitary stimulation, and the ones that do respond produce less estrogen than in earlier years. FSH and LH levels increase, and estrogen dramatically decreases. During her childbearing years, most of a woman's estrogen is estradiol produced by her ovarian follicles as they mature. As follicular stimulation declines and finally ceases, estrone—a weaker, less bioactive estrogen—is produced by the stroma of the ovary, adrenal glands, liver, muscle, bone, bone marrow, fibroblasts, and hair roots. Obese women have higher estrogen levels because this hormone is also synthesized in adipose tissue.

perimenopause
The time surrounding menopause, the permanent cessation of menstrual periods that marks the transition from reproductive to postreproductive life.

GERIATRIC
NOTES

Estrogen replacement after menopause was very popular until recently and was thought to be protective against stroke and heart attack. Recent research has indicated that hormone replacement therapy (HRT) significantly increases the risk of conditions such as breast cancer, heart attack, stroke, and blood clots and that these hormones should be used with caution and in low doses. Some women remain on HRT for many years after menopause to avoid the severe hot flashes that come with estrogen withdrawal. The EMS professional may encounter women in their 60s or older who are still on estrogen replacement therapy. EMS personnel should remember that these women are at higher risk for myocardial infarction, deep vein thrombosis, and stroke.

It is common for perimenopausal women to have unpredictable, irregular cycles and dramatic changes in bleeding patterns as ovarian function begins to fail. The first indication of impending menopause is often shortened menstrual cycles with a shortened follicular phase, resulting from the lower number of follicles.

A perimenopausal woman may fail to menstruate for months at a time, then have abnormally heavy menses. She may complain of insomnia, weight gain or bloating, mood changes, irregular menses, palpitations, loss of libido, difficulty concentrating, memory lapses, depression, fatigue, breast pain, and headache. Unintended pregnancies can occur during perimenopause, and the provider should remember that irregular bleeding may result from a pregnancy complication or impending spontaneous abortion.

PEARLS The irregular menses of perimenopause can sometimes cause heavy vaginal bleeding that can result in hypovolemia or anemia.

PEARLS Always consider pregnancy as a cause of amenorrhea or irregular bleeding in any woman, including those in perimenopause.

Hot flashes, caused by declining estrogen production, are characterized by a sensation of spreading warmth from trunk to face, often accompanied by red face and sweating. They last at most several minutes, but may disturb sleep when the woman awakens uncomfortably hot and diaphoretic. Some women opt to replace the lost estrogen and progesterone with artificial hormones. Others tolerate the discomfort of menopause knowing that the hot flashes and mood swings will eventually subside.

The uterus and ovaries become smaller in response to the lack of estrogen, and the pelvic-floor musculature becomes weaker. Bone loss occurs, making the postmenopausal woman vulnerable to fractures. Her risk for coronary artery disease also increases.

With loss of estrogen, the vaginal epithelium becomes thin and turns redder as small capillaries below the surface become more obvious. As menopause progresses, the vaginal tissue becomes pale, dry, and smooth because of a reduction in the number of capillaries. This can lead to dyspareunia (painful intercourse).

Menopause is a profound emotional and physical transformation. Some cultures honor menopause and esteem postmenopausal women for their insight and life experiences. The transition may be difficult for women who value youth and popular definitions of physical beauty above maturity and the wisdom of years. Other women gain greater knowledge and appreciation of themselves as they move though menopause, becoming more productive, authentic, creative, and sexually fulfilled.

Surgical Menopause

Surgical menopause usually results from bilateral oophorectomy (removal of the ovaries), a procedure usually performed to treat ovarian cancer or in conjunction with a hysterectomy (removal of the uterus). Surgical menopause can also result from ovarian failure following chemotherapy or radiation treatments or from surgical trauma, such as damage to the ovarian blood supply during hysterectomy.

Whereas natural menopause is a gradual process involving many years of hormonal and emotional adjustment, surgical menopause is abrupt. When ovaries are removed from a premenopausal woman, she moves suddenly from an estrogen-rich hormonal balance to nearly complete estrogen withdrawal. Without exogenous hormones, she will experience the physical symptoms of menopause with great intensity. Physically and psychologically, it can be difficult to recover from surgery while adjusting to a new hormonal balance and often an altered self-concept. Younger women who undergo surgical menopause usually remain on estrogen supplementation until the age of 45 or 50, when menopause would naturally occur. Women who undergo oophorectomy after menopause has occurred do not experience subsequent endocrine imbalance.

Conception and Fetal Development

This book presents a greatly simplified overview of fetal development. The EMS professional who is interested in learning more should consult one of the excellent texts that explore this complex topic in greater detail.

Fetal development texts tend to date development from conception. In obstetrical care, pregnancies are dated from the first day of the last menstrual period (LMP). Conception usually occurs about 2 weeks after the first day of the last period. So by this method of calculation, the first 2 weeks of the pregnancy occur paradoxically before the pregnancy has started.

The development of the unborn child occurs in three trimesters. The first trimester lasts 12 weeks from the beginning of the LMP. This encompasses the entire embryonic stage and the first 2 weeks of the fetal stage. During the first trimester, all organ systems and body parts are formed. The second trimester includes the 13th through 27th weeks after the LMP, or weeks 11–25 after conception. This period involves rapid growth and maturation of organ systems. The third trimester includes weeks 28 through 40–42 after the LMP, or weeks 26–38 after conception. During the third trimester, the fetus grows and gains weight. Essential body systems, such as the lungs and digestive tract, mature. Normal pregnancy lasts about 266 days (38 weeks) after ovulation, which is 280 days (40 weeks) after the LMP. This is 10 lunar months, or just over 9 calendar months.

Male and female gametes unite to create new human life possessing 46 chromosomes, the same number as either parent. In order to do this, egg and sperm must possess half that number. At ovulation, the ovum contains 23 chromosomes and stands ready to accept 23 more from the sperm that accomplishes fertilization. Each chromosome contains complex coils of DNA that hold the complete genetic blueprint for the new individual.

The ovum has no means of self-propulsion, so it passively relies on the action of the fallopian tube to direct it to the uterus. At ovulation, the fimbriated end of the tube closely applies itself to the ovary, and the fimbriae sweep the ovarian surface, raking the oocyte into the funnel-shaped infundibulum of the uterine tube. The walls of the fallopian tubes secrete fluid, and cilia create a current that flows to the uterus while peristaltic waves move the ovum along. In order to fertilize the ovum, sperm cells must swim in the opposite direction, whipping flagellated tails against the current. A single ejaculation deposits 200 million–500 million spermatozoa in the vagina. This is a staggering number: If each sperm cell were paired with one egg, there would be more than enough spermatozoa in a single ejaculation to impregnate one woman a day for 547,570 years—much longer than modern human beings have walked the earth. Of this quantity, only a few hundred sperm survive to make their way to the ampulla of the fallopian tube, where fertilization may occur. (A man with fewer than 10 million sperm cells per milliliter of semen is usually considered sterile, because only by producing large quantities of sperm is he likely to beat the odds against conception.)

The sperm alone determines the sex of the future child. The sex chromosomes of normal females, present in every somatic cell, are always XX; normal male cells carry an XY pair. Egg and sperm contain half the usual number of chromosomes. Thus a normal ovum always carries an X chromosome, but a normal sperm cell may carry an X or a Y. An egg fertilized by an X-bearing sperm will develop into an XX girl; an egg fertilized by a Y-bearing sperm will yield an XY boy. Because Y-bearing sperm swim slightly faster than their X counterparts, having slightly less genetic material on board, 125 males are conceived for every 100 females. More males are lost to miscarriage, however, so 106 males are born for every 100 females. Throughout life, males continue to suffer higher mortality than females. By age 18, the ratio is 1:1. Thereafter, women outnumber men.

Timing is critical. The ovum is fertilizable for only 12–24 hours after ovulation, and ovulation occurs but once a month. Sperm can survive in the female reproductive tract 48–72 hours (sometimes as long as 5 days), but are most able to fertilize within 24 hours of ejaculation. Optimally, upon arrival in the ampulla of the tube, the egg is mobbed by dozens or even hundreds of sperm. When one penetrates, the outer layer of the ovum becomes impenetrable to others.

At this moment, all of the future child's genetic potential is established. Maternal and paternal genes combine in pairs to determine hair color, approximate height and intelligence, susceptibility to certain diseases, and even certain broad personality tendencies. Over the course of a lifetime, environmental factors such as nutrition, upbringing, social interactions, and overall health will shape the expression of these genes; but the hereditary blueprint is drawn at conception, as sperm and egg meld to form a zygote genetically distinct from either parent.

About 30 hours after fertilization, the single-cell zygote splits into two identical cells, then four, then eight. By the time it reaches the uterus, about 4 days later, it is a cluster of identical cells (morula), encased in an elastic membrane, with the appearance of a mulberry.

When the conceptus enters the uterus, uterine fluid seeps through the membrane and fills the space in the center. As the fluid pocket enlarges and cell division continues, the conceptus, now termed a blastocyst, consists of a round, hollow structure with fluid in the center and cells on the outside. It generates new cells rapidly, and these cells differentiate into layers that will give rise to the placenta, the fetal membranes, and the embryo.

About one week after conception, the blastocyst implants in the endometrium of the uterus. The conceptus extends fingerlike projections into the endometrium, dissolving capillaries and uterine glands with enzymes and deriving sustenance from the eroded tissues. (Sometimes the mother will experience vaginal bleeding at the time of implantation.) At this phase of development, establishment of a life-support system takes priority over the growth of the embryo, and the tissues that will become the placenta develop most rapidly. As it proliferates, this placental precursor secretes human chorionic gonadotropin (hCG), a hormone that signals the body that pregnancy has occurred and prompts the corpus luteum to produce hormones that will sustain the pregnancy until the placenta is mature enough to assume the role. This is the hormone responsible for a positive pregnancy test.

Science still does not understand how the woman's immune system readily accepts the embryo and does not reject it as a foreign invader. After birth, any body part transplanted from child to mother would be immediately recognized as foreign; but as an embryo, its presence is not only accepted but also accommodated and nurtured by maternal physiology. Instead of trying to destroy the conceptus, as it would anything else that it recognizes as not self, the mother's body welcomes the new life, offering a favorable hormonal balance and engorged blood vessels to bring it sustenance.

The rapidly developing blastocyst continues to differentiate into an embryonic disc and the rudiments of a placenta and amniotic sac. Placental projections (chorionic villi) tap into lacunae—tiny pools of maternal blood and glandular secretions from eroded endometrium—and the embryo can now utilize maternal circulation for nutrition, oxygenation, and elimination of waste products. Maternal blood flows in and out of the lacunae, and the embryo takes what it needs. The system is designed so that maternal and fetal blood ideally never mix.

By the third week after conception (5 weeks after the LMP) the embryo organizes itself to map out major body systems. Three layers of cells form, and each layer gives rise to different structures and systems. The precursors to central nervous system, spine, and cranial nerves form. Other cells stand ready to give rise to the vertebrae, ribs, limb muscles, and a primitive cardiovascular system, in which a tubular heart pumps the earliest blood cells. Development is cephalocaudal, or head to tail. That is, before and after birth, the parts of the child closer to the head develop first—fingers appear before toes, purposeful hand control appears before walking.

Like a sheet of paper in the hands of an origami master, the embryonic disc folds and refolds, creating complex, specialized organs and body regions out of flat sameness. Cells migrate, physically moving to where they are needed, programmed to become lungs, limbs, or brain. This process is similar to building a ship at sea—the heart continues to beat and circulate blood even as it remodels itself from an S-shaped tube into a complex configuration of chambers, vessels, and valves.

In the early embryo, blood is first created in the yolk sac. The liver then takes over blood production. As the fetus nears term, bone marrow becomes the primary site for hemopoiesis. Fetal red blood cells have a shorter life span than those of adults—90 days as opposed to 120 days.

Weeks 4–8 after conception (6–10 weeks after the LMP) are the most crucial to normal development, for this is the time when all major organs and body systems form. While the three layers of the early embryo fold to give rise to the beginnings of organs and body regions, exposure to **teratogens** (substances that produce congenital anomalies) can cause devastating damage.

teratogen
Anything (such as ionizing radiation or a toxic substance) that interferes with normal embryonic or fetal development.

Expectant parents often wonder whether a binge of drinking or recreational drug use will damage the unborn baby. In truth, it is difficult to determine what substances damage human embryos at which times in their development. A toxic substance may do serious damage at some points of development and none at others. Animal studies do not always yield results applicable to human beings, but exposing pregnant women to damaging substances in the name of research is, of course, unethical. When a malformation occurs, it cannot always be traced to specific teratogens. Some damaged children are born with a normal appearance, but suffer learning disabilities or diseases later in life that may not be attributable to prenatal injury.

Some teratogens, however, are well recognized, though in most cases the degree of damage is variable. Maternal alcohol consumption and use of phenytoin (Dilantin) both can cause intrauterine growth restriction (IUGR), mental retardation, abnormally small head, and distinctive facial malformations in some exposed fetuses. Tetracycline can cause permanent tooth discoloration. Maternal infections such as rubella and cytomegalovirus can cause multiple anomalies. Persistent hyperglycemia in a diabetic woman can result in congenital heart defects, and elevated maternal temperature (caused by disease, use of hot tubs or saunas, or prolonged exercise) can damage the embryo. Even excessive intake of certain vitamins, notoriously vitamin A, can cause permanent malformations.

The 9th through 38th weeks of intrauterine development (11–40 weeks after the LMP) is termed the fetal period. During the embryonic period, the developing child lays the foundations for all its organs and body systems. Development during the fetal period involves rapid growth and further refinement of the body overall and maturation of organs until they are able to sustain life outside the maternal environment.

Developmental Highlights from Date of Conception

(Add 2 weeks when dating from LMP.)

- **Day 1.**   Fertilization; conceptus is a single cell.

- **Day 4.**   Conceptus enters uterus.

- **Days 6–7.**   Implantation in uterus.

- **Week 2.**   The conceptus differentiates into what will become the embryo, the placenta, and the amniotic cavity. A yolk sac serves as a temporary digestive and respiratory system while the placenta forms and is the first site for the production of blood cells. Chorionic villi, projections of the forming placenta, penetrate uterine tissues to form a means of gas and nutrient exchange between the embryo and the mother.

• **Week 3.** The embryo, now consisting of millions of specialized cells, maps out its major body systems. Every bulge, fold, and hollow present on the embryo now indicates cellular differentiation. The foundations of the brain, skeleton, muscles, sense organs, nervous system, and digestive tract are created. By 17–19 days, blood cells are forming, along with a tube-shaped heart and primitive blood vessels. About 21–23 days after conception, the heart begins to beat. The third week after conception begins the embryonic period. The mother has missed her menstrual period and may suspect that she is pregnant. Size (crown to rump) 2–3 mm.

• **Week 4.** The entire embryo begins to curve into a C-shape and grows rapidly. Limb buds form, as do the beginnings of the oral cavity, jaw, lungs, stomach, intestines, eyes, and ears. The liver begins to function. A beating heart can be seen by ultrasonography. At this stage of development, the embryo has a tail. Size (crown to rump) 4–6 mm.

• **Week 5.** The head is the fastest-growing part of the embryo at this point because of the rapid growth of the brain. The brain has differentiated, and cranial nerves are now present, as are the nerves responsible for muscular activity. The heart is developing chambers. Size (crown to rump) 8–11 mm. See Figure 1-9.

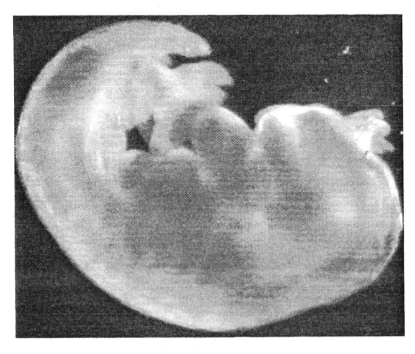

FIGURE 1-9
The Embryo at 5 Weeks.
At 5 weeks' gestation the embryo is differentiating all body systems and organs.
Petit Format/Nestle/Science Source

* **Week 6.**   A primitive skeleton forms, and muscles flesh out the frame. The beginnings of nipples form on what will be the chest. Digital rays appear in the hand plates—the beginnings of fingers—and the arms bend at the elbow. Twitching movement is possible. The liver begins to produce red blood cells, and lung tissue becomes more sophisticated. Oral and nasal cavities form, as do the upper lip and external ears. Size (crown to rump) 17–23 mm.

* **Week 7.**   The fingers of the hand begin to separate. The tongue, stomach, and diaphragm are present. Arm and leg movements are visible on ultrasound. Gonads differentiate into ovaries or testes. The intestines move outside the body into the umbilical cord to develop. Size (crown to rump) 22–31 mm.

* **Week 8.**   The end of the 8th week after conception marks the beginning of the fetal period because the beginnings of all major organ systems have been established. The fetus looks unmistakably human, but his head is still large, and his features are not in their final locations. His tail has finally disappeared. His fingers and toes are formed, and his muscles and nervous system have now developed enough to allow for movement. The heart is structurally complete, but will continue to grow and mature. There is approximately 7 ml of amniotic fluid surrounding the fetus. Size (crown to rump) is 40 mm, weight 2 g.

* **Week 10.**   The fetus's face has a very human appearance. His fingers and toes have nail beds. He moves vigorously *in utero*. Male and female genitals begin to differentiate—male fetuses produce testosterone that prompts masculine development. Genital tissue forms the clitoris in females and the penis in males. The intestines, which developed for a time outside the body, encased in the umbilical cord, have returned to the abdomen. His pancreas produces insulin and his kidneys produce urine. Hair follicles are beginning to form. Size (crown to rump) 53 mm, weight14 g.

* **Week 12.**   The fetus begins to show individuality. At this stage habits and facial expressions differ from one fetus to another. He moves vigorously *in utero*. He can suck his thumb and make a fist. He swallows amniotic fluid and urinates into the amniotic sac, in this way helping to regulate the volume of fluid surrounding him. He inhales and exhales amniotic fluid. The skin is thin, pink, and translucent. His skin is very sensitive, and he responds to skin stimulation and shows some postural reflexes. The thyroid gland secretes hormones, and the liver secretes bile. Genitals appear clearly male or female. Lungs assume mature shape. Size (crown to rump) 87 mm, weight 45 g. See Figures 1-10 and 1-11.

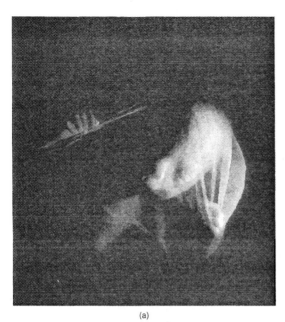

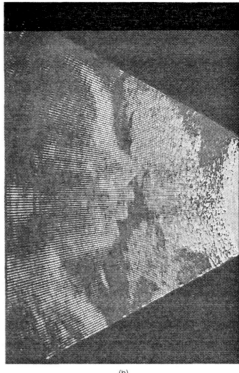

(a)

(b)

FIGURE 1-10

The Fetus at 4 Months and at 6 Months.

(a) A fiberoptic image of a 4-month fetus.

Lennart Nilsson/Albert Bonniers Forlag AB

(b) The profile of this 6-month fetus is clearly visible on a 2-D ultrasound scan.

Photo Researchers, Inc.

- **Week 16.** The eyes are in their final position on the face and can move slowly beneath their fused lids. Reflex response is more established. The fetus has unique fingerprints and footprints and distinctive patterns of scalp hair follicles. The fetus has taste buds, and research has shown that he will drink more amniotic fluid if it is sweetened, less if a bitter substance is added. His thyroid, gallbladder, and pancreas function, and his thymus produces the precursors of T-cells. The fetus can salivate. Bones continue to ossify and are visible on X-rays. Female fetuses have immature eggs in their ovaries. Male fetuses may experience erections of the penis. There is approximately 200–250 ml of amniotic fluid present. Size (crown to rump) 140 mm, weight 200 g. See Figure 1-12.

- **Week 20.** This is the midpoint of pregnancy. The mother is aware of fetal movement now, and the fetus is very active, somersaulting and responding to maternal activities. The fetus hiccups sometimes, giving

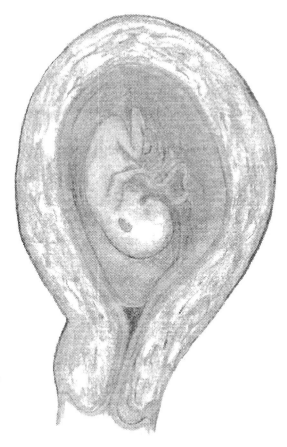

FIGURE 1-11
The 12-Week Fetus.
By 12 weeks' gestation,
the fetus is active,
though the mother can-
not yet feel his move-
ments.
Illustration by Bonnie U.
Gruenberg

his mother a sensation of rhythmic tapping. He can now hear sounds, and his handgrip is strong. Hair grows on the scalp and eyebrows, and lanugo, fine downy fetal body hair, covers the skin. *Vernix caseosa* (Latin for "cheesy varnish")—a white, tenacious, cold-creamlike substance secreted by fetal sebaceous glands—adheres to the body hair and protects delicate fetal skin. The fetus produces brown fat, which will serve as a valuable fuel source for heat production after birth. Most bones have hardened. The female fetus has a uterus and vagina, and her ovaries contain more ova than she will ever again have in her life. At 21–23 weeks, REM sleep—the phase of sleep associated with dreaming—is observable. Size (crown to rump) 190 mm, weight 460 g. See Figure 1-13.

viable
Able to live outside
the womb. The
threshold of fetal
viability is usually
considered 500 g
or 20 weeks of ges-
tation, though 24
weeks is generally
the practical limit.
Legal and popular
definitions are nu-
merous.

• **Week 24.**   Lungs mature to allow for gas exchange and begin to produce a surfactant, a substance that helps the alveoli to remain open between breaths. The fetus is now potentially **viable**, but achieves his greatest chances of life and health if he stays *in utero* until term. An infant born at this stage has about a 60% survival rate and, if he lives, is likely to suffer long-term health problems related to prematurity. His

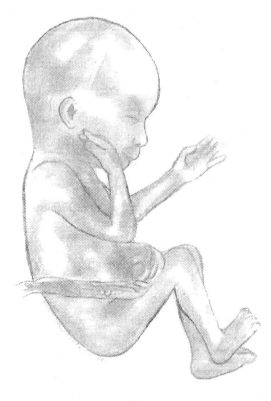

FIGURE 1-12
The 16-Week Fetus.
The 16-week fetus shows some of the reflexes he will have at birth. Some mothers report feeling movement at this stage.
Illustration by Bonnie U. Gruenberg

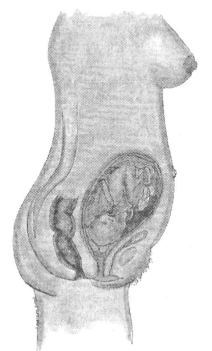

FIGURE 1-13
The 22-Week Fetus.
By 22–24 weeks' gestation the fetus in some cases could live outside the uterus if born prematurely, but further intrauterine maturation would greatly enhance his odds of survival. The 22-week fetus has thin, red, gelatinous skin and very little subcutaneous fat.
Illustration by Bonnie U. Gruenberg

The Woman and the Fetus 31

skin is thin, red, wrinkled, and translucent, and there is little subcutaneous fat. Reflexes such as sucking and startling are present, and he even makes the motions of crying while *in utero*. The fetus responds to light, even though eyelids are fused. Buds for permanent teeth appear in his gums. The female fetus has a prominent clitoris and labia minora. Size (crown to rump) approximately 230 mm, weight 820 g.

⦾ **Week 28.** The fetus can open his eyes, which are rimmed by eyelashes. Scalp hair is well developed. The spleen has become an important site for red blood cell production, but after 28 weeks the bone marrow dominates. The testes of the male fetus begin to descend into the scrotum. Movement is vigorous, and the fetus begins to prefer a head-down position. Size (crown to rump) 270 mm, weight about 1,300 g.

⦾ **Week 36.** By 36 weeks after conception, the fetus has put on subcutaneous fat, producing rounder contours and smooth, pink skin. He has a very strong grasp and goes though predictable periods of quiet sleep, REM sleep, and wakefulness. If born now, most babies will not require intensive care, and may discharge home within 48 hours of birth, like a full-term baby. Size (crown to rump) 350 mm, length (crown to heel) 19 in., weight 2,500–2,900 g (about 5.5–6.0 lb).

⦾ **Weeks 38–40.** Baby is full-term and well-prepared for life outside of his mother, able to breathe, suck, and digest breast milk. Vernix remains in the folds of the skin only. Fingernails have grown beyond the tips of the fingers. Some babies suck their hands so vigorously *in utero,* they are born with blisters on their skin. Boys' testes are in the scrotum. Size (crown to rump) 365 mm, length (crown to heel) 20–21 in., weight 3,400+ g (about 7–8 lb). See Figure 1-14.

The Placenta

The placenta, the fetus's life-support system, interfaces with the mother's circulation, allowing him to gain nutrients, oxygen, and other necessary substances from the maternal bloodstream and eliminate waste products. See Figure 1-15. It is an important endocrine gland that produces large quantities of essential pregnancy hormones, and it transfers maternal antibodies to the fetus to protect him from disease. As the liver does later, it synthesizes glycogen, cholesterol, and fatty acids early in pregnancy.

The placenta develops at the site of implantation, optimally in the upper part of the uterus. At delivery, the maternal side looks like a slab of roughened, segmented liver. The fetal side is shiny and pale, with a tree-like pattern of vasculature where the umbilical cord inserts and amniotic membranes trailing like a ruptured balloon. See Figure 1-16.

At delivery the umbilical cord appears blue, just as veins appear blue when viewed through the skin. After the cord stops pulsing, it

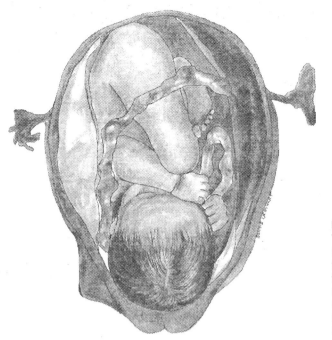

FIGURE 1-14
The 40-Week Fetus.
By 40 weeks the fetus takes up most of
the available space in the uterus and is
fully mature. His activities, circadian
cycles, and reflexes are essentially the
same as those he will exhibit as a newborn.
Illustration by Bonnie U. Gruenberg

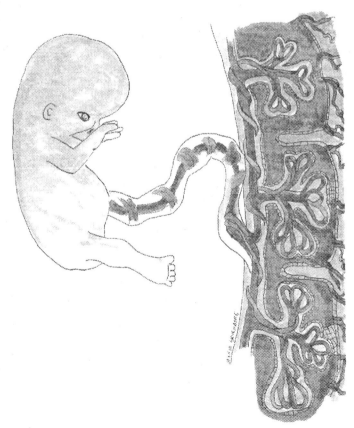

FIGURE 1-15
Placental Circulation.
The chorionic villi of the placenta
are bathed by the mother's blood,
allowing the embryo to pick up
oxygen and nutrition from the maternal circulation and dispose of
waste products by the same route.
The blood in the placenta and cord
belong to the embryo. Maternal
and fetal blood ideally never mix.
Illustration by Bonnie U. Gruenberg

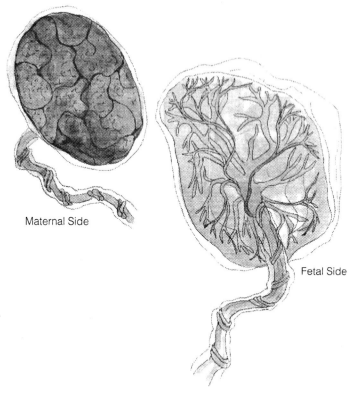

Maternal Side

Fetal Side

FIGURE 1-16
Placenta Front and Back.
The maternal side of the placenta looks similar to a piece of liver—red,
rough, and fleshy. The fetal side is smooth, shiny, and covered with
branching blood vessels and amniotic membranes.
Illustration by Bonnie U. Gruenberg

turns white and becomes thinner and softer. Blood vessels spiral along
its length, and a gelatinous material (Wharton's jelly) serves to prevent
them from crimping and knotting.

Fetal Circulation

Fetal circulation maximizes blood flow to and from the placenta. Although the lungs develop prenatally, and the fetus practices breathing
movements *in utero,* before birth the lungs are not vital organs. They require only enough circulation to allow them to grow. It is the multifunc-
tional placenta that sustains fetal life. The fetus's only source of oxygen
is the maternal bloodstream.

To bypass the fetal lungs and increase placental perfusion, a series of
shunts within the fetal circulatory system directs blood flow where it is

most beneficial. As blood enters the right atrium, much of it is diverted into the left atrium through an opening between the atria, the foramen ovale. From the left atrium, it is pumped to the left ventricle and out to the aorta with the next heartbeat. Branches from the aorta send blood to perfuse the brain, limbs, kidneys, and all other body parts.

Blood that does not pass though the foramen ovale passes from the right atrium through the tricuspid valve to the right ventricle with atrial contraction. The blood vessels that perfuse the fetal lungs are constricted. As the blood exits the right ventricles through the pulmonary artery, the constricted vessels resist filling, so the blood follows the easier path through the ductus arteriosus into the aorta.

By the time the blood in the lower aorta reaches the umbilical arteries, it is desaturated and returns to the placenta for oxygenation. Umbilical arteries are two slender vessels that spiral around the larger umbilical vein down the length of the umbilical cord to the placenta. Fetal blood circulates into the capillaries of the placental chorionic villi. Shaped like branching trees, chorionic villi extend into circulating pools of maternal blood, where they exchange blood gases, nutrients, immunological components, and other substances. Ideally, maternal and fetal blood never mix.

Oxygenated and nutrient laden, the blood returns to the fetus via the umbilical vein, which runs up through the umbilical cord and enters the fetal abdomen at the umbilicus. Inside the fetus, the umbilical vein divides into two branches—one circulates though the fetal liver on its way to the inferior vena cava via the hepatic vein, and the other, the ductus venosus, empties directly into the vena cava. From there it is carried back to the right atrium, mixing along the way with blood returning from the head and upper limbs. The cycle begins again.

The uterus is a low-oxygen environment, and the fetus must rely on whatever oxygen his mother can provide through the placenta. Profound changes take place at the moment of birth. Fluid is squeezed out of the respiratory tract as the baby moves though the vagina and out. He takes his first breath. The lungs fill with air for the first time, and the remaining lung fluid is absorbed. Oxygen floods his circulatory system from his own alveoli, and the tight blood vessels in the lungs suddenly relax.

Before birth, the fetus's heart circulates blood not only through his own body but also through the complex, branching network of umbilical and placental vessels. At birth, the cord is clamped, and suddenly the infant needs only to circulate blood through himself. Systemic blood pressure increases sharply.

Decreased pulmonary vascular resistance, loss of the placenta, and elevated blood pressure dramatically increase blood flow to the newborn's lungs. Blood moves into the pulmonary vessels instead of the ductus arteriosus, which begins to constrict. The foramen ovale closes, and circulation begins to follow the usual route.

Congenital Abnormalities

The causes of most birth defects are unknown, but many can be linked to environmental or genetic factors. Every human being has 46 chromosomes comprised of 30,000–35,000 genes that determine most aspects of our physical appearance and physiological function. A single abnormal gene can affect development catastrophically. Exposure to chemicals, medications, infection, or radiation can cause defects such as cleft lip and palate, clubfoot, and heart anomalies.

Some genetic diseases, such as cystic fibrosis, manifest only when one recessive gene from the mother pairs with the same recessive gene from the father. Both parents can be free of any sign of the disease, and commonly the disease will not manifest for generations. Conversely, conditions such as Marfan syndrome are genetically dominant—a parent with Marfan is likely to have a child with the disease. Other diseases are passed down silently through maternal lines and manifest primarily in sons, such as hemophilia.

Some anomalies occur when the developing embryo carries too many or too few chromosomes. One of the most common chromosomal abnormalities is Down syndrome, in which the baby is born with an extra chromosome 21. The child with Down syndrome has distinctive facial features, mental retardation that may be mild or profound, and frequently heart defects and other problems. The fetus with an extra copy of chromosome 13 or 18 has severe abnormalities and often dies *in utero* or shortly after birth. Missing or extra X and Y sex chromosomes may affect fertility, sexual development, cognitive function, and behavior.

Physical and Behavioral Changes of Pregnancy

Pregnancy causes profound alterations of maternal anatomy, physiology, and psychology, yet by 6 weeks after delivery most women have returned almost entirely to their prepregnant state. Most of the physical changes are progressive and relate to either hormonal alterations or the physical changes wrought by the developing fetus.

Metabolism

The fetus and placenta are metabolically very active and therefore generate large amounts of heat. The pregnant woman disperses this heat through increased respiratory and circulatory rate, increased plasma volume, and increased blood flow to the skin.

Reproductive System

Uterine enlargement is one of the most obvious changes in pregnancy. At the end of pregnancy, this organ has 500–1,000 times greater capacity than before pregnancy. Uterine enlargement is not due solely to the growing fetus and surrounding fluid; it also reflects a hormonally influenced increase in maternal muscle mass. Uterine walls thicken in early pregnancy, but thin to about 1.5 cm or less at term. By the end of pregnancy, the vascular system of the uterus contains one-sixth of the mother's total blood volume.

From the first trimester on, the uterus begins contracting, presumably to tone the muscles for labor. These contractions, known as Braxton Hicks contractions, are often painless, especially with primigravidas, but some women feel them as uncomfortable cramps. Research suggests that pregnant women are aware of only 10–17% of these uterine contractions. Runs of painful Braxton Hicks contractions can become false labor in the third trimester, but the contractions of progressing premature labor can be painless. It can be difficult to differentiate among Braxton Hicks contractions, false labor, and labor.

ON TARGET Preterm labor may be difficult to distinguish from Braxton Hicks contractions.

The uterus outgrows the confines of the pelvis at about 12 weeks' gestation and pushes the intestines out of place as it enlarges. It rotates to the right as it grows, displaced by the sigmoid colon on the left side of the abdomen. At term the uterus nearly reaches the liver and may displace the appendix as far as the right flank. The rising diaphragm, in turn, pushes the heart up and to the left, changing the cardiac silhouette seen in radiographs. As pregnancy advances, the uterus compresses the ureters at the pelvic brim, a situation that may allow urine to back up and distend the kidneys (hydronephrosis).

The abdominal wall supports the uterus and helps to keep its long axis upright in relation to the pelvic inlet. Repeated childbearing can slacken the abdominal wall, however, allowing the pregnant uterus to fall forward.

Throughout pregnancy, uterine blood flow increases to perfuse the growing placenta. The cervix and vagina may become so vascular and blood engorged that they turn purplish or bluish. The cervix and uterus soften. A plug of thick mucus forms in the cervical opening to seal it against infection. The vagina produces greater amounts of thick, white, acidic discharge to discourage bacterial growth. Hormones are secreted by the corpus luteum and placenta that loosen pelvic connective tissue.

Breasts

Breasts tingle and become tender during the first 2 months of pregnancy. They enlarge and become nodular and vascular as ductal networks begin to prepare for lactation. Colostrum, the yellowish, high-protein, antibody-rich fluid that sustains the infant for the first days of breast-feeding, may leak from the breasts by the end of the first trimester.

Nutritional Needs

The changes of pregnancy may mask underlying problems or mimic disease.

Protein requirements increase because the woman is building not only a fetus and placenta, but also breast tissue, blood, and uterine muscle. See Table 1-1. Increased iron intake is required for blood building in both mother and fetus and for stores laid down in the fetal liver. Folate is required for protein tissue construction; low folate levels can result in neural tube defects, such as spina bifida. If maternal intake of calcium is inadequate, calcium is obtained from the mother's long bones to nourish the fetus.

Cardiovascular System

The most significant changes in cardiac function occur in the first 8 weeks of pregnancy. Cardiac output increases as early as the 5th week of pregnancy, as a result of lower systemic vascular resistance and higher heart rate. In pregnancy, cardiac output increases 30–50% over nonpregnant levels. At term the placenta and uterus receive blood flow of about 600–800 ml per minute. Pregnancy increases the resting pulse by about 10 beats per minute. Blood pressure drops slightly during the first two trimesters, but returns to prepregnant levels by term. Postural hypotension can become pronounced due to low peripheral vascular resistance and increased venous capacitance.

Table 1-1 Distribution of Weight Gain in Pregnancy

Location	Average Weight (lb)
Fetus	7.5
Placenta	1.5
Amniotic fluid	2.0
Uterus	2.0
Breasts	1.0
Blood	3.0
Water	3.5
Fat	7.5

Based on normal weight gain of 25–35 lb (28–40 lb for women considered underweight, 15–25 lb for those considered overweight).

The paramedic may notice a loud, exaggerated splitting of the first heart sound and a third heart sound. Ninety percent of pregnant women have a systolic murmur, attributable to the increased intravascular volume, that disappears soon after delivery.

The cardiac apex moves upward and laterally, and a 12-lead EKG may suggest left axis deviation. ST depression and T-wave changes may be present in about 14% of healthy pregnant women. T-wave inversions may be seen in V_2, and small q waves in leads II, III, and aVF.

Maternal blood volume increases dramatically, usually 45–50% over prepregnant levels. This is important for several reasons. Extra blood is needed to perfuse the placenta and the increased vascularity of the reproductive organs, to protect against orthostatic and supine hypotension, and as a hemodynamic safeguard in preparation for blood loss during delivery. Blood clots more easily in pregnancy, minimizing the mother's risk of hemorrhage, but increasing her risk of venous thrombosis. Both plasma volume and erythrocyte count increase, but the fluid part of the blood increases disproportionately, producing what is termed a physiological anemia that peaks at about 28 weeks. Because of the greater blood volume, a pregnant woman can acutely lose 30–35% of her blood without a change in vital signs.

 PEARLS A pregnant woman can become significantly hypovolemic before her vital signs reflect volume depletion. Conversely, a pregnant woman's normally lowered blood pressure and elevated pulse may mimic shock when she is hemodynamically stable.

Respiratory System

Oxygen demands increase in pregnancy. As pregnancy advances, the encroaching uterus elevates the diaphragm. To compensate, thoracic circumference increases, and airway resistance declines. The woman's respiratory rate does not change, but her tidal volume, minute volume, and minute oxygen consumption increase significantly. Growing awareness of the desire to breathe is often seen in early pregnancy. About 60–70% of healthy pregnant women will complain of dyspnea during pregnancy, sometimes making it difficult for the EMS provider to distinguish pathological from physiological processes.

Urinary System

Kidneys enlarge and work harder during pregnancy as glomerular filtration rates increase by more than 50%. Compression of the ureters by the uterus causes them to dilate and become more vulnerable to infection. Urinary frequency is common in the first and last trimesters.

Gastrointestinal System

Gastric emptying and intestinal transit times are delayed in pregnancy by hormonal and mechanical factors. Constipation is common, and the iron supplements taken by many pregnant women can exacerbate it. Stomach sphincter relaxation and the pressure of the gravid uterus result in frequent heartburn. Rising hormone levels and blood-sugar fluctuations make nausea and vomiting common during the first trimester. There is also an alteration in gallbladder function; it seems likely that progesterone retards gallbladder contraction, leading to stasis and an increased formation of gallstones.

Musculoskeletal System

Progressive lordosis or "swayback" normally occurs in pregnancy as the woman compensates for the heavy uterus weighing down the front of the body. See Figure 1-17. Hormones loosen joints to maximize pelvic expansion during delivery, when an extra centimeter may be crucial, but they also loosen joints throughout the body. A pregnant woman's shoe size may increase even in the absence of pedal edema.

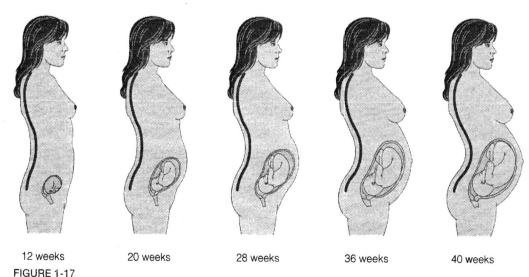

| 12 weeks | 20 weeks | 28 weeks | 36 weeks | 40 weeks |

FIGURE 1-17
Postural Changes of Pregnancy.
The posture of the pregnant woman changes with advancing pregnancy.

PEARLS The joint laxity of pregnancy predisposes the woman to subluxations and dislocations. EMS professionals should maintain a high index of suspicion when evaluating trauma victims—even relatively low-force mechanisms of injury can produce significant joint displacement in any articulation, including the spine.

Psychological Changes

Pregnancy prompts a woman to turn inward and try to understand herself, especially during the first trimester. Her emotions become labile. Her moods may shift unpredictably, and she may become hypersensitive and tend to overreact. She may feel vulnerable and distressed over her lack of control over her own bodily changes. Some women become more dependent, others become more demanding. Most women are ambivalent about their pregnancies at least some of the time, even if the baby is very loved and wanted. Eighty percent of women experience some disappointment, anxiety, or unhappiness about the pregnancy during the first trimester.

By the second trimester, the fatigue and nausea of early pregnancy have usually subsided, and the woman often feels in radiant good health. Her friends may remark on the "glow of pregnancy." By the second trimester the woman usually accepts the pregnancy, and her self-image begins to evolve from care receiver to caregiver in preparation for the mother role. When she first experiences quickening, or the perception of fetal movement, the coming baby begins to feel like a person separate from herself, and she shifts her primary concerns from herself to the baby.

The third trimester brings the physical discomfort of having a large fetus compressing abdominal organs and kicking vigorously at all hours. The woman generally focuses on preparing for the baby's arrival. The prospects of labor and delivery may become very frightening as they draw near, but often, by term, the woman is eager to start labor.

Psychologically, pregnancy is a time of crisis, whether the baby is wanted or not. The birth of a child engenders irreversible changes in the life of a woman, her partner, and other family members. The family budget must stretch to accommodate another member, and the infant may alter work schedules, recreation, and household responsibilities. First-time parents often find that starting a family involves a complete reordering of lifestyle and priorities.

Summary

A woman's reproductive life includes a series of profound physical and psychological transitions—puberty, menstruation, pregnancy, childbirth, perimenopause, and menopause. Although these phases are natural and usually proceed uneventfully, related conditions and complaints can arise that may pose a threat to the woman's health and sometimes her life. To render optimal care to female patients throughout their lifetimes, the EMS provider must understand the anatomy, physiology, and biochemical processes that are the underpinnings of these reproductive transitions. A solid foundation of knowledge inevitably provides valuable insight into the origin of symptoms when assessing patients in the field.

REVIEW QUESTIONS

1. A 20-year-old woman complains of sharp left-sided pain. Her LMP was about 15 days ago. She is experiencing odorless clear mucus discharge, but no itching or burning. What normal physiological occurrence could account for her symptoms?

2. Describe the changes that occur at birth as the fetal circulation transitions to neonatal circulation.

3. Briefly describe the main events that occur during of the first phase of the menstrual cycle, onset through ovulation.

4. Laurel is 12 weeks pregnant with her first child. You detect a grade 2 systolic murmur. Laurel says that she has no history of a cardiac murmur. Is a systolic murmur normal in pregnancy? Why or why not?

5. Briefly describe the functions of the placenta.

CHAPTER 2

Evaluating the Pregnant Woman

Objectives

By the end of this chapter you should be able to

- Recognize signs and symptoms that may indicate a woman is pregnant

- Obtain a brief obstetrical history and assessment of the present complaint

- Calculate a due date and approximate gestational age

- Assess a pregnant abdomen

- Identify which facility is best suited to managing a pregnant patient

- Consider the emotional, social, spiritual, and physical aspects of the pregnant patient

CASE Study

Heidi and Laura arrived at Tara's residence in response to a call for a "woman in pain." Tara did not volunteer details, was evasive, and whimpered incessantly, shifting her weight from foot to foot and rubbing her abdomen.

Through gentle, persistent questioning, Heidi determined that Tara was a 25-year-old with no chronic medical problems except occasional migraines. Tara complained of severe suprapubic pain over the last two days, so intense it doubled her over. She denied nausea, vomiting, diarrhea, fever, flank pain, or unusual vaginal discharge, but said that she "felt lousy," had a splitting headache, and sometimes felt pain in her epigastrium and sacrum. Tara also reported that she had been dribbling urine since the pain began. She was somewhat obese, but her appearance did not necessarily suggest pregnancy. She denied being or ever having been pregnant, stating that her last menstrual period was two months earlier, but that her periods had always been very irregular in timing and duration. She told Heidi that she was not sexually active and that she lived with her mother. She had been treated for depression and anxiety, but was not currently on any medications. Her only allergy was to codeine.

When they took Tara's blood pressure, the EMS providers obtained a reading of 150/90. Physical examination showed pitting pedal and pretibial edema to Tara's knees bilaterally, and her hands and face appeared puffy as well. There was no costovertebral angle tenderness. Heidi carefully palpated Tara's abdomen and was surprised to find it firm from pubis to about two finger widths below the xyphoid. She also noted that the suprapubic pain was intermittent, and that Tara's abdomen grew rigid when the pain was present.

"Tara, are you sure you aren't pregnant?" Laura asked carefully. "It looks to me like you are."

Tara avoided eye contact and fixed her gaze on the window, but admitted that she might be.

She told Laura that she had been at a party many months ago and had drunk herself to unconsciousness. "While I was passed out, I guess four or five guys had their way with me," she said. She had not sought prenatal care or modified her lifestyle, indulging in weekly drinking binges and occasional marijuana use. She denied drug or alcohol use in the past 24 hours.

Laura was unable to get fetal heart tones with a stethoscope, but between the 3-minutes-apart contractions she could palpate fetal movement. Laura could palpate a fetal head above the pubic bone. Tara denied rectal pressure or a need to push. Laura checked for crowning and saw no evidence of imminent delivery. The sanitary pad that Tara had applied two hours before appeared soaked with particulate, mustard-colored fluid. A second blood pressure yielded a reading of 210/100.

Questions

1. In her assessment, Laura identified problems that could prove life threatening for mother or infant. What are they? What other concerns should Laura have in managing this patient?

2. Upon initially meeting Tara, before discovering she was pregnant, what clinical impression do you think Laura and Heidi formed from Tara's complaint of suprapubic pain, urinary leakage, and headache?

3. In which position should Tara be transported?

Introduction

The EMS professional has only a few minutes in which to assess each patient, form a clinical impression, begin executing a management plan, and decide whether and where to transport. Often the responder meets the patient for the first time in an emergency situation and must rapidly synthesize the patient's story, her signs and symptoms, and other details into an accurate picture of the current problem. Patients often give sketchy or incorrect information, omit important facts, or report misleading symptoms due to miscommunication, fear, confusion, altered consciousness, social pressure, cultural or religious prohibitions, or the simple desire for privacy. This lack of concrete information can lead providers to draw erroneous conclusions about the patient's condition.

The obstetrical patient presents a unique set of challenges to the EMS professional. Prehospital providers must recognize signs of pregnancy, learn how pregnancy relates to pathological processes, and develop interview techniques that elicit and filter relevant information rapidly while gaining the patient's trust.

KEY TERMS

amenorrhea, p. 46	multipara, p. 51	primipara, p. 51
antepartum, p. 62	nulligravida, p. 51	supine hypotension syndrome, p. 53
gestation, p. 48	nullipara, p. 51	
multigravida, p. 51	primigravida, p. 51	

Signs of Pregnancy

In the centuries before blood and urine pregnancy tests, ultrasound machines, and radiography, it was not always easy to determine whether a woman was pregnant or to predict a due date. Sometimes on ambulance calls, it seems that very little has changed. The EMS provider often encounters women who have had no prenatal care, do not know when they are due, claim they are pregnant when they are not, or deny pregnancy despite advanced labor. When a woman is unconscious or otherwise unable to answer questions, the provider must look for physical evidence that suggests or determines pregnancy. Most of the signs of pregnancy that can be observed by an examiner, however, are ambiguous or attributable to other causes. Determining whether a patient is pregnant and when she is due can be challenging.

Presumptive Signs of Pregnancy

Presumptive changes are experienced by the woman and may indicate pregnancy.

amenorrhea
Absence or cessation of menstruation.

- **Amenorrhea.**   For women with regular menses, **amenorrhea** (lack of menstruation) is often the first sign that pregnancy has occurred. Although pregnancy is the most common cause of secondary amenorrhea (periods that cease after normal menarche), amenorrhea can be caused by many other conditions, including emotional upset, endocrine disorders, perimenopause, menopause, and malnutrition. A woman may also experience bleeding during pregnancy that can be mistaken for menses.

- **Fatigue.**   Fatigue is common in the first trimester, but typically subsides by 14 weeks gestation.

- **Nausea and vomiting.**   "Morning sickness" most commonly manifests during the first trimester. Nausea and vomiting are not necessarily limited to mornings; but in pregnancy, fasting between dinner and breakfast causes hypoglycemia, which is a possible trigger of the classic nausea experienced before rising. Nausea and vomiting may persist throughout the day, triggered by odors, meals, fluctuations in blood sugar, or pregnancy hormones, but by 14 weeks symptoms usually improve. Women with complications such as hyperthyroidism, hydatidiform mole (see chapter 3), and multiple gestation often experience more intense nausea and vomiting with their pregnancies.

- **Increased urination.**   In early pregnancy, the growing uterus leans across the bladder, causing urinary frequency. Late in pregnancy, the baby "drops" and moves lower in the pelvis, compressing the bladder. This pressure causes an increased urge to void and involuntary urine leakage when the baby moves suddenly.

PEARLS Pregnancy is often associated with frequent urination, especially in the first and third trimesters. Pregnancy predisposes women to urinary tract infections, which can also cause urinary frequency and urgency. A pregnant woman with a urinary tract infection may or may not have dysuria, hematuria, or foul smell to the urine.

- **Breast changes.**   In pregnancy, breasts feel larger, fuller, nodular, tense, and tender. The nipples enlarge and darken. Montgomery's tubercles (enlarged sebaceous glands) appear as bumps on the areola. The pattern of veins on the breast becomes more noticeable. Many of these changes may also occur with pituitary tumors and disorders, hypothyroidism, and medications such as oral contraceptives, amytriptyline

(Elavil), chlorpromazine (Thorazine), cimetidine (Tagamet), monoamine oxidase inhibitors (Nardil, Parmate), haloperidol (Haldol), opiates (codeine, morphine), and metoclopramide (Reglan).

- **Colostrum in breasts.** Throughout pregnancy the breasts prepare to make milk for the infant. Colostrum, a yellowish first milk rich in protein and antibodies, can often be expressed by the 12th week of pregnancy. Other medical conditions (including those listed under breast changes) can also cause discharge from the nipples in the non-pregnant woman. A serous or yellowish discharge is fairly common if patients have fibrocystic changes of the breast. Blood-tinged or bloody discharges may indicate malignancy.

- **Quickening.** Quickening (perceptible fetal movement) begins as flutters and wriggles and progresses to definite kicks and rolls. The fetus is active long before the mother can discern movement. Perception of fetal activity is related to the amount of fluid present and to maternal awareness and emotional state. Quickening is felt usually at 18–20 weeks for a primigravida and usually 2 weeks sooner for a multigravida. It is not considered a positive sign because intestinal gas and vigorous peristalsis can mimic fetal movement—and with pseudocyesis (false pregnancy), the woman may imagine the kicks of a fetus.

- **Skin changes.** The higher estrogen and progesterone levels of pregnancy stimulate melanocytes (pigment-producing cells) throughout the body. Nipples darken, and the linea nigra, a dark line running from pubis to umbilicus, appears. Some women develop chloasma, irregular brownish discoloration of the face. Striae (stretch marks) commonly appear on the enlarging breasts and abdomen and sometimes on the buttocks and thighs.

Probable Signs of Pregnancy

The examiner can directly observe the probable signs of pregnancy.

- **Positive pregnancy test.** Pregnancy tests can detect the presence of human chorionic gonadotropin (hCG) in the urine or blood with great accuracy. Over-the-counter urine tests are as accurate as office urine tests, and almost as accurate as blood tests if performed correctly. They are not infallible, however; so a positive test is considered only probable evidence of pregnancy and should be interpreted in the context of history and physical symptoms.

- **Braxton Hicks contractions.** Braxton Hicks are uterine contractions that occur throughout pregnancy and can be palpated by an examiner during the third trimester. Often they are painless, and the woman is unaware that they occur. At other times, they can be very painful and at term may be so frequent as to resemble labor.

○ **Abdominal enlargement.**   At about the 4th month of pregnancy, the uterus grows too large for the pelvis and tips forward, producing the distinctive curve of the pregnant abdomen. Women who have had numerous pregnancies tend to have poor abdominal tone and may present a pregnant contour earlier in gestation.

○ **Palpation of fetus.**   After the 20th week, the examiner may palpate the fetal outline; but because uterine fibroid tumors can feel very similar to a fetus, this is considered only a probable sign.

Positive Signs of Pregnancy

Positive signs of pregnancy cannot be attributed to any other condition.

○ **Fetal heart tones.**   The fetal heart begins to beat about 4 weeks after conception and sustains a rate of 120–160. The examiner can usually locate the fetal heartbeat with a Doppler device between 9 and 12 weeks' **gestation**, and with a fetoscope or good stethoscope after the 20th week, especially if the woman is fairly thin and the fetus is lying with his back in an anterior position.

○ **Fetal movement felt by examiner.**   In the third trimester, fetal kicks become clearly identifiable.

○ **Ultrasound, MRI, or radiograph showing fetus.**   Visualization is unmistakable evidence of pregnancy.

gestation
The time from conception to birth.

Taking a Relevant History

In managing any patient, the EMS professional must rapidly differentiate normal from abnormal, insignificant from significant, and benign from life-threatening. History taking and assessment must be rapid but also thorough and insightful—especially if the situation encountered upon arrival differs significantly from that conveyed by the caller or dispatcher. Become familiar with the signs of pregnancy and always consider it a possibility when assessing a female patient of childbearing age. Ask, "Is there any chance you might be pregnant?" remembering that some women will deny pregnancy at any stage of gestation. Questioning her in private sometimes yields more accurate answers.

During the first minutes of the encounter, the EMS provider should assess for potentially life-threatening conditions and get an accurate sense of the patient's current circumstances.

Useful questions include

- How far along are you? When is your due date? How accurate do you think your dates are?
- How many pregnancies have you had? How did they end? Were they vaginal births, cesarean sections, spontaneous or elective abortions?
- Are you in pain? Can you describe the pain?
- Are you having contractions?
- Any vaginal bleeding or leakage of fluid? What color is the fluid?
- Is the baby moving as much as usual?
- Have you had prenatal care? How often do you see your provider? When was your last visit?
- Have you ever had a sonogram? Early in the pregnancy or later on?
- Do you know for sure how many babies you are carrying?
- Any complications in your pregnancy so far? Do you have any medical problems that started before your pregnancy? Any other issues I should know about?
- Have you had severe headaches, visual disturbances, or unusual swelling of your hands, feet, or face?
- Are you experiencing difficulty eating, urinating, or moving your bowels?
- Any fever or other illness?
- Do you take any medications, herbs, supplements, or vitamins? What do you take them for?
- Do you smoke, drink alcohol, or use recreational drugs?
- Are you allergic to anything?

Obstetrical History

Last Menstrual Period (LMP)

Most calendar pregnancy-dating methods are based on a 28-day menstrual cycle, but in reality normal menstrual cycles range from 23 to 35 days, and many women have irregular cycles. Not every pregnancy can be accurately dated using a calendar and a menstrual record.

Accurate dating is further complicated by the fact that women sometimes spot blood when the embryo implants, and this implantation bleeding can be mistaken for a light period. Therefore, it is important to determine the patient's last *normal* period, base calculations on that, and consider the potential for inaccuracy.

PEARLS Implantation bleeding occurs when the embryo penetrates the uterine lining during the implantation process and ruptures blood vessels, resulting in vaginal bleeding that may be as heavy as a menstrual period. It normally subsides after a day or two. Implantation bleeding usually occurs in the 5th or 6th week following the last normal menstrual period. If implantation bleeding is mistaken for the LMP, the pregnancy may be more than a month farther along than expected.

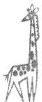 **PEDIATRIC**
NOTES

A girl may ovulate before menarche. If she is sexually active, she can become pregnant before she has her first menstrual period.

When Is She Due?

Because it is difficult to determine when a woman conceives, health care providers date pregnancies from the first day of the last period. If a woman has regular 28-day menstrual cycles and knows exactly when the last one started, she should be due 40 weeks, or 280 days, after that date. However, menstrual cycles vary in length, many women keep poor records of menses, and fully half of American pregnancies are unplanned. Even if the time of conception is known, the date of actual onset of spontaneous labor can vary by weeks.

When a woman seeks care early in her pregnancy, gestational age can be pinpointed fairly closely (plus or minus about a week) by ultrasound scanning or by measuring blood levels of hCG. Sonographic dating methods become progressively inaccurate with rising gestational age. Third-trimester ultrasounds allow a 3-week margin of error in either direction.

 ON TARGET Although accurate dating can be difficult, it is extremely important as a predictor for infant health. Infants are at significantly greater risk for illness or death when born before 37 weeks' or after 42 weeks' gestation.

A gestational wheel (made of two paper discs that align to calculate the relationships among LMP, due date, and gestational age) is a useful tool to keep with the obstetrical kit in the ambulance. It is easy to determine a due date from a menstrual period if the patient has regular 4-week cycles. Simply subtract 3 months from the first day of her last period, then add 1 week and 1 year. This is called Naegele's Rule. Therefore, a woman who began her last menses on January 1 would be due October 7.

This date is usually termed the estimated date of confinement, or EDC, based on an old term dating to when women were put to bed for a long period after childbirth. The due date is also referred to as estimated date of delivery (EDD) or estimated date of birth (EDB). All are prefixed

nulligravida
A woman who has never been pregnant.

nullipara
A woman who has never delivered beyond 20 weeks' gestation.

primigravida
A woman who is pregnant for the first time.

primipara
A woman who has had one delivery beyond 20 weeks' gestation. This term is also used informally to indicate a woman giving birth for the first time.

multigravida
A woman who is or has been pregnant for at least the second time.

multipara
A woman who has had two or more deliveries beyond 20 weeks' gestation. This term is often used in actual practice to indicate a woman who is giving birth for at least the second time.

with the word *estimated* for a good reason: Few women spontaneously deliver on their due dates, even when those dates are accurate. A pregnancy is generally considered term from 3 weeks before to 2 weeks after the due date.

How Many Times Has She Been Pregnant?

Gravida indicates the number of times a woman has been pregnant. This is the number of pregnancies, not the number of babies or how the pregnancy ended. For example, any woman with a history of two pregnancies is considered *gravida 2*, whether she has been pregnant twice and gave birth to two children, has been pregnant twice and gave birth to two sets of triplets, or has been pregnant twice and had two abortions.

Para indicates how many of those pregnancies ended with the birth of a fetus (or fetuses) that had reached the point of viability, whether or not they were born alive. If a woman has had 2 pregnancies that ended in first-trimester miscarriages, she is *gravida 2 para 0*. If a woman is pregnant for the second time and had a full-term live baby the first time, she is *gravida 2 para 1*.

Using a single number to express parity is limiting—it does not convey much of the information that health care providers need to know. In most systems, parity is expressed in four digits.

- **First digit.** Number of full-term babies the woman has delivered. "Full term" in this context means 37 weeks' gestation or longer.
- **Second digit.** Number of preterm infants born, that is, between about 20–24 (legal definition varies by state) and 37 weeks.
- **Third digit.** Number of pregnancies ending in spontaneous or elective abortion.
- **Fourth digit.** Number of children currently living to whom the woman has given birth.

Therefore, a woman halfway through her fourth pregnancy who has two living children, one of whom was premature, and a history of one spontaneous abortion is *gravida 4 para 1112*. The pregnant mother of premature toddler twins who has had no other pregnancies is *gravida 2 para 0202*.

A **nulligravida** is a woman who has never been pregnant, and a **nullipara** has never given birth. A **primigravida** is a woman who is pregnant for the first time. The correct definition of **primipara** is a woman who has delivered once before, but it is commonly used to reference to a woman giving birth for the first time. A **multigravida** has been pregnant two or more times. The correct definition of **multipara** is a woman who has had two or more deliveries, but in common usage the term often refers to a woman giving birth for at least the second time.

Evaluating the Present Complaint

In most cases, the EMS provider encounters a pregnant patient because she or someone else has called for an ambulance in response to a problem. The person who reports the problem or passes the initial report along sometimes misunderstands or omits important details. A call for a woman in labor may turn out to involve a 60-year-old with psychiatric problems who only *thinks* she is having a baby.

Most complaints and pains, obstetric or not, can be evaluated using the OLDCART mnemonic:

Onset.   When did this begin? What were you doing? Was the onset gradual or rapid? In what order did the symptoms occur?

Location.   Where does it hurt? Did the pain start there or has it moved? Is it localized or does it radiate?

Duration.   How long have you had the symptoms? Do they come and go? Have you experienced them before?

Characteristics.   Quality and quantity of the pain—Sharp? Dull? Frequency? On a scale of 1–10, with 10 being the worst pain you have ever had and 1 being barely there at all, what number would you give this pain?

Associated symptoms.   What other symptoms are you experiencing?

Relieving/aggravating factors.   What makes your symptoms better? What makes them worse?

Treatment.   Have you treated the symptoms (with medications, herbs, remedies, hot soaks, etc.)? Did the treatment help or make things worse?

When presented with a patient who has a conspicuously curving abdomen, it is easy to focus on that and fail to notice serious conditions not necessarily related to her pregnancy. In most cases, the best way to care for the fetus is to concentrate on stabilizing the mother. As with any other patient, an EMS professional must remember to evaluate ABCs (airway, breathing, circulation) first and look for potentially life-threatening conditions in the mother before turning attention to the gravid abdomen.

It is also important to notice the woman's surroundings and mode of living. Her primary care provider usually does not have the opportunity to come into her home and observe her lifestyle. The EMS professional is in a unique position to spot hazards and problems in the patient's home or work environment.

The provider should not assume that a woman is pregnant simply because her girth is enlarged. Many conditions can cause an abdomen to distend, including tumors, ascites, and obesity. An overweight woman or an athlete with strong abdominal muscles can effectively hide a pregnancy through much of gestation, especially if she is tall. The responder will sometimes encounter a woman who shows obvious signs of pregnancy and denies any possibility of conception.

Universal Precautions

Gloves should be worn for procedures and assessments that may involve exposure to body fluids. Goggles and a gown will help protect the provider from fluid splashes at a birth. HIV and other disease organisms can be present in blood, semen, vaginal secretions, breast milk, and amniotic fluid, and all these fluids can be present at a birth or in certain complications of pregnancy.

Vital Signs

Increased progesterone levels decrease systemic vascular resistance by 21% as compared with the nonpregnant state. This produces a parallel drop in blood pressure during the first half of pregnancy that usually returns to the nonpregnant baseline by term. The diastolic value typically drops 16–20 mmHg, but changes in the systolic pressure are less dramatic. Low readings such as 86/60 may be found in young women and women who exercise regularly. Mildly high blood-pressure readings are a much greater cause for concern in pregnant women than in nonpregnant women of childbearing age. A reading of 140/90 can indicate the onset of a life-threatening hypertensive disorder, especially if accompanied by generalized edema and symptoms such as malaise, headache, or epigastric pain. (See Hypertensive Disorders in chapter 3 for a more thorough discussion.)

A pregnant woman greater than 20–24 weeks should avoid lying flat on her back. When a woman lies supine, up to 13–15 lbs of uterus, fetus, amniotic fluid, and placenta (about the weight of a bowling ball) are positioned directly over the aorta and vena cava, the two vessels primarily responsible for cardiac output. As pregnancy advances, the uterus becomes heavy enough to compress these vessels, especially the vena cava, against the spine. If blood return to the heart is compromised, the woman can experience signs of cardiogenic shock—pallor, anxiety, hypotension, tachycardia, and even syncope, a condition termed **supine hypotension syndrome.** Her cardiac output may be reduced by 30%. Research suggests that vena caval compression can produce placental abruption. Supine positioning can also cause respiratory compromise by limiting lung expansion and diaphragm excursion, and it may elevate blood pressure in the hypertensive patient.

ON TARGET Left lateral positioning may be the single most effective intervention an EMS provider can perform to increase placental perfusion in any pregnant patient beyond 20 weeks' gestation.

supine hypotension syndrome
A drop in blood pressure that occurs when a pregnant woman lies on her back, allowing her uterus and its contents to compress her vena cava against her spine.

PEARLS The EMS provider should avoid placing a pregnant trauma victim supine on a backboard. In some situations, supine positioning is more dangerous to the mother–fetus dyad than the trauma that necessitated the backboard. It may be appropriate to wedge a pillow (4–6 in. thick) under her right hip to tip her slightly to the left. Alternatively, the provider can tip the entire backboard to the left 15–30°.

Transporting in the position that yields the best maternal vital signs without monitoring the fetal heart rate may result in an adequately perfused mother with a distressed fetus. The fetus can become compromised long before maternal vital signs become abnormal. Left lateral recumbent positioning should be considered for most transports not requiring spinal immobilization. Research supports utilizing the left lateral position for maximizing cardiac output and placental perfusion, especially if fetal heart rate is not monitored.

Fetal distress can occur while maternal vital signs remain stable; if a woman is ill or injured enough to necessitate ambulance transport, the provider should administer oxygen. Oxygen therapy may benefit the majority of pregnant patients with an acute complaint. Intravenous fluids, usually normal saline or lactated Ringer's, are often indicated as well.

Evaluating the Pregnant Abdomen

• **Observe for bruises, scars, and injuries and ask the patient to explain them.**   You may be the only provider to recognize that she has been physically abused. Scars may reveal clinically significant surgeries, such as appendectomy or previous cesarean section.

• **Palpate the fundal height (upper margin of the uterus).**   In the ambulatory care setting, this is usually measured in centimeters. See Table 2-1. Measuring from pubic bone to fundus, the number of centimeters measured should approximately equal the weeks of gestation after about 22–24 weeks. See Figure 2-1.

In the field it may be simpler to describe the fundal height in relation to the pubic bone, umbilicus, and xyphoid. See Table 2-1. For example, if her uterus is at the level of her umbilicus, she is probably about 20–22 weeks' pregnant. See Figure 2-2. The chief disadvantage of this method is the wide variation in finger widths and torso heights. A small woman with a large baby or a tall woman with a deep pelvis may measure differently and still be perfectly normal. A primigravida may have stronger muscle tone and carry her baby

Table 2-1   Relative Fundal Height

12 weeks	The uterus is just palpable over the top of the pubic bone.
16 weeks	Halfway between pubis and umbilicus.
20–22 weeks	Uterus is at level of umbilicus.
24 weeks	1–2 finger breadths above umbilicus.
32 weeks	3–4 finger breadths below xyphoid process.
36–38 weeks	1 finger breadth below xyphoid process.
40 weeks	2–3 finger breadths below xyphoid process if lightening occurs.

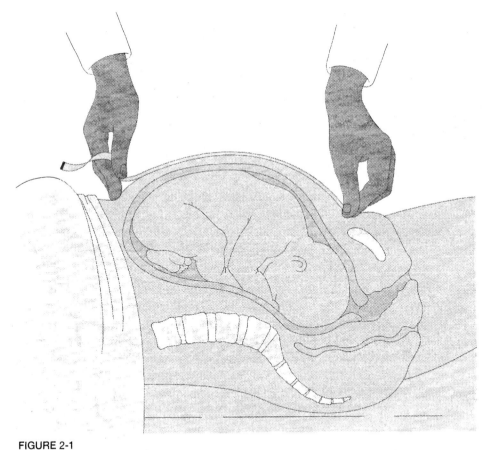

FIGURE 2-1
Determining Gestational Age by Measuring the Maternal Abdomen.
Gestational age can be approximated by measuring from pubic bone to fundus—the number of weeks of gestation approximately equals the measurement in centimeters after about 22–24 weeks.

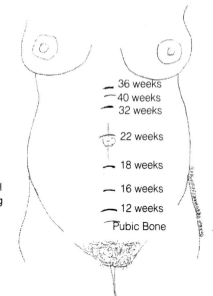

FIGURE 2-2
Approximating Gestational Age by Anatomical Relationships.
It is possible to approximate gestational age by determining relationships among the fundus and the pubis, umbilicus, and xyphoid. This is not absolute—actual fundal height can be influenced by the length of the maternal torso, whether the mother carries her fetus low or high, and other factors.
Illustration by Bonnie U. Gruenberg

higher, whereas the multiparous woman may carry the fetus deep in the pelvis and measure small. Measuring by bodily landmarks is, however, useful for a rough approximation of gestational age. See Figure 2-3.

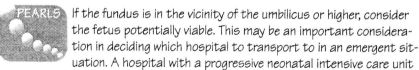

PEARLS If the fundus is in the vicinity of the umbilicus or higher, consider the fetus potentially viable. This may be an important consideration in deciding which hospital to transport to in an emergent situation. A hospital with a progressive neonatal intensive care unit (NICU) is better able to support an infant born at the cusp of viability; a small community hospital will usually transfer such babies immediately.

• **Fetal heart tones.** Refer to local protocols regarding monitoring of fetal heart rates; most EMS response services do not routinely auscultate fetal heart tones or carry Dopplers or fetoscopes. However, auscultation of the fetal heart tones may provide clinically useful information that can affect outcomes.

The embryo's heart begins to beat only 4 weeks after conception, but usually cannot be detected until 10–12 weeks with a Doppler device or 20 weeks with a fetoscope. Fetuses between 12 and 18 weeks' gestation may be too active to locate for more than a few seconds at a time. Heart tones are often best heard though the fetal back. After about 20 weeks, direct the Doppler or fetoscope towards the firmest part of the

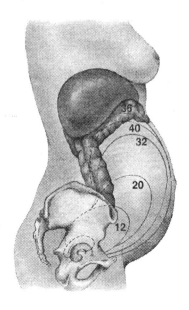

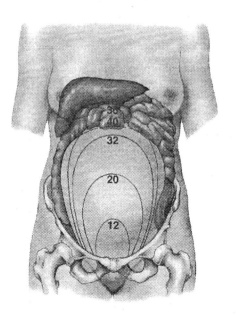

FIGURE 2-3
Expansion of the Gravid Uterus by Weeks.
The uterus displaces abdominal organs as pregnancy advances.
Illustration by Bonnie U. Gruenberg

abdomen to detect heart sounds. See Figure 2-4. A stethoscope may be used after about 20 weeks' gestation, but the audibility of heart sounds often depends on fetal position and maternal body size. The fetus may not be detectable with a Doppler at 12 weeks if the uterus is retroflexed (tilted backward) or the placenta is anterior; in both cases the Doppler must penetrate more tissue to locate the heartbeat.

Evaluating the Pregnant Woman   57

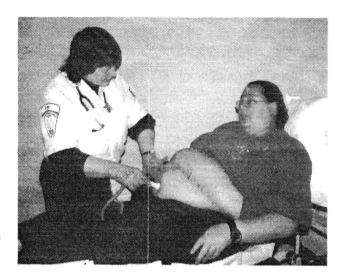

FIGURE 2-4
Obtaining Fetal Heart Tones with a Doppler Device.
A Doppler device is useful for listening to fetal heart tones and is much more effective than a stethoscope in the back of a moving ambulance.
Photographed by Bonnie U. Gruenberg

ON TARGET The EMS professional is not usually required to auscultate fetal heart tones in the field; but by mastering and applying this skill, the provider can potentially improve outcomes for pregnant patients and their unborn children.

It can be extremely difficult to hear fetal heart tones in an ambulance. Extraneous noise makes the task more difficult, and if the baby is positioned with his back toward his mother's spine, or if the mother is obese, finding a heartbeat can be very challenging. The absence of fetal heart tones in the field does not necessarily mean that there *are* no fetal heart tones. Clarifying this important point to the patient may spare her needless fear and grief.

The normal fetal heart rate ranges from 120 to 160 beats per minute. When the fetus is active, the rate can increase for several minutes. A persistently high baseline, over 160, can indicate a compromised fetus. A high baseline can also be seen if the mother is on certain labor-stopping or asthma medications, such as terbutaline. Hypoxia and infection can also cause fetal tachycardia. A low baseline, 110–120, is sometimes normal for a particular fetus. Heart rates range lower and show less variation when the fetus is sleeping. Significant dips in heart rate, or decelerations, can occur if the umbilical cord is compressed or if blood flow to the fetus is compromised. (See chapter 7.) Decelerations (drops in heart rate) may also occur in response to fetal head compression in second-stage labor.

PEARLS A fetus may develop a tachycardic heart rate in response to maternal infection before the mother shows any signs or symptoms of illness.

Always make sure that you are not accidentally auscultating the maternal pulse. Sometimes the maternal heart rate elevates into the fetal ranges during labor, when in shock, or with other bodily stressors, and fetal distress may drop the fetal heart rate into the normal maternal range. A pulse oximeter applied to the maternal finger or external cardiac monitoring can conveniently clarify whether the rate auscultated is maternal or fetal.

A fetus with a persistently low heart rate or repetitive decelerations with slow recovery needs to be in an appropriate facility as soon as possible. The mother should be transported on her side or hands and knees (whichever results in a fetal heart rate that most nearly approaches normal). Administer high-flow oxygen and isotonic crystalloid intravenous fluids at a rapid rate (normal saline or lactated Ringer's) unless there is pulmonary edema. As usual in emergency obstetrics, a focus on treating whatever is wrong with the mother maximizes fetal well-being.

The location of fetal heart tones with a stethoscope can also help determine fetal position. See Figure 2-5. If the heart sounds are strongest low in the abdomen, the fetus is often in a cephalic (head-first) presentation. If they are above the umbilicus, especially if you feel a hard, firm mass in the fundus, the fetus may be breech. A Doppler device obtains heart tones by bouncing sound waves, and so may pick up a fetal heart rate in other locations. This makes it unreliable for determining fetal position.

A "whooshing" quality to the heart sounds may indicate that you are auscultating the funic souffle (the sound of blood in the umbilical cord) or the placental souffle (blood rushing through the placenta). As long as a fetal rate distinct from the maternal pulse is reflected, either is suitable for evaluating the fetal heart rate. Sounds of the fetal heart itself are usually crisp and have a clicking quality.

• **Palpate for position.** Sometimes it may be possible to accurately palpate fetal position, important if delivery may be imminent. Leopold's maneuvers are a four-step systematic method for determining fetal position. A modification of Leopold's (as follows) can be useful in the field.

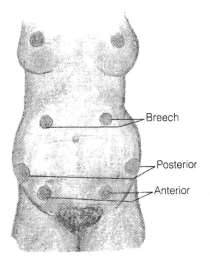

Breech

Posterior

Anterior

FIGURE 2-5
Determining Fetal Position by Location of Heartbeat.
When auscultated with a stethoscope or fetoscope, the fetal heart is best heard in the locations shown here, depending on fetal position. A Doppler works by bouncing sound waves and so may pick up a fetal heartbeat in other locations.

Evaluating the Pregnant Woman

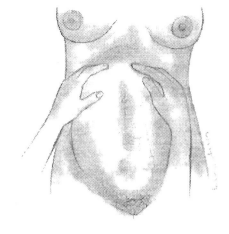

FIGURE 2-6
Modified Leopold's Maneuvers I.
Palpate the fundus with both hands.
Feel for a head (which is round and
can be bounced between your fingertips) or a rump (which is irregular
and moves the whole body when
balloted between your fingertips).
Illustration by Bonnie U. Gruenberg

First, palpate the fundus. See Figure 2-6. The fetal head will feel
firm and hard, and can be bounced between the hands. The fetal rump
will feel irregular, and the entire body will move if it is displaced. The
fetus may keep his feet up alongside his head, so the presence of feet
beside the mass in the fundus does not guarantee that it is a rump. Fetal
positioning is easier to feel close to term, but may be palpated as early
as 30 weeks, earlier if the provider is experienced and the woman thin.

Next, walk your hands across the abdomen from one side to the
other, pressing firmly with your fingertips. See Figure 2-7. If the fetus
is breech or cephalic, you will probably feel that one side of the abdomen is firmer than the other. The firm fetal back may be felt as early
as 20–24 weeks, but often is hard to palpate before 28–30 weeks.

Next, press the finger pads of both hands firmly but gently into
the right and left lower abdomen, just above the pubic hairline, palms

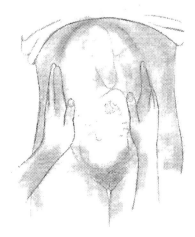

FIGURE 2-7
Modified Leopold's Maneuvers II.
Hold one hand flat against the side of the
abdomen, then palpate the length of the
other side with the flats of your fingertips.
Repeat on opposite side. The fetal back
will feel firm, and opposite the back the
abdomen will feel softer, often with small
parts palpable (knees, feet, etc.).
Illustration by Bonnie U. Gruenberg

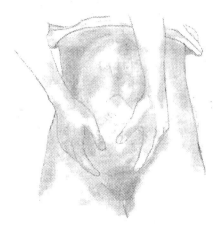

FIGURE 2-8
Modified Leopold's Maneuvers III.
Palpate above the pubic bone to determine what is entering the pelvis. If the head is engaged, it may be difficult to differentiate the upper margin of the pubic bone from the fetal head.
Illustration by Bonnie U. Gruenberg

facing the abdomen. See Figure 2-8. A head will feel like a hard, round coconut, sometimes deep in the pelvis, other times close to the surface and almost contiguous with the upper margin of the pubic bone. If the fetus has descended into the pelvis, it is possible the head may not be palpable at all, just the shoulders. A rump descending into the pelvis in a breech presentation will usually feel irregular, and softer and smaller than the head, but often fetal presentation is difficult for even experienced practitioners to determine, so do not spend too much time on this assessment.

If the abdomen is soft above the pubic bone, soft in the fundus, and firm on both the right and left sides, suspect a transverse presentation. In a transverse presentation, the fetus lies at right angles to the mother's spine, his head on one side of her abdomen and his rump on the other. This position is not uncommon in the earlier part of pregnancy, and most babies will turn to vertex by 32–34 weeks. This position is not deliverable vaginally.

• **Fetal movement.** Between 16 and 20 weeks, the mother usually feels quickening, or the first stirrings of fetal movement. After the first few weeks, she should feel movement daily. After about 26 or 28 weeks, normal fetal movement is usually described as more than 10 kicks in 2 hours and is considered a reassuring sign of fetal well-being. This is true whether the examiner palpates the movement or the mother reports it. Her obstetrical provider may instruct her to record "kick counts" or chart fetal movement patterns every day.

• **Contractions.** Uterine contractions are felt best by the examiner high in the fundus, where the greatest muscle contraction occurs. They are usually felt more strongly by the mother low in the pelvis or in the sacral area. A strong contraction feels much like a tightly flexed bicep when palpated.

- **Uterine tone.** A rigid uterus may occur in some emergencies, such as placental abruption.

- **Uterine tenderness.** A tender uterus, discovered by palpation, may be present in some emergencies, such as placental abruption, uterine rupture, and chorioamnionitis.

- **Vaginal bleeding.** Although many women experience benign vaginal bleeding at some point in their pregnancies, this symptom must always be taken seriously. In early pregnancy it can indicate an imminent loss of the fetus. Later in pregnancy, vaginal bleeding can indicate life-threatening emergencies such as placenta previa or placental abruption.

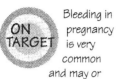

Bleeding in pregnancy is very common and may or may not be significant, but the EMS provider should always consider it a potential emergency and treat accordingly.

If a woman is bleeding, the EMS provider should obtain a history and quantify the amount of blood loss. Does she have any conditions that could account for the bleeding, such as placenta previa or cervical dysplasia? When did the bleeding begin? How many pads is the patient soaking in an hour? Look at the pads yourself if possible. If the patient says that she is saturating three pads an hour, find out whether she is referring to maximally absorbent overnight pads or thin panty liners that hold minimal moisture. Note whether the blood is bright red, brown, or pinkish; whether it has an odor or contains mucus; and whether the flow has slowed or increased. Save any clots or tissue passed and bring it with you to the hospital.

Where to Transport

In some circumstances, it may be beneficial for the EMS crew to bypass certain hospitals to bring the patient to a facility that offers comprehensive services for high-risk pregnant women and neonates. In other cases, transport to the nearest hospital for stabilization can be lifesaving. The EMS provider should learn which local and regional hospitals offer obstetric and neonatal intensive care and the local protocols regarding transport to these facilities. When in doubt, consult with medical control.

Some infants will require prolonged care at a hospital with a neonatal intensive care unit if they are to survive or have a good prognosis. Many serious conditions are diagnosed ultrasonographically during the **antepartum** period, and the parents may plan to deliver at a facility that specializes in the treatment of high-risk children. A fast-moving labor may force the woman to deliver a high-risk infant elsewhere, and then transport to an appropriate facility may occur after birth.

A hospital with level I neonatal intensive care facilities can manage normal newborn and maternal care, identify high-risk pregnancies, and provide basic emergency services. A level II facility can handle most

antepartum
A noun or adjective referring to the period of pregnancy before labor or delivery; prenatal.

maternal and neonatal complications. A level III facility offers the full range of maternal and neonatal services and can provide care for critically ill infants. At least one full-time neonatologist is on staff. In addition, there are regional facilities that provide special services for the sickest of babies, manage rare conditions and diseases with high mortality rates, and often perform fetal surgery and other procedures to begin treatment for certain anomalies while the fetus is still *in utero*. When in doubt about which facility is most appropriate, seek the advice of your medical control. It may be appropriate to consider air transportation.

Incorporating a Patient-Centered Approach

The effective EMS provider approaches each patient with respect and consideration, recognizing that childbearing is a function of a woman's most intimate bodily processes. Even in emergencies, the caregiver should treat every patient as an autonomous and multidimensional individual. Whenever possible, emergency care should address not only the woman's physical condition but also her emotions, social bonds, spirituality, cultural practices, lifestyle, and environment.

Consent is not informed unless the woman understands the procedures being proposed or performed, their rationales, and any associated risks. Ask permission before making physical contact. Many women have a history of sexual or physical abuse, and abrupt violation of personal boundaries can feel like an assault to them. Respect modesty within the boundaries of the situation. Whether the patient views your ministrations as helpful or invasive depends largely on the attitude you project as you provide treatment.

Pregnancy effects enormous physical, psychological, and emotional changes in a woman's body. Not only is her body indelibly altered by the experience, but childbearing is also a developmental milestone that changes a woman's self-perception, social dynamics, and indeed the course of her life.

Cultural and Religious Considerations

The American population has great ethnic, cultural, religious, and linguistic diversity. It is difficult to generalize about how a particular culture or a particular individual within that culture may respond to obstetric emergencies because generalizations lead to stereotyping. Can you say that generalizations about *your* gender, race, ethnicity, and culture universally hold true for *you*—or for anyone you know?

Ethnocentrism is the belief that the values of one's own cultural group are the best or the only acceptable ones—or, perhaps more often, the failure to consider other cultures or beliefs. Virtually everyone engages in ethnocentrism to some degree at least some of the time. EMS professionals who are unaware of their own cultural biases filter each encounter through their own attitudes and values, and then become frustrated or judgmental when the patient does not react as expected. Before culturally sensitive care can be implemented, it is essential for providers to evaluate their own biases, attitudes, and prejudices and make a sincere effort to respect the values and beliefs of others.

It is ultimately the woman's right to make her own health care decisions. Always consider the patient's uniqueness and seek to determine what is important to her. The sensitive provider will take each patient's background and beliefs into consideration, and try to adapt caregiving to include cultural and religious variations. It is useful to recognize that certain groups have beliefs, aversions, or folk medicine that may play a role in assessment and treatment choices. For example, some patients have a cultural tendency to express pain openly, but some do not, and those who are very vocal may not be merely dramatic, but may indeed feel intense pain.

Antenatal Testing

The obstetric provider often orders numerous tests to assess for fetal abnormalities or pregnancy complications, and to monitor the well-being of mother and fetus. Some common tests include

- **Ultrasound.** This involves bouncing high-frequency sound waves off body structures and has proved valuable for assessing the growth and well-being of the fetus. Ultrasound can accurately date pregnancies, especially in the first trimester, and identify multiple gestation, ectopic pregnancy, bleeding behind the placenta, structural anomalies, fetal position and presentation, placenta previa. It can sometimes detect placental abruption, fetal demise, and many other conditions. It can estimate fetal weight and monitor growth, assess fetal well-being, and calculate blood flow through the umbilical cord. Procedures such as amniocentesis or breech version are done with ultrasound guidance. Ultrasound scans can be done transabdominally or transvaginally. See Figure 2-9.

- **Nuchal translucency screening.** This assessed is ultrasonographically. If a structure on the fetal neck is measured at about 13 weeks of gestation, an abnormal reading can indicate Down syndrome.

- **Chorionic villus sampling.** This is a first-trimester procedure in which a small piece of the placental tissue is removed through the cervix or abdomen, and the fetal chromosomes are studied.

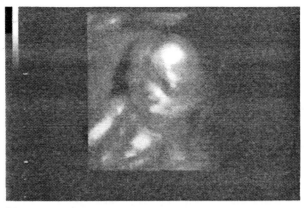

(a)

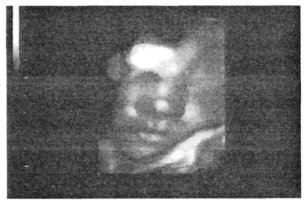

(b)
FIGURE 2-9
Three-dimensional Ultrasound Images of Fetuses in Utero.
(a) A 19-week fetus with the umbilical cord draped around his
neck. (b) A 37-week fetus with his hand at his cheek.

- **Amniocentesis.** This involves inserting a large needle through
the maternal abdominal wall under ultrasound guidance and withdrawing a sample of amniotic fluid. Fetal cells are then grown in a
laboratory and studied for chromosomal defects. Amniocentesis is
also used to assess fetal lung maturity.

- **Alpha fetoprotein test.** In an alpha fetoprotein test (also known
as a quadruple marker or multiple marker screen), blood is drawn
from the mother at 15–20 weeks' gestation to measure the levels of
four different substances. Abnormal results may indicate Down syndrome, neural tube defects, or other anomalies.

- **Glucose tolerance test.** At 26–28 weeks, a pregnant woman is
given a 50-g glucose challenge (usually in the form of carbonated

beverage), and her blood is drawn an hour later to determine her blood glucose level. If the reading is above 140, she returns for a second test to ingest 100 g of glucose after fasting. Her blood sugar is drawn before drinking the solution, then at three 1-hour intervals. If two or more of the four readings are elevated, she is considered to have gestational diabetes.

• **Group B strep carrier screening.**   At about 36 weeks' gestation, most women are tested for the presence of group B strep in their vaginas. Group B streptococci are part of the vaginal and intestinal flora in about one-third of all women at any given time. If the baby is infected by group B strep at birth, he may develop a life-threatening illness such as meningitis or pneumonia. To prevent illness in the newborn, women who test positive for group B strep receive antibiotics in labor.

Summary

The prehospital provider usually enters an emergency knowing little or nothing about the patient, her condition, or her environment and has little time in which to assess and treat. History taking is as much art as science; signs and symptoms of illness in the pregnant patient are often ambiguous or conflicting; and the EMS provider must rapidly sort through irrelevant details to recognize the true problem. The OLDCART mnemonic is a highly effective checklist for eliciting information about the present complaint. When assessing, treating, and transporting the pregnant patient, the insightful EMS provider will adopt a holistic perspective that considers the patient's lifestyle and individual needs.

REVIEW QUESTIONS

1. List the probable signs of pregnancy and reasons that these are not definitive evidence of pregnancy.

2. Describe use of the OLDCART mnemonic in evaluating a complaint.

3. Why should EMS provider avoid placing a pregnant women in the supine position?

4. While auscultating the fetal heart rate with a Doppler, you notice decelerations to 60 that begin at the peak of each contraction and continue for about a minute after the contraction is over. What should you do?

5. What are three ways to approximate estimated due date in the field?

Pregnancy
Complications

Objectives

By the end of this chapter you should be able to

- Implement treatment for vaginal bleeding during pregnancy

- Assess and treat the patient with suspected ectopic pregnancy

- Understand the causes of disseminated intravascular coagulation in pregnancy

- Understand common etiologies of pelvic and abdominal pain in pregnancy

- Understand how to assess and transport the patient with hyperemesis gravidarum

- Recognize signs and symptoms of preeclampsia

CASE
Study

Michael and Kayla arrived at the maternity unit to transport a pregnant woman with a life-threatening condition 300 miles to a hospital nearer her home. Because it was likely that her infant would require months of intensive care, delivery at a distant hospital would limit the time she could spend with the baby during his stay in the NICU.

Estella Alces had presented to the emergency department the night before and was discharged after evaluation. Estella was a 23-year-old primigravida at 30 weeks' gestation who had recently immigrated to West Virginia from Argentina. She had driven 5 hours to go camping with friends when she developed substernal chest pain radiating to the back. She had a history of symptomatic mitral valve prolapse and was on propranolol, a beta blocker. Upon arrival at the hospital, the ED evaluated her heart, lungs, and vital signs and found no pathology. She was normotensive and well oxygenated. The staff evaluated the well-being of her fetus and saw no abnormalities on the fetal heart tracing or sonogram. Her CBC was unremarkable except for moderate thrombocytopenia—her platelet count was 75,000 (normal is 150,000–450,000).

Dr. Presque, the on-call obstetrician, had been informed when the patient arrived, but after evaluating her symptoms the ED discharged the apparently healthy and now asymptomatic woman without further word to the obstetrician. The ED attending physician noted the thrombocytopenia and discharged her with a copy of her labs, advising her to share them with her own physician when she returned from vacation. He assumed that her blood work indicated gestational thrombocytopenia, a common and usually benign condition of pregnancy.

When Dr. Presque looked over her blood work the next morning, she was alarmed to see the low platelet count. She called the lab to ask whether it still had Estella's blood sample and whether enough blood remained to perform a hepatic function panel. A few hours later, the report showed that Estella had severely elevated liver enzymes. Dr. Presque and staff immediately began to make phone calls in hope of locating Estella so that she might return to the hospital.

Questions

1. What was Estella's diagnosis?
2. What are the signs and symptoms of this condition?
3. What could happen to Estella if she were not treated for this condition?
4. What should Michael and Kayla consider when transporting this patient?

Introduction

Most pregnancies proceed with only minor discomforts and concerns, but when serious complications do arise, it is often the EMS provider who is summoned. Prehospital care of the woman with a high-risk pregnancy involves requires rapid assessment, judicious management, and prompt transport to an appropriate health care institution. To achieve optimal outcomes for mother and fetus, the EMS professional must become familiar with the etiology, diagnosis, consequences, and management of the most common pregnancy complications.

Antepartal Bleeding—First Half of Pregnancy

Bleeding in early pregnancy does not always herald a miscarriage. Sometimes the bleeding proves to originate from the rectum or urinary tract rather than the vagina. Causes of vaginal bleeding in pregnancy include vaginal or cervical infection, cervical polyps, cervical cancer, cervical or vaginal trauma, ectopic pregnancy, and hydatidiform mole. A woman may spot after intercourse or after an office vaginal exam because even gentle cervical manipulation may rupture small blood vessels. A woman who fails to produce sufficient progesterone may experience vaginal bleeding—treatment with supplemental progesterone sustains the pregnancy until the placenta has matured and can manufacture adequate amounts. Implantation bleeding results from vascular disruption as the embryo burrows into the endometrial tissue. Implantation bleeding can be scanty or profuse; it often occurs 5–6 weeks after the last menstrual period and lasts a day or two.

Spontaneous Abortion

Spontaneous abortion is the clinical term for what is commonly termed a miscarriage. The usual definition is the loss of a pregnancy before the fetus reaches 20 weeks or 500 g. This boundary can blur in practice. It is common for dates to prove incorrect, and occasionally a baby weighing less than 500 g will survive.

It is difficult to determine what percentage of pregnancies end in spontaneous abortion. In about 30% of miscarriages, the woman is unaware that she is pregnant and experiences simply a delayed, heavy menstrual period. Ten to 17% of pregnancies spontaneously terminate between 4 and 20 weeks of gestation. Twenty-five to 50% of conceived embryos never implant. Forty-year-old women lose twice as many pregnancies as 20-year-old women.

Most women who suffer spontaneous abortion wonder whether they did something to cause it. In most situations, this is not the case unless they have exposed their fetuses to damaging drugs or toxins. About half of spontaneous abortions are due to chromosomal errors. Others are related to problems with maternal anatomy or hormones, or to maternal diseases such as diabetes, infections, placental abnormalities, uterine scarring, or immune dysfunction. Often the cause of a pregnancy loss will remain unknown.

Threatened Abortion

About one-third to one-half of women who experience vaginal bleeding in the first trimester will lose the pregnancy. Bleeding may be red (fresh) or brown (old), scanty or profuse. The patient may complain of cramping in the back or abdomen. Many women say that the accompanying pain equals or surpasses the contractions of labor. *Always consider ectopic pregnancy a possibility unless the conceptus has been sonographically confirmed in the uterus.*

Field treatment usually involves basic care and transport, but it is important to be vigilant for a decline in the patient's condition. Most local protocols support the following management strategies:

- **Get a complete history, including a history of the present problems.** The OLDCART checklist works well for this purpose (see chapter 2). Could this be an ectopic pregnancy? If the patient is certain of her blood type, document this information and relay it to the hospital staff. If she is Rh-negative, she will need a shot of anti-D immunoglobulin (RhoGam); without it her body may manufacture antibodies that could attack the next fetus she conceives. Because the blood type of the fetus is usually unknown, RhoGam is given to all bleeding or miscarrying pregnant women with a negative Rh blood type.

- **Monitor vital signs carefully.** If the patient is bleeding significantly, frequent vital signs are necessary. If you suspect hypovolemia, take orthostatic vital signs by measuring her pulse and blood pressure in left lateral position, then in a high Fowler's position or, better yet, standing. A 15-mmHg drop in the blood pressure and 20-beat-per-minute increase in the heart rate indicate that blood volume is significantly low. If your patient is volume-depleted, she may faint in an upright position, so keep her safety in mind at all times. If she shows signs of shock, orthostatic vital signs should not be obtained, and she should be kept flat and on her left side.

- **Watch for signs of shock.** If the patient is pale, clammy, and restless, treat her like any other patient in hypovolemic shock. Position her flat on her side, apply high-flow oxygen, and start at least one large-bore

IV of a crystalloid solution such as lactated Ringer's or normal saline in a sizable vein—two if she is actively hemorrhaging. Second-trimester pregnancy losses carry a significant risk of severe hemorrhage.

- **Draw blood.**   A blood draw in the field can expedite the processing of the patient's lab work after she arrives at the hospital. Check your local protocols to determine whether it will be accepted by the lab.

- **Count pads to measure bleeding.**   Blood loss may vary. To measure blood loss, look at the pads the patient has been discarding and determine their thickness and how saturated they are. If she is not wearing a pad, note whether blood has soaked through her underpants or outer clothing, whether it has soaked through the sheet or into the mattress, or whether it is enough to puddle on the floor. Often much of the evidence will have been flushed away before your arrival, so try to quantify any amount she lost in the toilet. Remember to consider other sources of blood in the toilet, such as hemorrhoids or rectal fissures. If she passed any clots or tissue, bring them along to the hospital.

  If she is passing large amounts of blood that does not clot, or if she is bleeding from other bodily orifices or her intravenous access sites, consider DIC (see later). DIC is most likely to occur with septicemia or with second-trimester abortion.

- **Fetal heart tones.**   If you carry a Doppler on the ambulance, you can obtain fetal heart tones if the patient is beyond 12 weeks' gestation. Heart tones can be difficult to find in the field, especially in the first half of pregnancy. The decision to auscultate heart tones in a patient less than 18–20 weeks should be weighed carefully. The presence or absence of fetal heart tones will not change your plan of care; if you fail to hear a heartbeat you will increase maternal anxiety.

- **Provide emotional support.**   Losing a pregnancy can be frightening or heartbreaking, not only for the pregnant woman but also for her family and friends. Statements that acknowledge their feelings and show genuine concern are generally the most comforting. Explain procedures clearly and honestly, give the patient your focused attention, and listen to her concerns. Reassure her that bleeding and cramping do not necessarily mean that she is losing the pregnancy and that there is nothing that she could have done to prevent miscarriage.

abortion
The spontaneous or induced termination of pregnancy before fetal viability.

Inevitable Abortion

When **abortion** is certain to occur, it is termed inevitable. The woman reports abdominal or back pain and bleeding, and sometimes a gush of fluid from the vagina. This condition progresses to either complete abortion or incomplete abortion.

Complete Abortion

products of
conception
(conceptus)
The results of con-
ception—not only
the embryo or
fetus, but also the
placenta, mem-
branes, amniotic
fluid, and other
substances and
structures.

Complete abortion is the spontaneous loss of all of the **products of conception,** as evidenced by an empty uterus upon ultrasound exam. After the uterus is empty, bleeding should diminish. Most cases of complete abortion occur very early in pregnancy, and nature completes the process without incident.

Incomplete Abortion

In incomplete abortion, part of the products of conception is not expelled. Usually it is the placenta or part of the placenta that is retained. Bleeding can be profuse because the uterus is unable to clamp down and maintain hemostasis if placental fragments remain. The woman must have a dilation and curettage (D&C) operation to complete the process and stop the bleeding. See Figure 3-1.

Missed Abortion

In a missed abortion, the products of conception are retained *in utero* after the fetus has died. Expulsion occurs days or weeks later. The introduction of ultrasound has revealed that almost all spontaneous abortions present this way, making this term obsolete. A blighted ovum is a condition in which the gestational sac and placenta develop with no embryo.

Septic Abortion

In septic abortion, infection invades the uterine cavity during the abortion process. Septic abortion may occur after conception with an intrauterine device (IUD) in place; with prolonged, undiagnosed rupture of membranes; or after attempts by unqualified individuals to end a pregnancy. The woman presents with pain, fever, and foul-smelling vaginal discharge.

Elective Abortion

Elective abortion occurs when the woman chooses to end her pregnancy for nonmedical reasons. This is often documented as voluntary interruption of pregnancy (VIP). The EMS provider may encounter women

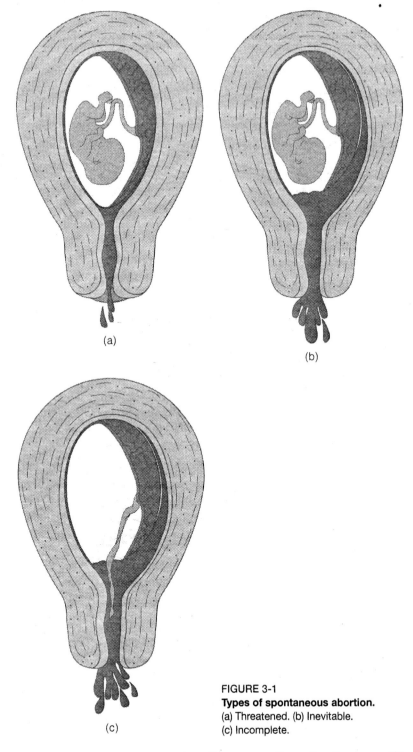

(a)

(b)

(c)

FIGURE 3-1
Types of spontaneous abortion.
(a) Threatened. (b) Inevitable.
(c) Incomplete.

Pregnancy Complications   73

experiencing complications of this procedure. About 88% of VIPs in the United States are performed during the first trimester, and nearly all are performed before 15 weeks of gestation, most by surgical suction. The procedure has a low rate of complications. When abortion is performed by a qualified provider, the mortality and morbidity risk to the mother is significantly less than her risk would be if she carried the pregnancy to term. There are currently several legal methods of abortion in the United States, and in 2000, the FDA approved a pharmacological means.

Surgical abortion is accomplished by opening the cervix and extracting the products of conception—fetus, amniotic sac, placenta, and other structures—with suction or curettage. Less commonly, abortion is accomplished by inducing labor later in gestation, but before viability. Abortion performed very early in pregnancy confers a much lower risk of complications than at later stages of gestation.

By FDA guidelines, medical (nonsurgical) abortion can be induced by a clinician with mifepristone (RU 486, or Mifeprex) orally no later than 49 days after the LMP. Mifepristone blocks the action of progesterone, a hormone necessary to maintain pregnancy. One to 3 days later, a dose of misoprostol (Cytotec, a prostaglandin) is administered. Abortion usually occurs within 4 hours, but may take 24 hours or longer. Medical abortion is 97% effective, is considered very safe to the mother's health, and allows the loss to take place in the privacy of the woman's own home.

All around the world, individuals without medical training induce abortion. Complications frequently follow and may be life threatening. Some procedures involve the insertion of a foreign body through the cervix, often a urinary catheter, which may cause hemorrhage or sepsis along with the loss of the pregnancy. If a rigid object is used, the uterus, bowel, or bladder may be perforated or otherwise damaged. Tablets of potassium permanganate have been inserted vaginally to produce abortion, resulting in deep vaginal ulcerations that bleed copiously. Chemicals or soap solutions have been forced into the uterus, sometimes causing emboli, hemolysis, and death.

Women who attempt to terminate a pregnancy by themselves or with unlicensed personnel are at great risk for serious complications. With the surge of interest in botanical medicines, herbal preparations such as pennyroyal, oil of juniper, and black and blue cohosh are widely available and hold some appeal for women seeking a "natural" means of abortion. Herbal abortifacients can cause incomplete abortion or bleeding and cramping without loss of pregnancy. Misoprostol is widely used as a gastrointestinal drug, and some women dose themselves to abort pregnancy without medical supervision. In most cases this practice causes incomplete abortion or failed abortion.

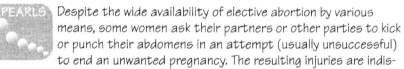

Vaginal bleeding and cramping, often with passage of blood clots and small bits of tissue, are the anticipated effects of medical abortion. The patient's bleeding will resemble a heavy period for about 2 days, then will subside to a lighter flow or spotting until 3–10 days after the procedure. One in 100 women, however, will experience prolonged or heavy bleeding that may necessitate an emergency response, and infection may occur. The woman with complications will likely need a surgical abortion to complete the process.

Treat the hemorrhaging elective abortion patient similarly to the woman with a profusely bleeding spontaneous abortion (see earlier). The patient may be reluctant to discuss her abortion with family members present and when questioned may not disclose the true reason for bleeding. She also may withhold information if her abortion was performed by nonmedical personnel or if she thinks that her caregivers do not approve of abortion.

The topic of abortion inspires strong emotions and judgments in many caregivers. As always, EMS professionals must remain supportive and act in the patient's best interests regardless of the choices she has made.

Therapeutic Abortion

Therapeutic abortion is the termination of pregnancy when carrying to term would endanger the woman's health or result in an infant with profound anomalies. Therapeutic abortion may also end a pregnancy in which the fetus is not viable, such as one with severe deformities or metabolic defects incompatible with life. In the case of a woman who conceives a large number of embryos, the parents and physician may decide to abort several of the embryos to improve viability for those that remain, a procedure called selective reduction. Some authorities consider rape or incest grounds for therapeutic abortion.

Certain maternal conditions can prompt some women to consider therapeutic abortion, from severe hypertension and cardiac disease to endocrine disorders, HIV, and coagulopathies. Invasive cervical cancer is treated with surgery or radiation, both of which will kill a previable fetus; but delaying treatment until the fetus is viable may result in the death of the mother. Therapeutic abortion is performed in the same manner as elective abortion and carries the same risks.

Hydatidiform Mole

Hydatidiform mole, known as a molar pregnancy or gestational trophoblastic disease, occurs with 1 in every 1,000 conceptions in the United States. Some parts of Asia have a rate that is significantly greater. In a complete molar pregnancy, conception involves a defective egg that has no nucleus, which is fertilized by two sperm or by a sperm that duplicates its own chromosomes. Consequently, there is no maternal genetic input and no embryo, only a malformed placenta that proliferates as rapidly growing, grapelike fluid-filled vesicles. See Figure 3-2.

A partial molar pregnancy usually begins when two sperm fertilize a normal egg. An embryo begins to develop, but soon dies, and the abnormal placental tissue fills and distends the uterus as with a complete mole.

In both kinds of molar pregnancy, the uterus becomes larger than expected for gestational dates. The molar tissue produces the pregnancy hormone hCG at a rate much greater than the placenta of a normal pregnancy, often triggering severe nausea and vomiting in the woman. The woman begins to experience vaginal bleeding, which is often the color of prune juice, but may be bright red. Sometimes the woman will show

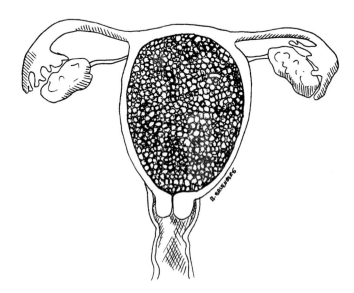

FIGURE 3-2
Hydatidiform Mole.
The hydatidiform mole distends the uterus with thousands of fluid-filled vesicles.
Illustration by Bonnie U. Gruenberg

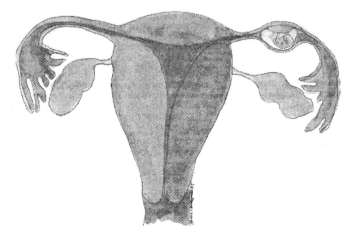
signs of preeclampsia before 24 weeks. (In viable pregnancies, preeclampsia typically develops after this time.) A history of severe nausea and vomiting is common. About 10% show signs of hyperthyroidism—hypertension, warm skin, tremors, and tachycardia.

Treat the woman with suspected hydatidiform mole like any other woman in early pregnancy with vaginal bleeding. Diagnosis is made by ultrasound, and the mole is removed by surgical evacuation. Women who have had a molar pregnancy run a slight risk of later developing choriocarcinoma, an aggressive cancer of the uterus.

Ectopic Pregnancy

In a normal pregnancy, conception occurs in the fallopian tubes. Propelled by cilia, the dividing cell mass reaches the uterus within about a week. There it implants in thick, hormonally primed, vascular uterine tissue, the endometrium, and taps into the mother's bloodstream for life support.

Ectopic pregnancy occurs when the embryo embeds somewhere outside the uterus (*ectopic* meaning "out of place"). The most common site is the fallopian tube (95%), but occasionally the embryo will implant on the ovary (4%), on the cervix (1%), or even in the abdominal cavity (<1%). See Figure 3-3. None of these structures is suitable for supporting a growing embryo, and the fragile, vascular fallopian tube is especially vulnerable. An embryo implanted in the thin wall of the tube outgrows the available space at about 6–8 weeks' gestation, often causing the tube to rupture and creating the hemodynamic equivalent of a shotgun blast to the abdomen. Tubal rupture can initially present as a small tear in the tube with minimal pain and bleeding that grows gradually worse, or as massive hemorrhage into the woman's abdominal cavity. Immediate surgery is usually indicated for ectopic pregnancy,

FIGURE 3-3
Ectopic Pregnancy.
The most common site of implantation for an ectopic pregnancy is in the fallopian tube. A tubal pregnancy is not viable and will endanger the mother's life and future fertility if the fallopian tube ruptures.
Illustration by Bonnie U. Gruenberg

Pregnancy Complications 77

although early unruptured ectopics are often managed with embryo-killing medications such as methotrexate.

The incidence of ectopic pregnancy in the United States has tripled since 1970 to 1 in every 44 live births. It is the leading cause of first-trimester maternal death.

Some women are more susceptible to ectopic pregnancy. Scarred tubes with damaged cilia are less effective in moving an embryo to the uterus. Chlamydia, the most common sexually transmitted infection in the United States, and gonorrhea, another common STI, can scar the fallopian tubes. Other risk factors are previous pelvic or tubal surgery, prior ectopic pregnancy, history of infertility, smoking, maternal age over 35, the presence of an intrauterine device (IUD) for contraception, altered hormone levels, and congenital anomalies of the fallopian tubes. Only about half of women with ectopic pregnancy have one or more of the risk factors.

Tubal ligation is also a risk factor for ectopic pregnancy. Sterilization is the most popular method of contraception in the United States and around the world. Almost 50% of American women choose tubal ligation by the age of 44. Tubal ligation involves destruction of the fallopian tubes in some fashion. Sometimes an opening remains in the scarred tube, wide enough to let sperm through to fertilize the egg, but not large enough let the zygote pass to the uterus. The embryo implants in the tube, and ectopic pregnancy results. EMS providers should also be aware that women may experience ectopic pregnancy 10 years or more after tubal ligation. The woman may insist that she cannot be pregnant. Women who have undergone tubal reanastomosis (reversal of tubal ligation to achieve pregnancy) are also at greater risk for ectopic pregnancies.

Ectopic pregnancy is so potentially life threatening that the EMS provider should suspect this condition in *any* woman whose symptoms and history even remotely fit the clinical picture. To further complicate matters, the clinical picture is variable, and diagnosis may be difficult. Emergency room physicians fail to correctly diagnose ectopic pregnancy more than 40% of the time on the patient's first visit, and missed ectopic pregnancy is one of the leading causes of emergency physician malpractice lawsuits.

The woman with an ectopic pregnancy may not know that she is pregnant and may not show signs or symptoms of pregnancy. Ectopic pregnancy usually becomes symptomatic by 6–8 weeks of gestation, but can cause symptoms as early as 5 weeks' gestation or (rarely) as late as 14–16 weeks.

The classic presentation is a woman of childbearing age with a history of amenorrhea (cessation of menses) presenting with diffuse abdominal pain that later localizes as severe, knife-like pain on one side of the lower abdomen. A ruptured ectopic pregnancy rapidly progresses to hypovolemic shock with rapid, weak pulse; confusion and restlessness; pale, clammy skin; collapsed neck veins; and low blood pressure, sometimes even syncope. Her abdomen is tender to palpation and may be rigid or distended. Rebound tenderness, nausea and vomiting, and diarrhea are often present. Free blood in the abdomen often irritates the phrenic nerve (which runs under the diaphragm) causing referred pain to the right shoulder. Sometimes (but not always) she may have vaginal bleeding with or preceding the other symptoms, but the degree of shock usually exceeds that accounted for by visible blood loss.

Many women with ectopic pregnancy, however, do not fit the classic picture. Some present with only syncope. Some experience little more than nausea and vomiting. Many look and feel fine except for unilateral pelvic pain. Some display only profound shock. Vital signs may be normal if rupture has not yet occurred. In most cases, pain onset is abrupt and severe; but in some cases, the woman may have chronic discomfort with irregular spotting for days before becoming acutely symptomatic. A rare finding is Cullen's sign, a blue tint beneath the umbilicus indicating free blood in the abdomen. There may be few available clues to support a clinical impression of ectopic pregnancy, but any woman of childbearing age with the symptoms described should be presumed to have an ectopic pregnancy until proven otherwise.

Other problems can present similarly. Differential diagnoses include spontaneous abortion, ruptured ovarian cyst, appendicitis, salpingitis (infection of the fallopian tube), torsion (twisting) of the ovary, round-ligament pain, torsion or degeneration of a uterine fibroid, kidney stone, abscess, and urinary tract infection.

Field treatment for a suspected ectopic pregnancy must be swift and efficient. Rapid transport to a hospital with the capacity for immediate surgery is essential. Bilateral intravenous lines should be established and isotonic crystalloid solution such as lactated Ringer's or normal saline run at a rate consistent with the patient's level of shock. Hospital laboratory studies may be expedited if the EMS crew draws blood while establishing intravenous access. The EMS provider should administer oxygen, initiate cardiac monitoring, and treat for shock.

Antepartal Bleeding—Second Half of Pregnancy

Placental Abruption

Also known as abruptio placentae, this condition occurs when the placenta prematurely separates partially or entirely from the uterine wall after 20 weeks of gestation. Abruption complicates 1 in 75–90 births and can be catastrophic. The ensuing hemorrhage carries a 20–35% mortality rate for the fetus (up to 100% if the placenta separates completely) and can cause significant harm to the mother. Abruption may or may not present with vaginal bleeding—the blood may remain trapped behind the placenta and never leave the body.

Hypertension strongly predisposes pregnant women to placental abruption. Other risk factors include multiparity, age over 35, smoking, poor nutrition, cocaine use, and chorioamnionitis. Abruption is associated with overdistention of the uterus, as in the case of multiple pregnancy or polyhydramnios (increased amniotic fluid volume). Blunt external trauma, especially from motor vehicle accidents and maternal battering, is also an important cause of abruption. (See Trauma in Pregnancy, chapter 4.)

Presentation varies with degree and location:

• **Marginal abruption.** The edge of the placenta separates, causing bleeding that flows between the fetal membranes and the uterine wall and exits through the vagina. This presentation is called a revealed hemorrhage. The placenta may or may not continue to separate.

• **Central abruption.** The center of the placenta separates, but the margins remain intact. Free blood accumulates between the placenta and uterine wall, but none escapes to exit the vagina. This presentation is known as a concealed hemorrhage. Signs and symptoms usually include sharp, tearing pain; rigid, board-like abdomen; and change in uterine size and shape. See Figure 3-4.

• **Combined abruption.** This condition has features of both marginal and central abruptions; some of the blood escapes, and some remains hidden behind the placenta.

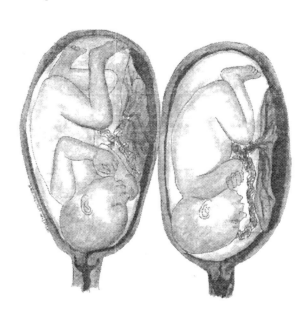

FIGURE 3-4
Placental Abruption.
A marginal placental abruption may result in vaginal bleeding. A central abruption may conceal blood loss within the uterus.
Illustration by Bonnie U. Gruenberg

- **Complete abruption.** Complete separation of the placenta causes profuse vaginal bleeding and shock while depriving the fetus of oxygen. Immediate surgery is necessary to save the life of the fetus.

Signs and symptoms can vary from subtle to dramatic. Vaginal bleeding may be profuse, scanty, or nonexistent and may be dark or bright red. Abruption may be excruciating, uncomfortable, or painless. The patient may have contractions. With a concealed hemorrhage it is common for the uterus to remain very tender, rigid, and board-like between contractions; but if the placenta is on the posterior wall of the uterus, these signs may not be present. Sometimes with a concealed hemorrhage, the uterus may enlarge and change shape. Shock may be disproportionate to visible blood loss.

Fetal movements often become less frequent or stop up to 12 hours before any obvious signs of abruption, but in a large, sudden abruption the woman may report violent fetal movement followed by stillness. Fetal heart tones may be faster than usual (above 160), bradycardic (under 120), generally within normal ranges with periodic decelerations, or absent. In a large abruption, only immediate surgery can save the baby from severe neurological damage or death. Chief risks to the mother are shock and disseminated intravascular coagulation (DIC).

EMS field treatment for placental abruption consists of treatment for hypovolemic shock and rapid transport to a hospital with the capacity for immediate cesarean section. If the fetus is preterm, transport to a hospital with a neonatal intensive care unit if possible. Vital signs, fetal heart tones, and assessments of uterine tone, contractions, and vaginal bleeding should be performed frequently. Some providers mark the fundal height on the maternal abdomen with a pen in order to monitor changes caused by trapped blood.

Bilateral large-bore intravenous lines should be established and blood drawn in accordance with local protocols to expedite hospital laboratory studies. The patient will need type and cross matching for blood products at the hospital and may require transfusion. Infuse normal saline or lactated Ringer's at a rate consistent with her condition. If shock is developing, aggressive fluid therapy is indicated. High-flow oxygen and left lateral positioning may improve the delivery of oxygen to the fetus.

Disseminated Intravascular Coagulation (DIC)

DIC is a life-threatening derangement of the clotting cascade triggered by underlying disease or trauma. Obstetrical causes include abruptio placentae, eclampsia, intrauterine fetal demise, amniotic fluid embolism, septic shock, and trauma. Serious infections are the most common cause of DIC. During DIC, the body forms and dissolves fibrin clots throughout the circulation, causing simultaneous uncontrolled bleeding and clotting. DIC begins when an event triggers the formation of innumerable microscopic clots throughout the body, which use up the clotting factors. The body responds by attempting to dissolve the unneeded clots. The by-products created by this widespread clot forming and clot dissolving interfere with the ability of the blood to coagulate, and the patient begins to hemorrhage.

The woman with DIC will present with bleeding from body orifices and breaks in the skin including venipuncture sites, nose, mouth, GI tract, and vagina. Bruising, purpura, and petechiae are commonly noted on the skin. DIC may lead to stroke, myocardial infarction, end-organ dysfunction, shock, and death. Definitive treatment in a hospital setting includes removing the cause, if possible, and transfusion of blood products. In some circumstances, DIC is treated with heparin to interrupt the clotting cascade.

Field treatment includes rapid transport with an advanced life support (ALS) crew to a hospital with the capacity to deal with a critically ill obstetrical patient. If the fetus is preterm, a hospital with a capable neonatal intensive care unit will give the baby a better chance of survival. EMS personnel should establish bilateral large-bore intravenous lines, draw blood for rapid laboratory tests upon arrival, administer high-flow oxygen, begin cardiac monitoring, and implement left lateral flat positioning. The crew member with the greatest skill in venipuncture should establish venous access to minimize skin punctures that may bleed profusely as DIC progresses, and isotonic crystalloid intravenous solution should be infused at a brisk rate as permitted by local protocols. Vital signs should be reassessed frequently along with fetal heart tones, uterine tone (Is it soft or rigid? Are contractions regular?), and vaginal bleeding.

Placenta Previa

Placenta previa is a condition in which the embryo implants in the lower uterine segment instead of the uterine fundus. At or near term, the placenta partially or completely covers the cervical os (cervical opening). When the cervix begins to thin and dilate in preparation for labor, placental villi are torn from the uterine wall, and bleeding results. There are three variations of this condition:

- **Marginal placenta previa.** The placenta encroaches on the edge of the cervical os. Marginal previa may resolve as the pregnancy progresses. See Figure 3-5.
- **Partial placenta previa.** The placenta partially covers the cervical os.
- **Total placenta previa.** The placenta occludes the cervical os. See Figure 3-6.

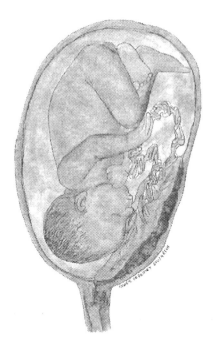

FIGURE 3-5
Marginal Placenta Previa.
A marginal placenta previa occurs when
the edge of a low-lying placenta
encroaches on the cervical os.
Illustration by Bonnie U. Gruenberg

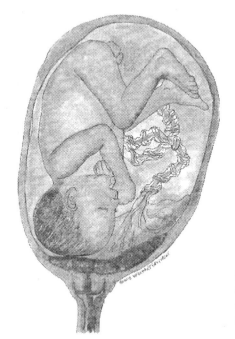

FIGURE 3-6
Complete Placenta Previa.
A complete placenta previa is im-
planted directly over the cervical os.
Illustration by Bonnie U. Gruenberg

Placenta previa most commonly presents with painless bleeding that may be scanty or profuse. Sometimes it accompanies or is preceded by contractions. Typically, the first bleeding episode is slight, and each subsequent hemorrhage is more copious.

Even in the hospital, vaginal exams are not performed on women who present with third-trimester vaginal bleeding unless the placental location has been confirmed on ultrasound; if an examiner were to put a finger through the placenta, uncontrolled hemorrhage would result. The woman with placenta previa will probably undergo a cesarean delivery if she is near term. If the fetus is still immature and her bleeding is slight, her provider may admit her and observe for further bleeding while the fetus continues development. Occasionally the woman is discharged home and instructed to call if further bleeding occurs.

Field treatment for any vaginal bleeding in the second half of pregnancy calls for history and assessment (including serial vital signs and fetal heart tones), rapid transport, at least one large-bore intravenous line with isotonic crystalloid intravenous solution hanging (flow rate dependent on her condition and vital signs), transport in left lateral position, oxygen as indicated, and frequent reassessment.

 Positive diagnosis of the source of vaginal bleeding can be made only by an obstetrical provider, usually in a hospital setting. In prehospital care, it is not necessary to distinguish between placental abruption and placenta previa. Field treatment is the same for either condition.

Pelvic and Abdominal Pain

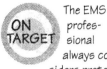 *The EMS professional always considers preterm labor as a possible cause of abdominal discomfort in women between 20 and 37 weeks' gestation.*

The presence of pelvic pain does not necessarily herald loss of the pregnancy. Most pregnant women feel discomfort at various points in the pregnancy, and usually these aches and pains are inconsequential. In most cases, field care will consist of taking a good history, positioning for comfort, giving nothing by mouth, and perhaps establishing IV access and drawing blood. If a patient is hypovolemic, consider a fluid bolus. As always, follow local protocols.

A few of the most common etiologies follow.

Ligament Pain

Round ligaments are like stretchy guy wires that hold the uterus in position. They run from the lateral aspect of the uterus to the pubic bone bilaterally. During the second trimester, the uterus outgrows the pelvis and falls forward, putting stress on these ligaments and causing crampy spasms on one side or the other of the pubic bone, along either or both sides of the uterus, and up to the level of the umbilicus. The right side is more commonly affected because the uterus rotates to the right as it grows. As the uterus continues to expand and have toning contractions, the ligaments continue to stretch. Round-ligament pain is one of the most common discomforts in pregnancy. The pain is sharp and can be severe, but it does not indicate any pathological process. It is often triggered by coughing or sudden movement. A woman can avoid triggering spasms by splinting the area with her hand when she moves suddenly. Sometimes she will find relief if she curls toward the pain and flexes her thigh on the painful side. Warm baths, application of heat, and wearing a maternity belt can improve symptoms.

Appendicitis

During pregnancy, the growing uterus displaces the appendix, and at term the appendix is located above the right iliac crest in most women. Appendicitis presents initially as epigastric or periumbilical pain in pregnant and nonpregnant women, but can later localize to either the right upper or lower quadrant. The patient with appendicitis may also complain of fever, chills, nausea and vomiting, rebound tenderness (test for increased pain with cough), and rigid abdomen.

Urinary Tract Infection

Pregnancy predisposes women to urinary tract infections, which can range from inconvenient to life threatening. Pregnancy hormones relax smooth muscle in the ureters, which can kink and allow urine to pool and support bacterial growth. Sometimes urinary tract infection mimics or triggers preterm labor.

Cystitis, or bladder infection, presents with frequent urination, lower pelvic cramping (especially while voiding), a burning sensation with urination, and sometimes a low-grade fever. Urine may be cloudy, bloody, or bad smelling.

pyelonephritis
Inflammation of the kidney and renal pelvis, usually from infection.

Pyelonephritis, or kidney infection, is often preceded by a bladder infection and occurs in about 2% of pregnancies. Symptoms include sudden onset of high fever, shaking chills, hematuria, nausea, vomiting, urinary pain and urgency, flank or low back pain, costovertebral angle (CVA) tenderness, and malaise. During pregnancy the right side is most likely to be affected because the intestines push the uterus to the right and compress the right ureters and kidney.

Check for costovertebral angle (CVA) tenderness by firmly tapping down the back from scapula to pelvis with a closed fist. If the patient winces upon percussion of where her lower ribs meet the spine, she has CVA tenderness.

Sometimes the woman with pyelonephritis will experience swelling of the kidney and ureter that can reduce urine output and cause severe pain and even small bowel ileus. Pyelonephritis can also lead to preterm labor and life-threatening maternal sepsis. It is treated by intravenous antibiotics and bed rest in the hospital.

Hydronephrosis and Renal Calculi

Most cases of renal colic present in the second or third trimester of pregnancy. Hydronephrosis is fluid buildup in the kidneys when urine flow is obstructed in the urinary tract. Hydroureter is distention of the ureter with urine. During pregnancy, these conditions most commonly result from smooth muscle relaxation of the ureter due to progesterone and HCG, coupled with compression of the ureter at the pelvic brim by the heavy uterus, obstructing urine flow. Physiologic hydronephrosis and hydroureter of pregnancy is seen in 90% of pregnancies and is usually asymptomatic.

The woman with symptomatic hydronephrosis often presents similarly to the patient with pyelonephritis or renal calculi, exhibiting severe flank pain that may be acute or chronic, but usually without fever. If hydronephrosis threatens kidney function, the patient may require percutaneous or stent drainage. Rarely, hydronephrosis can exacerbate hypertension or cause renal failure.

Hydronephrosis can persist for months, sometimes causing intractable pain for the pregnant woman. Many patients are managed on narcotic medications and taught techniques to reduce pressure on the kidneys and ureters, such as urinating while positioned on hands and knees in a bathtub. Pain from hydronephrosis may increase if the condition worsens or if she develops a urinary tract infection.

Renal calculi can form in pregnant women and present as in nonpregnant patients, with a typical flank-loin-abdomen distribution and often with severe pain. Uncommonly, kidney stones can lead to premature labor or preeclampsia. Urinary obstruction with concurrent infection is unusual, but carries a high risk of spontaneous abortion and premature labor.

Whereas calculi can affect either side, physiologic hydronephrosis is usually more pronounced on the right. Pain from appendicitis, cholecystitis, perforated intestine, preterm labor, and other conditions may present similarly in the pregnant women, so consider differential diagnoses carefully.

Chorioamnionitis and Pelvic Inflammatory Disease

When disease-causing microorganisms ascend from the vagina into the upper reproductive tract, they can cause infection in the mother, fetus, placenta, or membranes. **Chorioamnionitis,** or infection of the fetal membranes, is most likely to develop if the mother has had prolonged rupture of the amniotic sac. Ruptured membranes can present as a leak so subtle that the woman may not be aware of it or as an unmistakable gush. When the membranes are no longer intact, vaginal microorganisms may ascend and cause infection. Women who have undergone **cerclage** (a suture that secures the cervix in an attempt to prevent premature delivery) are at higher risk for chorioamnionitis.

The woman with chorioamnionitis will present with abdominal pain, uterine tenderness, fever, foul-smelling vaginal discharge, and a generalized feeling of illness. The fetus usually shows signs of distress—often tachycardia—before the mother becomes symptomatic. Chorioamnionitis is always an emergency and is potentially life threatening to both mother and fetus. Chorioamnionitis may also contribute to cerebral palsy in the infant.

Pelvic inflammatory disease, or PID (infection of the upper genital tract), may also occur in pregnancy and is most commonly caused by chlamydia or gonorrhea. PID can be life threatening to the fetus.

Cholecystitis/Cholelithiasis

Gallstone formation is accelerated in pregnancy, and as many as 6% of pregnant women develop cholelithiasis (gallstones). Progesterone slows the emptying of the gallbladder, increases the proportion of cholesterol present in the bile, and the bile salt pool decreases. Symptoms are the same in pregnant and nonpregnant women, and include

- Nausea
- Vomiting
- Right upper quadrant tenderness

chorioamnionitis
Infection of the fetal membranes.

cerclage
A suture that secures the cervix in an attempt to prevent premature delivery.

- Lancing or cramping epigastric pain that radiates to the right upper quadrant, around the back, or to the right scapula
- Sudden onset of colicky pain or a deep ache, building to peak intensity in 15–60 minutes, then receding over several hours.

Symptoms are aggravated by eating a greasy meal, and pale or gray stools may occur if the bile duct is completely obstructed. Laparoscopic cholecystectomy (removal of the gallbladder) is sometimes performed in the first or second trimester but is usually avoided during the third trimester.

Other Pain

leiomyoma (fibroid)
A benign tumor of
the uterine smooth
muscle.

Pregnant women have intestinal gas or diarrhea cramps just like the rest of the population. A woman may have benign fibroid tumors within her uterus, which can cause bleeding and pain, especially if they become twisted. Any woman who has had uterine or abdominal surgery may have adhesions—scar tissue—that bind and anchor her organs painfully as they try to expand and shift position. Abdominal pain in a pregnant woman can indicate placental abruption, uterine rupture, preeclampsia, or trauma. Pancreatitis, peptic ulcer disease, gastric reflux, ruptured or twisted ovarian cysts, and degenerating fibroid tumors (**leiomyomas**) of the uterus can also cause abdominal pain.

Low Back Pain

lordosis
Exaggerated for-
ward curvature of
the lumbar spine
(considered nor-
mal in pregnancy);
"swayback."

Low back pain affects 50–90% of women during pregnancy, especially with prior history of back problems, lack of exercise, increasing parity and age, poor posture, or improper lifting. When the pregnant abdomen moves out of the pelvis, abdominal muscles become stretched and lose tone, and become less effective at maintaining neutral posture and stabilizing the pelvis. Elevated levels of the hormone relaxin, which loosens joints, increases mobility of the lumbar spine. The pregnant woman develops progressive **lordosis,** and her center of gravity shifts backward and down, increasing the workload of the muscles of the back.

The hormones of pregnancy transform the previously rigid pelvic joints into a series of hinges with the ability to stretch open during childbirth. These changes in the pelvis can cause back pain. The symphysis pubis widens throughout pregnancy, placing stress on the sacroiliac joints. Increased mobility of the sacroiliac joints can cause discomfort when the associated ligaments are stretched.

When evaluating the pregnant patient with back pain, always consider the possibility of hydronephrosis, pyelonephritis, pancreatitis, pelvic deep vein thrombosis, or renal calculi. Preterm labor can present as back pressure or pain. Fever, sensory loss, motor weakness or paralysis, or incontinence may indicate a neurologic emergency.

Syncope

Syncope is not unusual in the pregnant patient, and it is a common reason for an emergency response. It is frequently caused by hypoglycemia, prolonged standing, orthostatic hypotension, vena caval compression from supine positioning, overheating, or a vagal response. Early in pregnancy consider ectopic pregnancy as an etiology. Syncope infrequently can be attributed to pathological conditions such as stroke or arrhythmia, long QT syndrome, hypertrophic cardiomyopathy, or Wolf Parkinson White syndrome. The syncopal patient may show brief tonic-clonic activity with bradycardia and hypotension, but quickly recovers. (A true seizure would be followed by a postictal state and would not show these cardiovascular changes.)

Hyperemesis Gravidarum

hyperemesis gravidarum Severe, persistent nausea and vomiting; an extreme form of pregnancy-related "morning sickness" that can cause weight loss, ketosis, dehydration, and hypokalemia or other electrolyte imbalance and sometimes requires hospitalization.

Hyperemesis gravidarum is severe, persistent nausea and vomiting with weight loss, dehydration, hypokalemia, or ketonuria. Unlike morning sickness, which is generally confined to the first trimester and does not often interfere with nutrition, hyperemesis can occur at any point in the pregnancy and can result in ketosis and dehydration.

Hyperemesis appears multifactorial. It can be related to vitamin B deficiency, endocrine imbalances such as hyperthyroidism, allergies, psychological disturbances, and conditions that increase the levels of human chorionic gonadotropin (hCG), for example, multiple gestation and hydatidiform mole. Severe cases can lead to hypokalemia that can disrupt kidney function and heart rhythm, hypovolemia and syncope from dehydration, acidosis or alkalosis, muscle wasting, and severe protein and vitamin deficiencies. Wernicke's encephalopathy can uncommonly occur from severe thiamine deficiency, presenting with altered consciousness, double vision, constant eye movement, and poor muscle coordination. Hyperemesis gravidarum can cause irreversible metabolic changes or even death, but both are extremely uncommon.

Symptoms usually develop between 4 and 9 weeks' gestation, and include

- Intractable vomiting.
- Poor appetite.
- Poor nutritional and fluid intake.

- Weight loss greater than 5% of prepregnant weight.
- Dehydration (dry mucous membranes, orthostatic hypotension, concentrated urine, possible syncope especially in hot weather, poor skin turgor).
- Ketonuria.
- Advanced cases may show jaundice, bleeding gums, peripheral neuropathy, arrhythmia, changes in level of consciousness.

Morning sickness is common in pregnancy and can make a woman *feel* unable to hold anything down, but it does not result in the dehydration, ketosis, and weight loss experienced in hyperemesis gravidarum. Differential diagnoses are infectious disease such as hepatitis, drug reaction, intestinal obstruction, peptic ulcer, food poisoning, diabetes, and gastroenteritis. Treatment involves intravenous rehydration and electrolyte, glucose, and vitamin administration with no oral intake for 48 hours. This regimen can be accomplished at the hospital or through home nursing services. Antiemetics are used to suppress nausea. After vomiting ceases, food is gradually reintroduced. Refractory cases may require nasogastric feedings or total parenteral nutrition.

Emergency medical personnel should focus on the ABCs when caring for the patient with hyperemesis gravidarum. Carefully assess the severity of her condition and consider other possible causes. Check glucose levels. If she is dehydrated, infuse lactated Ringer's or normal saline at a rate consistent with her condition. If she is severely affected, monitor for arrhythmias and be prepared for the possibility of coma. If she shows signs of Wernicke's encephalopathy, your medical control may advise intramuscular thiamine administration. If the patient is hypovolemic, position for shock—on her left side if pregnancy is advanced. Try to avoid exposing her to strong smells or excessive motion that may trigger vomiting, and maintain a clear airway if she does vomit.

Hypertensive Disorders

Pregnancy-Induced Hypertension (Preeclampsia)

Pregnancy-induced hypertension (PIH) is a widely studied and poorly understood condition that remains responsible for 15% of maternal deaths in the United States, second only to embolism. It involves systemic vasospasm that can lead to poor perfusion and eventually tissue ischemia, affecting placental blood flow and the maternal cardiovascular, renal, neurologic, hepatic, and hematologic systems. Often used synonymously with the term *preeclampsia* (and once called toxemia),

PIH complicates 6–8% of pregnancies and may be superimposed on underlying chronic hypertension. It is more common in African Americans, women with multiple gestation, teenagers of lower socioeconomic class, diabetics, and women over 35. Other maternal risk factors are nulliparity (or first baby with a new partner), family history of PIH, underlying chronic hypertension, chronic renal disease, and antiphospholipid syndrome (an autoimmune clotting disorder). The fetus of a woman with PIH may suffer growth restriction and hypoxia or experience the challenges of premature birth.

Dietary, immunological, genetic, and hemodynamic factors have been implicated in PIH, but researchers do not fully understand the disease or its etiology. Central to the condition is vasospasm, which leads to increased resistance to blood flow with resultant hypertension that can lead eventually to multisystem organ damage. Hypertension can lead directly to cardiac failure, brain hemorrhage, or pulmonary edema. Kidneys damaged by restricted blood flow are poor filters that allow proteins to escape the bloodstream while allowing toxins to remain; in some cases kidneys may fail altogether. A poorly perfused liver may produce fewer blood proteins, the lack of which allows fluid to escape from blood vessels and cause edema. Liver damage also elevates hormone and toxin levels (the liver metabolizes both) and interferes with clotting and other vital processes. Abnormal liver-function tests with elevation of liver enzymes are often seen with PIH, and occasionally the liver will become necrotic or rupture. Central nervous system involvement can cause convulsions, coma, altered mental status, and cortical blindness. The woman with PIH may experience significant third-spacing as fluid moves from her intravascular space to the interstitial space, causing edema and intravascular depletion. The woman may also experience placental abruption or DIC.

Preeclampsia is a condition classically distinguished by a triad of hypertension, proteinuria, and generalized edema developing in the second half of pregnancy; but symptoms can vary widely between individuals. Preeclampsia is a progressive disorder, and in its mild or early form symptoms can develop subtly and appear benign.

Hypertension in pregnancy is defined as a sustained elevation of blood pressure to 140/90 or above. Research once suggested that an increase of 30 mmHg systolic and 15 mmHg diastolic over baseline was diagnostic of PIH, but this concept is outdated. Generally, blood pressure elevation that begins after 20 weeks is considered preeclampsia. Hypertension before 20 weeks is usually a manifestation of preexisting chronic hypertension. The exception is the patient with hydatidiform mole—whereby the patient exhibits signs of preeclampsia during either the first or early in the second trimester.

Generalized edema may be present, but because edema is commonplace in pregnancy and one-third of women with preeclampsia never demonstrate edema, the presence of edema is no longer seen as important to diagnosis. Proteinuria, measured routinely with a dipstick at office visits or more precisely though 24-hour urine collection, is not evaluated in the prehospital setting, but a reading of +2 or greater on dipstick or greater than 300 mg of protein in a 24-hour urine is significant.

While the woman with mild preeclampsia may be managed at home on bed rest, *severe* preeclampsia is an emergency situation. Severe preeclampsia may develop suddenly and presents with

proteinuria
Abnormal amounts of protein in the urine.

hyperreflexia
Exaggerated patellar reflexes, sometimes a sign of preeclampsia.

- Hypertension with a systolic pressure of 160 mmHg or greater and a diastolic pressure of 110 mmHg or greater.
- **Proteinuria.** Abnormal amounts of protein in the urine.
- Oliguria: Urine is dark, concentrated, and scanty.
- Visual disturbances: Blurred or double vision, flashing lights, or spots before the eyes. Visual disturbances can indicate impending seizure. Loss of vision may precede cerebral hemorrhage.
- Hyperreflexia: Exaggerated patellar reflexes.
- Epigastric pain: Liver ischemia, swelling, or rupture can cause epigastric pain or tenderness in the right upper quadrant.
- Nausea and vomiting.
- Pulmonary edema.
- Poor blood clotting.
- Fetal distress or poor growth; decreased amniotic fluid.
- Headache: Can be bitemporal, frontal, occipital, or diffuse; but it is progressive and does not respond to over-the-counter remedies.
- Seizures (eclampsia).
- Anxiety, malaise, or restlessness.
- Cerebral hemorrhage.

The only cure for preeclampsia is delivery of the fetus. Some authorities advocate immediate induction if preeclampsia is severe, regardless of gestational age. Others support allowing pregnancy to continue in the hospital until the fetus demonstrates lung maturity, maternal or fetal distress develops, or a gestational age of 34 weeks is achieved.

Eclampsia

When preeclampsia progresses to seizures or coma, the condition is termed eclampsia. The usual presentation is tonic-clonic seizures lasting less than a minute following signs of severe preeclampsia. Partial seizures or complex partial seizures also can occur, and some patients will move directly into coma without observed seizure. Coma can also result from a brain hemorrhage or brain swelling without hemorrhage.

Convulsions can occur antepartum, during labor, or postpartum. Most patients who develop eclampsia show marked edema, significantly increased blood pressure, and increased proteinuria prior to seizing; but up to 30% do not. Therefore, rather than trying to determine which patients are at the highest risk, the EMS professional should remain alert when transporting any preeclamptic woman.

EMS Treatment and Transport of the Woman with PIH

Preeclampsia and eclampsia are life threatening to both mother and fetus. It is important to take a comprehensive history, including assessment for the signs of severe preeclampsia mentioned earlier using the OLDCART checklist (see chapter 2), and to carefully document the information gleaned to serve as a baseline for hospital personnel.

Blood pressure can vary greatly with position. Pressure will usually diminish if she rests on her left side, and lower pressure increases perfusion of her organs and placenta. See Figure 3-7. Therefore, it is preferable to take a baseline blood pressure while she is seated, then to transport her on her left side with subsequent vital signs taken in that position, taking care to use the proper-sized cuff. See Figure 3-8. Document position with each blood pressure. Record the fetal heart tones, if taken. If she is complaining of dyspnea or coughing, assess for pulmonary edema and transport in Fowler's position. Assess and document patellar reflexes.

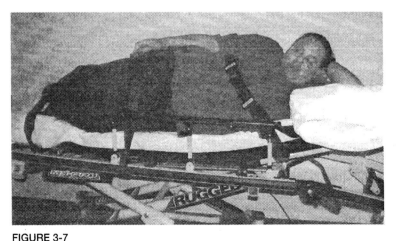

FIGURE 3-7
Left Lateral Position.
Placental perfusion is maximized when the pregnant woman is in a left lateral position.
Photographed by Bonnie U. Gruenberg

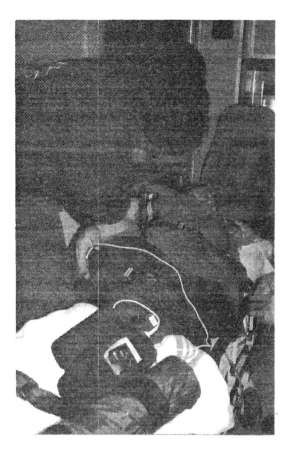

FIGURE 3-8
Transport of Woman with Severe Preeclampsia.
The woman with severe preeclampsia should be
transported in left lateral position, on oxygen, with
intravenous access in place and minimal noise,
jostling, or stimulation. Vital signs should be
assessed frequently.
Photographed by Bonnie U. Gruenberg

Make an effort to reduce environmental stimulation in order to decrease the potential for seizures. The PIH patient should be transported without flashing lights or sirens. Dim the interior lights and
speak quietly. Separate the patient from family members if they are ag-
itating her.

Establish an intravenous line of normal saline and run it at a KVO
(keep vein open) rate, and draw blood if required by protocol. Local
medical control may order an antihypertensive medication to reduce her
blood pressure. Magnesium sulfate is sometimes used in prehospital
care of preeclampsia to raise the seizure threshold, and it is the anticonvulsant of choice in the hospital.

If the woman begins to seize, protect her from injury (as in any
other seizure) and do not attempt to restrain her. Keep her airway
clear. Some protocols allow the paramedic to administer a bolus of
magnesium sulfate (2–5 g diluted in 50–100 ml normal saline given
slow IV push) for eclampsia. Some protocols allow for diazepam
(Valium) to stop the seizure, but apnea or cardiac arrest may result

from rapid administration. Suctioning may be necessary to maintain the airway. Give oxygen to ensure adequate oxygenation, and support respirations in the unlikely event that spontaneous breathing does not resume when the seizure breaks. Monitor cardiac rhythm and vital signs.

The seizure will be followed by a postictal period, and she may become agitated as she regains consciousness. The provider should monitor the woman and fetus for signs of abruption following the seizure, including auscultating the fetal heart, checking for vaginal bleeding, and palpating the uterus for rigidity. Listen to the mother's lungs frequently, because aspiration and pulmonary edema commonly occur with eclampsia.

The woman with preeclampsia can decompensate rapidly, moving from mild, ambiguous symptoms to full-blown eclampsia, organ damage, and fetal death in a very short time. Keep potential complications in mind while treating her, and monitor for the earliest indication of decompensation, such as signs of abruption or central nervous system dysfunction. Monitor her level of consciousness—remembering that magnesium sulfate can make a woman groggy, cause slurred speech and affect muscle tone.

If you must assist delivery of a preeclamptic patient, remain vigilant for changes in her condition and take steps to keep her stimulation level and blood pressure as low as possible. Position her on her side for delivery, and do not coach forceful pushing or prolonged breath holding with each contraction. If a woman responds to natural urges, a woman will usually push frequently for very short intervals, as in defecation. This moves the baby down at a reasonable rate and results in better placental oxygenation and improved maternal blood pressure (see Pushing Techniques, chapter 6). Administer low-flow oxygen to maximize fetal oxygenation.

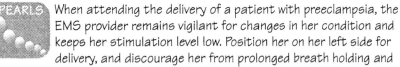

PEARLS When attending the delivery of a patient with preeclampsia, the EMS provider remains vigilant for changes in her condition and keeps her stimulation level low. Position her on her left side for delivery, and discourage her from prolonged breath holding and forceful pushing. Instead, coach her to push in short grunts, as in defecation.

Because a woman with preeclampsia third-spaces fluids from her blood vessels to her interstitial spaces, she may not have the intravascular reserve to tolerate blood loss after delivery. Remember that a woman with PIH is at high risk for eclamptic seizures for 48 hours after delivery and occasionally may seize within 2 weeks postpartum.

HELLP Syndrome

The medical community has yet to agree on whether HELLP syndrome is a separate category of preeclampsia or a variant of severe preeclampsia. HELLP syndrome is a multiple-organ-failure syndrome that is life threatening to mother and fetus. Unlike preeclampsia, it is diagnosed only through laboratory studies. The acronym describes the physiologic

Table 3-1   Danger Signs in Pregnancy and Possible Causes

Sudden gush of fluid	Premature rupture of membranes, urinary incontinence, vaginal infection.
Vaginal bleeding	Placenta previa, placental abruption, bloody show, polyps, lesions of cervix or vagina. Sometimes a woman will spot after a recent vaginal exam or intercourse.
Abdominal pain	Preterm labor, placental abruption, appendicitis, round ligament pain, gallbladder, urinary tract infection, renal calculi, hydronephrosis, pancreatitis.
Dizziness	Many causes, some of them benign. May relate to hypertension, medications, low blood sugar, or orthostatic hypotension.
Visual disturbances	Preeclampsia.
Severe vomiting	Hyperemesis gravidarum, gastroenteritis, or other gastrointestinal disorder. May occur with appendicitis, head injury, or other condition. Patient requires hospital evaluation if intake and output are poor.
Edema of hands, feet, or face	Preeclampsia. Pedal edema is often normal in pregnancy.
Severe headache	May be related to preeclampsia or may result from tension headache, migraine, or head injury.
Severe leg pain	Thrombophlebitis; or may be leg cramps.
Seizure	Preeclampsia; or may result from preexisting seizure disorder or head injury.
Epigastric pain	Preeclampsia, gallbladder inflammation, heartburn.
Reduced urine output	Preeclampsia, poor fluid intake, renal dysfunction.
Painful urination	Urinary tract infection, vaginal or vulvar infection.
Absence of or decrease in fetal movement	Fetal compromise or death, maternal distraction, medication, maternal obesity.
Preterm contractions	Premature labor; may also be triggered by urinary tract infection or dehydration, uterine irritability.
Elevated temperature, chills	Infection.

abnormalities that define the syndrome: **H**emolysis, **E**levated **L**iver enzymes, and **L**ow **P**latelets.

The patient may present with the same symptoms as the preeclamptic—epigastric pain, chest pain or right upper quadrant pain, headache, nausea and vomiting, and malaise—but sometimes with very few physical manifestations. Sometimes HELLP syndrome will develop before signs of preeclampsia appear. The patient with HELLP syndrome is often transferred by ambulance from a community hospital to a tertiary-care facility, and in that case the EMS professional will know the diagnosis and laboratory findings. Otherwise, in the field, HELLP is indistinguishable from any other case of preeclampsia and sometimes not recognizable at all. Definitive treatment of antepartum HELLP involves delivery of the fetus, even if remote from term. Rarely, HELLP may develop postpartum.

Triaging the Pregnant Woman

Pregnancy alters the functioning of the healthy woman's body and can worsen certain preexisting conditions. Some potentially life-threatening conditions occur only during pregnancy. Table 3-1 lists potential danger signs and symptoms and their possible etiologies.

Summary

While a majority of pregnancies proceed without complication, a significant percentage develop problems that could become life threatening. Many complaints are difficult to diagnose even in a hospital. Conditions such as urinary tract infections, deep vein thrombosis, and cholecystitis occur in the nonpregnant population, but pregnancy can increase both the incidence and severity of these problems. Disorders such as hyperemesis gravidarum and preeclampsia develop only in pregnant women. Because of the intimate connection between mother and fetus, most conditions that prove catastrophic to one party necessarily affect the life and well-being of the other.

Complications of pregnancy can present a formidable challenge in the field. The mastery of basic principles remains paramount. For the present discussion, the most important of these are

- Any female of apparent reproductive age may be pregnant.
- Any pregnancy may have undiagnosed complications or may become complicated without warning.

1. Describe the signs and symptoms of placental abruption and how it can be differentiated from placenta previa.

2. Describe the field management of a patient with first trimester bleeding.

3. Describe potential complications of preeclampsia.

4. What are some nonobstetric causes of abdominal or pelvic pain that may be experienced by the pregnant patient?

5. List some conditions that present with similar signs and symptoms to ectopic pregnancy.

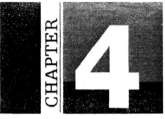

Threats to Mother and Fetus

Objectives

By the end of this chapter you should be able to

- Evaluate and transport the pregnant victim of trauma

- Understand cardiopulmonary resuscitation for the pregnant woman

- Manage the pregnant patient who has chronic preexisting conditions such as asthma or diabetes

- Treat the pregnant women who is actively seizing

- Recognize signs of preterm labor

- Understand the effects of substance abuse on the pregnant woman and her fetus

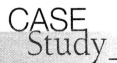

Samantha was driving her old Volvo down the dark road at about 50 mph when her headlights illuminated an adult moose. She jerked the steering wheel sharply to avoid a collision with the massive animal, bounced across a meadow, and struck a tree. Another driver called 911 on his cell phone.

The ambulance crew arrived to find Samantha conscious and alert, but terrified that she had injured her unborn baby in the impact. Paramedics Sean and Mick took a quick history and learned that Samantha was a primigravida at 32 weeks' gestation. She had no history of medical problems, and her pregnancy had been uneventful. The car did not have an air bag, but she was wearing a seat belt (placed properly across her hips and lower abdomen, and between her breasts) and had felt it tighten against her body upon impact. Samantha was not sure whether she had struck her abdomen on the steering wheel. Damage to the car was minor and confined to the front end with no damage to the steering wheel. It appeared that the wet meadow had slowed the car considerably before impact. There was no star on the windshield, and she denied striking her head or losing consciousness. She had not felt fetal movement since the accident, and she complained that her belly felt tight and firm. She was moving all extremities and had no complaints of pain anywhere.

Questions

1. After a primary and secondary survey, how should Sean and Mick assess Samantha's gravid abdomen and the fetus within it?
2. Given the mechanism of injury and the stage of gestation, Samantha is at greatest risk for what complications of pregnancy?
3. Describe the technique for immobilizing a pregnant trauma patient on a backboard.
4. How should Mick and Sean manage Samantha en route?

Introduction

In addition to complications that may develop as a result of pregnancy, such as those discussed in Chapter 3, preexisting maternal conditions can also put the pregnancy at risk and exacerbate the underlying disease process. The EMS provider must recognize potential insults to the pregnancy and the woman's well-being related to maternal conditions, teratogen exposures, and trauma. This chapter discusses threats to pregnancy and the emergency management of their sequelae.

KEY TERMS

Trauma in Pregnancy

Trauma, the leading nonobstetric cause of death among pregnant women, complicates 1 in 12 pregnancies. The severity of the trauma does not always predict the likelihood of adverse fetal outcome; 60–80% of fetal losses occur after relatively minor maternal trauma. If the mother dies, the fetus is likely to die, too. If the mother survives the trauma, placental abruption may occur and put the fetus at risk for hypoxia or death. Major maternal trauma involving multiple fractures and life-threatening injury carries a high fetal mortality rate.

Three causes are responsible for most of the trauma suffered by pregnant women.

• Motor vehicle accidents account for 60–80% of blunt trauma and are the most common cause of significant trauma in pregnancy. Almost 10% of motor-accident victims suffer significant injuries, but only about 2% of those injuries are critical. Pregnant pedestrians stuck by motor vehicles comprise another 10–12% of trauma patients.

• Domestic violence is a problem in all races, ages, and socioeconomic groups. Abuse often escalates in pregnancy. Frequently the woman will attribute her injuries to other mechanisms and deny that anyone has been injuring her.

• Falls account for 10–26% of trauma to pregnant women and commonly result from alterations in balance or orthostatic hypotension. Most falls occur in the third trimester.

Vulnerability to Trauma

During the first trimester, the uterus is well protected within the bony pelvis. The fetus is small and cushioned by a thick uterus and abundant fluid. In the second trimester, the uterus rises to a more vulnerable position in the abdomen, but the fetus is still fairly well protected.

Even small injuries can be catastrophic during the third trimester, because the uterus becomes larger and thinner walled and is increasingly vulnerable to blunt trauma, penetration, or rupture. The well-perfused uterus bleeds copiously when injured and can be a major source of blood loss in trauma. The third-trimester fetus occupies more space within the uterus and is surrounded by a proportionally smaller fluid volume. His head may be deep in the pelvis, where maternal pelvic fractures can cause head trauma.

Toward the end of pregnancy, the placenta is a massively perfused, comparatively rigid organ attached to the elastic uterine wall. If the uterus is subjected to abrupt accelerations or decelerations, even without blunt trauma, the placenta may shear off the uterine wall. Maternal **catecholamines** released by stress or injury can constrict vessels and decrease placental perfusion, causing fetal hypoxia.

Physiological changes associated with pregnancy greatly affect a woman's response to trauma. In the second and third trimesters, cardiac output increases by 40%, and uterine blood flow increases from 60 to 600 ml/min. Blood vessels in the pregnant uterus remain maximally dilated and have no mechanism for increasing perfusion when cardiac output is decreased. A drop in cardiac output can quickly result in decreased placental blood flow, and as a result the fetus may become severely compromised even when the mother's condition is stable. A pregnant woman also has a reduced oxygen reserve caused by diaphragm elevation and an increase in oxygen consumption associated with the fetus, placenta, and uterus.

The blood volume of a pregnant woman increases by 50% through the course of her pregnancy, creating a dilutional anemia in which blood has more liquid and therefore fewer red cells by volume than that of a nonpregnant woman. Despite her greater blood volume, the pregnant trauma victim may appear hypovolemic in the absence of serious injury because of the mild tachycardia and hypotension considered normal in pregnancy. The systolic blood pressure of a young healthy pregnant women may normally range from as low as 80 to 90.

An injured mother's body seeks to protect itself at the expense of blood flow to the fetus. Catecholamines can constrict vessels and shunt blood away from the placenta to perfuse maternal vital organs. A pregnant woman may lose 30% of her blood volume before her vital signs reflect hypovolemia, and she may not appear shocky until her blood loss is great enough to endanger the fetus. Once shock becomes obvious, fetal mortality may be as high as 85%.

Consequences of Trauma in Pregnancy

Preterm labor or preterm rupture of the membranes. This result can follow even minor trauma. All women beyond 18–20 weeks who have experienced trauma should be monitored at length for the presence of contractions, and those of earlier gestational age should be observed and evaluated. Research indicates that posttraumatic monitoring (including fetal monitoring) should extend to a minimum of 24 hours if during the first 4 hours there are more than three uterine contractions per hour, persistent uterine tenderness, a nonreassuring fetal monitor strip, vaginal bleeding, rupture of the membranes, or any serious maternal injury. The pregnant trauma victim may insist that her injuries are minor and that monitoring is not necessary, and it is the responsibility of the EMS provider to convince her that transport and observation are in her own and her baby's best interest.

Placental abruption. Direct trauma, shearing forces, or maternal shock can cause the placenta to detach from the uterine wall. See Figure 4-1. Most placental abruptions are seen within 24 hours of the accident; but it is important to remember that abruption can occur more than 5 days after trauma and follow even very minor injuries. Approximately 1–3% of all minor trauma results in fetal death, usually from placental abruption. Generally, every pregnant trauma patient beyond 18–20 weeks should be evaluated and monitored in an obstetrical unit.

Uterine rupture. This occurrence is rare but carries nearly 100% fetal mortality.

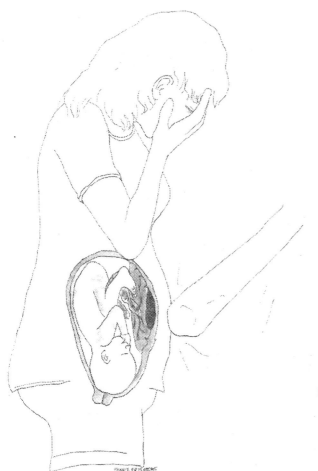

FIGURE 4-1
Effects of Blunt Trauma on the Fetus.
Blunt trauma can cause placental abruption, a condition that may cause fetal death, but the fetus is unlikely to be directly injured by the impact.
Illustration by Bonnie U. Gruenberg

Threats to Mother and Fetus 103

Penetrating trauma.   Trauma such as gunshot or stab wounds may directly injure the fetus. Maternal pelvic fracture may also cause direct injury to the fetus.

Hemorrhage.   Maternal hemorrhage decreases placental perfusion. A pregnant woman may lose 1,000–1,500 ml of blood before showing signs of shock. Once hemorrhage has progressed to shock, the mother may survive the ordeal; but the baby will usually die. Fetal blood loss can result in fetal anemia or death, and fetal blood may enter the maternal system. If the mother's blood type is Rh-negative, exposure to Rh-positive fetal blood may cause her to make antibodies that can attack the red blood cells of her unborn child.

Aspiration.   Slowed gastric emptying and the physical pressure of a large uterus on the organs of digestion increase the chance that the woman will aspirate stomach contents. If she is unable to maintain her own airway, be aggressive with intubation.

> **ON TARGET**   Placental abruption is most likely to occur within 24 hours of the trauma, but can occur more than 5 days later and follow even very minor injuries.

Managing the Trauma Victim

As with any trauma, perform a primary survey.

- **Airway.**   Open, protect, and secure the airway while protecting the cervical spine. A secure airway enables oxygenation and protects against aspiration.

- **Breathing.**   Administer oxygen and assist ventilation when breathing is inadequate. Reduced oxygen reserve and increased oxygen consumption put the pregnant woman and her fetus at increased risk for hypoxemia, so oxygen therapy should be aggressive.

- **Circulation.**   Control bleeding, establish intravenous access with a large-bore catheter, and administer a fluid bolus as indicated. Every liter of estimated blood loss should be replaced by three liters of lactated Ringer's, if available, or 0.9% normal saline. Lactated Ringer's is the solution of choice for trauma because it is more physiologic and less acidic than normal saline, but saline is also useful as a temporary volume expander. Vaginal bleeding often indicates placental abruption or uterine rupture; but abruption can occur without external bleeding, and vaginal bleeding can have other etiologies, such as bloody show in labor. If cardiac activity is abnormal or ineffective, follow ACLS guidelines or begin CPR as indicated.

- **Disability.**   Assess the patient neurologically. Is she alert and oriented? Does she have movement and sensation in all limbs?

- **Exposure.**   Remove clothing and examine for further injury, taking care to protect her from the environment.

The maternal secondary survey is the same as with any nonpregnant patient.

Perform a rapid primary survey of the fetus using the mnemonic FETAL. Assess for

Fetal heart rate or presence of fetal movement.

Estimated gestational age based on maternal or family report, abdominal measurement, or proximity of the uterus to the umbilicus. Is she sure there is only one fetus?

Trauma—observe for evidence of direct injury or penetrating trauma to uterus.

Abdominal palpation for tenderness and presence of uterine contractions.

Loss of amniotic fluid or vaginal bleeding.

The fetus is best served by making the care of the mother your priority. Fetal injuries can vary. A maternal pelvic fracture can injure the fetal head and brain if the fetus has descended into the pelvis. Penetrating trauma can puncture any part of the fetus. Blunt trauma is more likely to damage the uterus and placenta and indirectly affect the fetus than to cause direct harm to the unborn child.

Pregnant victims of major trauma should be treated like other trauma victims, but with accommodations for the physiological and anatomic changes of pregnancy. The pregnant trauma patient should be positioned in the left lateral position rather than supine whenever possible. If she lies flat on her back with her uterus compressing her vena cava, her blood pressure may drop precipitously, and she may experience the symptoms of shock, making it unclear whether injury or position is causing her symptoms. Supine positioning can reduce cardiac output by 30% and may trigger sinus bradycardia or sinus arrest. See Figure 4-2. This response may be even more pronounced in hemodynamically compromised patients. In

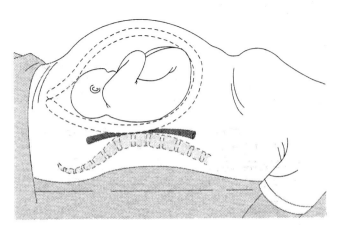

FIGURE 4-2
Vena Caval Syndrome.
When a pregnant woman greater than 20 weeks' gestation lies supine, her vena cava (and, to a lesser extent, her aorta) is compressed between the gravid uterus and the spine, reducing cardiac output by up to 30%.

cases in which supine immobilization on a backboard is essential, a wedge of pillows, blankets, or an equipment bag should be placed under the right side of the board to tilt the backboard at a 15–30° angle (raise the right side of the board 4–6 in.). High-flow oxygen by mask should be in initiated at the earliest opportunity. If she cannot support her own ventilations or maintain her airway, assist ventilation and be agressive with intubation.

Remain alert for the possibility of internal hemorrhage that could compromise the fetus long before signs are apparent in the mother. If internal injuries are suspected or if significant bleeding is present, bilateral large-bore intravenous lines should be established with isotonic crystalloid solution, preferably lactated Ringer's. Fluid resuscitation should be aggressive. Assess for uterine tenderness, vaginal bleeding, contractions, and fetal movement, and auscultate the fetal heartbeat if possible. Initiate cardiac monitoring when appropriate. Obstetric patients beyond 20 weeks' gestation who suffer multiple trauma should be transported to a facility that can provide comprehensive trauma and obstetrical care even if the patient appears stable.

RhoGam
A blood product (anti-D immunoglobulin) given to Rh-negative women in pregnancy and postpartum to prevent harm to Rh-positive babies (Rh isoimmunization).

> **PEARLS** Any pregnant woman with an Rh-negative blood type (such as AB negative) will need to receive an injection of anti-D immunoglobulin (RhoGam) if any fetal cells have entered her system.
> **RhoGam** is commonly to administered to Rh-negative women after any episode of vaginal bleeding or suspected abruption. A blood test (Kleihauer-Betke) can quantify the amount of fetal cells that entered the maternal bloodstream in case of trauma. If the obstetrical provider fails to administer RhoGam, the mother may produce antibodies that can cause hemolysis in a Rh-positive fetus.

Cardiac Arrest in Pregnancy

ON TARGET The three most common obstetric causes of maternal death are thromboembolism, pregnancy-induced hypertension, and hemorrhage.

Cardiac arrest in pregnancy is a rare but devastating occurrence. The three most common obstetric causes of maternal death are thromboembolism, pregnancy-induced hypertension, and hemorrhage. Most cardiac arrests in pregnant women result from nonresuscitatable causes such as multisystem trauma, intracranial hemorrhage, or massive pulmonary embolism.

Even if the cause of the cardiac arrest is survivable, the odds of successful resuscitation for the mother and fetus are low. Perfectly performed CPR on a nonpregnant patient results in cardiac output that is only 25–33% of normal. With the gravid uterus compressing the aorta and vena cava of the pregnant women, third-trimester CPR may result in cardiac output that is 10% of normal. The fetus's best chance for survival without deficit is delivery by cesarean section within 4 minutes of maternal cardiac arrest.

When cardiac arrest occurs, the priority is restoring maternal circulation. The pregnant woman and her fetus can tolerate only about 4–5 minutes of maternal cardiac arrest before irreversible damage begins to occur. The fetus requires strong and uninterrupted blood supply to maintain oxygenation; any decrease in placental perfusion can have dire consequences. Although babies have been resuscitated after as much as 30 minutes of maternal cardiac arrest, survival with intact neurological function is more likely if the infant is delivered within the first 5 minutes.

Anatomical changes of pregnancy work against successful resuscitation of the woman in cardiac arrest. Flared ribs, raised diaphragm, increased body fat, and breast enlargement make performing chest compression on a pregnant woman more difficult. She is very likely to vomit because of the pressure of the gravid uterus on the stomach. The pregnant woman has less functional respiratory reserve and becomes anoxic more quickly than the nonpregnant patient after respirations cease.

In general, pregnant women in cardiac arrest should treated like any other patient in that condition. ALS should be started, and the patient should be intubated early in the resuscitation process. *Do not* waste time looking for fetal heart tones; their presence or absence will not change treatment. Cricoid pressure may decrease the chance of aspiration in a nonintubated patient. Advanced cardiac life support (ACLS) guidelines should be followed as if the woman were not pregnant. It is difficult to apply an apical defibrillator paddle with the patient inclined laterally; adhesive electrodes are easier to use. Palpate for pulses during CPR compressions. If you can feel a carotid pulse but not a femoral pulse, placental perfusion may be inadequate.

Modifications for the pregnant patient can make resuscitation more effective. In the supine position, the weight of the gravid uterus on the vena cava significantly reduces cardiac return. In patients of greater than 20 weeks' gestation, one rescuer should manually displace the gravid uterus from the midline while CPR is in progress. Alternatively, employ a 15–30° left lateral tilt. Tilt should not exceed 30°, or the woman will tend to roll into full lateral position and thwart effective resuscitation attempts. If the crew consists of two people, a pillow wedged under the right flank and hip to displace the uterus to the left can take the place of the extra pair of hands. The patient can also be tilted onto the rescuer's knees to provide a stable position for CPR. Placing the patient on a backboard will facilitate this position.

While performing CPR, try to determine the cause of arrest and take steps to counteract the problem. If the arrest is secondary to a magnesium sulfate overdose given to treat preeclampsia, administer calcium chloride. If it is hypovolemia, infuse lactated Ringer's or normal saline though bilateral intravenous lines.

The objective of field care is to prevent or at least delay the arrest until the patient has arrived at the hospital. When transporting a patient with a life-threatening condition, use left lateral positioning (or left lateral tilt in the setting of trauma), aggressive airway management, oxygenation, and intravenous fluid replacement, in conjunction with rapid transport and any treatments appropriate to her particular condition. When the pregnancy is greater than 24 weeks, chances for survival are much greater for mother and fetus if she arrests in the ED rather than in the field. In a hospital setting, if the pregnant woman cannot be resuscitated within 4 minutes, immediate **perimortem cesarean delivery** is usually performed not only to save the fetus but also to improve chances of maternal survival.

perimortem cesarean delivery
Surgical delivery performed when the mother is in cardiac arrest.

Pregnancy and Chronic Diseases

Many women with serious health problems choose to bear children despite risks to themselves and their babies. Some consciously plan families and seek prenatal care from high-risk obstetrical specialists to ensure the best possible outcome. Others neglect their diseases, become pregnant accidentally, fail to seek prenatal care, or do not comply with the recommendations of obstetrical providers. The EMS professional encounters both varieties of high-risk patients, usually when they are in the middle of a health crisis. It is important to understand how pregnancy affects common chronic diseases.

Asthma

Asthma complicates 4–6% of pregnancies, remaining stable in about half of pregnant women, worsening in 20–35%, and improving in 20–35%. Perinatal mortality is no higher for an asthmatic woman than for a woman without the disease, although chronic hypoxemia can lead to intrauterine growth restriction. Exacerbations are mostly likely to occur early in the third trimester. Pregnant women with asthma are usually managed on the same medications they used before pregnancy, including bronchodilators and steroids. Steroid-dependent women with severe asthma are more likely to develop gestational diabetes and PIH. The infant of a mother with asthma has a 58% lifetime risk of developing the disease.

In the field, usual protocols for asthma exacerbations should be followed in the pregnant patient. Assess the severity of the attack, noting the

presence of agitation or lethargy and whether she is using accessory muscles. A pregnant woman in a severe episode may have a pulse greater than
120 and an audible wheeze, although a serious asthma episode may also
produce minimal wheezing if air movement is severely decreased.

Provide oxygen—high flow for moderate or severe distress, low
flow for mild distress. Establish an intravenous line of D5W or normal
saline. Albuterol (Proventil), metaproterenol (Alupent), or isoetharine
(Bronkosol), administered in normal saline via nebulized inhaler, are all
category B and considered safe for pregnant women. Terbutaline
(Brethine) is effective at relaxing bronchospasms, but is not ideal as a
field drug because it takes 30–60 minutes to become therapeutic.

Diabetes

Women with diabetes, an endocrine disorder of carbohydrate metabolism, are at risk for numerous complications of pregnancy. Chronically
elevated blood sugar increases the woman's risk of preeclampsia,
preterm labor, and polyhydramnios. Her fetus is at higher risk for either
IUGR or macrosomia (excessive size). Pregnant women with diabetes
are more likely to suffer infection, especially of the urinary tract, and
kidney dysfunction.

The woman with diabetes before pregnancy who has high glucose
levels early in the first trimester is much more likely to miscarry than the
woman with normal glucose levels. Her fetus has a four to eight times
greater chance of a structural anomaly, including cardiac malformations,
neural tube defects, absent kidneys or other urinary tract malformations,
fistula between the trachea and the esophagus, and imperforate anus.
Later in pregnancy, elevated blood sugar leads to **fetal macrosomia**, increasing the risk for cephalopelvic disproportion (head too large for maternal pelvis), birth trauma, and shoulder dystocia. In addition, fetal
lungs may be slow to mature, and the infant may become hypoglycemic
after delivery.

fetal macrosomia
Excessively large
fetus, with a birth
weight of at least
4,000–4,500 g
(8 lb, 13 oz to 9 lb,
15 oz) or greater
than the 90th per-
centile for gesta-
tional age.

Some women may develop gestational diabetes, or elevated glucose
levels during pregnancy. Obstetrical providers routinely screen most
women for this condition between 26 and 28 weeks of gestation, earlier if
she has a history of gestational diabetes in prior pregnancies. If a woman
can maintain normal blood-sugar levels by making dietary changes, she
may manage her disease by logging blood glucose readings and carefully
following her prescribed diet. If diet alone fails to keep glucose readings
within normal limits, she may be started on insulin. Half of all women
with gestational diabetes go on to develop type 2 diabetes later in life.

The EMS provider should be aware that some pregnant diabetic
women experience wide swings in blood sugar from significantly hyperglycemic to seriously hypoglycemic, sometimes within the space of

hours. Unstable blood glucose is most often seen in women who are learning to use insulin or those noncompliant with treatment.

When confronted with an unresponsive pregnant woman, the EMS provider should always consider hypoglycemia a possible cause. Hypoglycemia can cause mood changes, tachycardia, sweating, pallor, and headaches, sometimes progressing to changes in level of consciousness, coma, and seizures. Hypoglycemia in pregnancy is treated just as it is in the nonpregnant woman, with oral carbohydrate administration if she is conscious (20 g, obtainable from approximately 12 oz of orange or apple juice, 15 oz of milk, 14 oz of carbonated soft drink, or sugar paste) and, if unconscious, intravenous D-50 or IM glucagon.

Symptoms of hyperglycemia are increased urination, thirst, hunger, and fatigue, progressing to coma, deep (Kussmaul's) respirations, and an acetone scent to the breath. As with any hyperglycemic patient, hydrate intravenously (0.9% normal saline, 1 L infused over an hour) and transport rapidly.

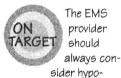

The EMS provider should always consider hypoglycemia or hyperglycemia as a possible cause of coma or altered mental status in the pregnant woman.

Cardiac Disease

Pregnancy can worsen preexisting heart problems, and some cardiovascular disorders may present for the first time during pregnancy. The most common cardiovascular disorders to arise during pregnancy are hypertension, valvular disease, arrhythmias, cardiomyopathies, aortic dissection (particularly in patients with Marfan syndrome), and ischemic heart disease. Previously benign congenital heart anomalies may become symptomatic during pregnancy. The woman with a cardiac disorder may decompensate suddenly even if closely monitored by her physician and compliant with recommendations for rest, stress reduction, weight restriction, and prophylactic antibiotics. Pregnancy places women with artificial valves or atrial fibrillation at increased risk for embolism, and their obstetrical providers may prescribe heparin or Lovenox through the pregnancy.

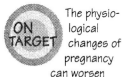

The physiological changes of pregnancy can worsen preexisting heart problems, and some cardiovascular disorders present for the first time during pregnancy.

The physiological changes of pregnancy increase the workload of the heart. Pregnant women have 50% more blood circulating through their vessels, and this increased intravascular volume increases cardiac output. Cardiac output increases further between 28 and 34 weeks, when blood volume expands rapidly; during labor; and immediately postpartum. Every contraction of labor increases cardiac output by about 20–30%. For days or weeks postpartum, fluid shifts can cause sudden fluctuations in cardiac output and can cause the woman to decompensate.

The growing uterus shifts the heart up and forward, frequently causing a 15° left axis deviation on electrocardiograms by the end of pregnancy. The electrocardiogram may also show flattened or inverted t-waves in lead III, and Q waves in lead III and AVF. Ectopic beats are also frequently seen in pregnancy, but a patient with pulse irregularities should have cardiac monitoring, if available.

When transporting the laboring patient with a history of cardiac disease or a pregnant patient with cardiac symptoms, advanced life support is recommended. Evaluate vital signs frequently, initiate intravenous access, and employ cardiac monitoring. Provide oxygen—4 L/min by cannula if she is not experiencing dyspnea, high flow by mask if she has dyspnea or signs of pulmonary edema.

Many of the usual diagnostic and treatment modalities normally indicated for cardiovascular disorders pose significant risk to the fetus. Reduction in cardiac output, however, may pose even greater risk to the fetus. If the patient is stable, in many cases rapid transport is the best option. Administration of potentially harmful medications is safer in a hospital setting with fetal monitoring. If the patient is unstable, field treatment is often the best option. As always follow local protocols and consult medical control with any concerns.

Arrhythmias in the pregnant woman are generally treated as they are in the nonpregnant state, but with a few differences. Adenosine is relatively safe in pregnancy and is the first-line drug for treating supraventricular tachycardia (SVT), although it can trigger heart block or bradyarrhythmias that could compromise the fetus. Verapamil is also useful for treating this condition. Lidocaine is generally safe in pregnancy, but uterine artery constriction can occur at high blood levels. Procainamide, which has not been shown to injure the fetus, is the first-line drug for undiagnosed wide-complex tachycardia. Cardioversion poses little risk to the fetus and should be used when necessary. Amiodarone can potentially cause birth defects, so it should be avoided in the first trimester and used in the second and third trimesters only for arrhythmias unresponsive to all other measures; consult medical control before using this drug.

The pregnant woman who reports a history of cardiac problems should not be allowed to perform Valsalva pushing in labor (see chapter 6). Instead, the woman should push with little grunts, expelling air gently as she bears down. This method reduces stress on the heart. A left lateral position is beneficial unless she has dyspnea, when the semi-Fowler's is preferable.

Seizure Disorders

When a pregnant woman is found seizing, the rescuer's first thought is often eclampsia. Although it is important to consider this possibility, remember that some pregnant women have preexisting seizure disorders and can seize at any time. Seizures can also accompany head injury, alcohol withdrawal, or stroke. Some seizures due to vascular abnormalities occur only during pregnancy.

About 20% of patients with seizure disorders show a worsening of seizures during pregnancy. The physiologic changes of pregnancy—changes in electrolyte balance, respiration, and intracellular volume—may lower the seizure threshold, and fatigue and emotional stress may contribute to more frequent seizures. It may be difficult to maintain therapeutic levels of anticonvulsant medications during pregnancy because of nausea, vomiting, changes in blood volume, or a patient's reluctance to take anticonvulsant medications in pregnancy. Women with seizure disorders have a higher risk of spontaneous abortion and perinatal mortality. Most anticonvulsants have the potential to cause anomalies in the infant; but because maternal seizures can cause fetal acidosis, hypoxia, and placental abruption, most women are maintained on anticonvulsants throughout pregnancy.

Prehospital treatment of the seizing pregnant woman includes

- Attending to ABCs; maintain open airway.
- Administering high-flow oxygen via nonrebreather mask.
- Initiating IV of normal saline 0.9% at a KVO rate.
- Drawing blood when the IV is started as per local protocols.

If seizures do not stop within 5 minutes,

- Administer diazepam 5–10 mg IV slowly (not faster than 1 ml/min) or as local protocols dictate.
- Determine glucose level. If severely hypoglycemic, administer 25 g 50% dextrose IV.
- Transport.

If the patient may have eclampsia (look for high blood pressure or history of hypertension with this pregnancy, brisk reflexes, generalized swelling, history of severe headache, epigastric pain, or visual disturbances before seizure),

- Keep the patient in the left lateral recumbent position.
- Transport rapidly.
- Avoid bright or flashing lights, sirens, jostling, or any other excessive sensory stimulation.
- Contact medical control for antihypertensive agent orders.
- Monitor urinary output if possible.
- Contact medical control and consider magnesium sulfate. Loading dose is 4–6 g in 100 ml of lactated Ringer's or normal saline over 30 minutes.

Infusion is usually run at 2 g/h. Assess for decreased patellar reflexes and respiratory depression. Magnesium sulfate may stop labor contractions. It may be reversed by calcium chloride IV over 5 minutes. Magnesium sulfate may increase postpartum bleeding.

- Cardiac monitoring, vital signs, fetal heart tones, level of consciousness, patellar reflexes, respiratory rate, and oxygenation status every 5 minutes. If patellar reflexes are absent, shut off magnesium sulfate infusion and contact medical control immediately.

- Evaluate for pulmonary edema. If it occurs, contact medical control and consider morphine sulfate 2–5 mg IV push over 1–2 minutes or furosemide 20–40 mg IVP over 2–3 minutes.

- Contact medical control for any questions or problems.

If the woman is not actively seizing upon arrival,

- Open airway and suction PRN.
- Proceed with secondary survey.
- Place in recovery position if postictal.
- Apply cardiac monitor and pulse oximeter.
- Determine glucose level and treat if necessary.
- Transport.

Thromboembolism

Thromboembolism is the leading cause of maternal mortality in the United States, claiming more lives than hemorrhage, infection, or hypertension. Pregnant women are especially prone to thrombus formation; the blood of a pregnant woman coagulates easily, the veins of her lower extremities tend to dilate, and the pressure in them is higher than usual. Deep-vein thrombosis (DVT) is the formation of a blood clot in a deep vein, usually in the leg, but sometimes in the pelvis or elsewhere. If this clot dislodges, it can move to the lung and cause a life-threatening pulmonary embolism.

Thromboembolism can occur in any trimester, especially postpartum, and more commonly after cesarean birth. Risk factors include varicose veins in the legs, obesity, hereditary tendency to clot excessively, recent surgery, injury to the leg, and history of DVT. Bed rest and prolonged periods of inactivity (even a long plane flight) can precipitate DVT. The woman will present with pain, heat, and redness and swelling in one of her legs and perhaps a palpable rigid, distended leg vein; and the affected leg may be considerably more swollen than the other. She

Homan's sign

Pain in the calf upon dorsiflexion of the foot.

may have a fever. Flexing the top of the foot toward the shin may increase the pain (**Homan's sign**).

Do not allow the woman with suspected DVT to walk to the ambulance. Transport her with her heel on a pillow and no pressure on the affected vein. Do not massage the leg, and use caution when palpating the swelling—rubbing the leg may dislodge the clot and send it to the lungs.

Symptoms of pulmonary embolism include chest pain and shortness of breath or sometimes shock or cardiac arrest. Suspected pulmonary embolism should be treated as in the nonpregnant patient—with high-flow oxygen, intravenous access with normal saline, cardiac monitoring, pulse oximeter, and rapid transport. Consider intubation and respiratory support if she is unable to maintain an airway.

HIV Infection

Only 0.17% of all pregnant women in the United States carry HIV, but certain localities have much higher rates. HIV is contracted by sexual contact or by direct exposure to blood and body fluids. The virus can also be passed from a pregnant woman to her fetus. In the United States, about 25% of babies born to mothers with HIV will contract the disease. (In Africa, the number approaches 40%.) The patient with HIV is more likely to give birth to a growth-restricted infant, and maternal infections may be more likely to develop.

Administration of certain medications during pregnancy reduces the baby's risk of contracting HIV by as much as 70%. Elective cesarean section at 38 weeks' gestation also decreases transmission of the virus from mother to baby and is usually offered as a delivery option. The American woman with HIV is discouraged from breastfeeding because she may transmit the virus through her milk. In developing countries, however, because the risk of malnutrition is greater than the risk of HIV infection, breastfeeding is encouraged.

Universal precautions should be taken with all patients regardless of HIV status.

Rh Incompatibilities and Hemolytic Disease

Human blood is typed A, B, AB, or O, and at least 85% of the population has a blood antigen named the Rh factor, for the rhesus monkey in which it was first identified. People with the antigen are Rh-positive; people lacking it are Rh-negative.

Blood type becomes important in pregnancy because it is the mother's bloodstream that brings oxygen and nourishment to the developing fetus. The mother's blood does not ordinarily mix with that of the fetus, and mother and fetus may have different blood types.

Occasionally, however, fetal blood enters the maternal system because of trauma or abruption or during placental separation in a normal delivery. If the mother is Rh-negative and the fetus is positive, exposure to foreign blood can cause the mother to manufacture antibodies against Rh-positive blood. If her next fetus is Rh-positive, these antibodies cross the placenta and attack and destroy fetal red blood cells, causing profound anemia and even death of the fetus. Historically, this condition has killed innumerable babies.

Today, the Rh-negative pregnant woman is typically injected with anti-D immunoglobulin (RhoGam) antepartum and postpartum to prevent her from forming antibodies that might endanger subsequent fetuses. She should also receive RhoGam following trauma, spontaneous abortion, and medical procedures such as amniocentesis.

It is helpful for the EMS provider to be aware of Rh incompatibility because women often resist treatment after falls, miscarriage, and minor accidents. The EMS provider can explain that this is another good reason to seek prompt treatment.

Hemolytic disease can also occur secondary to ABO incompatibility between mother and fetus. The most common scenario is the mother with O blood type carrying a baby with A or B blood. The anti-A and anti-B antibodies that naturally occur in individuals with O blood type cross the placenta and attack fetal red blood cells, causing **hemolysis.** Usually the amount of hemolysis is minor, although it is probably greater for subsequent offspring. Affected babies show hyperbilirubinemia (jaundice) within 24 hours of birth, and the jaundice is usually resolved with phototherapy.

hemolysis
Destruction of red blood cells.

Preterm Labor

Premature delivery, the birth of an infant before 37 completed weeks of gestation, affects about 1 out of every 8 infants born in the United States. Although advances in medicine have improved survival of preterm infants and have pushed back the age of viability to 22–24 weeks' gestation, the incidence of preterm delivery in the United States has actually increased by 27% in the last 20 years. Prematurity complicated 9.4% of births in 1981, but by 2001, rates of preterm births had increased to 11.9%. This increase may be attributed to more multiple births (caused by in vitro fertilization and other infertility treatments) and a greater willingness to deliver babies early when maternal complications occur (encouraged by better neonatal intensive care).

More than 60% of newborn morbidity and mortality is related to premature birth. The lower the birth weight, the more likely an infant is to die or suffer serious impairment.

Risk factors for preterm delivery include

- Previous preterm delivery—the more previous preterm deliveries, the higher the risk for this pregnancy.

cervical incompetence
Tendency of the cervix to open painlessly in the second or third trimester of pregnancy.

- Uterine anomalies, **cervical incompetence** (tendency of cervix to open painlessly in the second or third trimester), certain cervical surgeries such as loop electrosurgical excision procedure of the transformation zone (LEEP), and cone biopsy.
- Excessive uterine enlargement, as in multiple pregnancy or **polyhydramnios.**

polyhydramnios
Excessive amounts of amniotic fluid.

- Maternal infection—vaginal and urinary tract infections increase the risk of preterm delivery.
- Low socioeconomic status, lack of adequate prenatal care, domestic violence.
- Tobacco, cocaine, or alcohol abuse.
- Short interval between pregnancies.
- Fetal anomalies.
- Chronic health problems such as hypertension, diabetes, or clotting disorders.
- Poor nutrition, poor weight gain, and being underweight or obese at the beginning of the pregnancy.
- Emotional stress.
- Physically strenuous work, long working hours, prolonged standing.
- Age less than 17 or greater than 35.
- African American ancestry.
- Frequent preterm contractions, premature rupture of membranes, vaginal bleeding.

Preterm labor appears to be a long-term, multifactorial process rather than an acute condition. Preterm labor is diagnosed when a woman has regular uterine contractions accompanied by dilation and thinning of the cervix and descent of the fetus. Some women have cramping throughout the second and third trimesters without cervical change (and often go to or beyond their due dates), so preterm labor cannot be identified on symptoms alone. Preterm labor is diagnosed when a patient has persistent uterine contractions coupled with effacement (thinning) and/or dilation (opening) of the cervix.

Because the diagnosis of preterm labor can be made only by an obstetrical provider through vaginal or sonographic examination, the EMS crew should take seriously every complaint of preterm cramping or contractions.

Signs and symptoms of preterm labor may be vague. The woman may complain of contractions, generalized crampiness, pelvic pressure, rectal pressure, or back pain, but half of all women in preterm labor report no pain at all. The patient may have diarrhea and intestinal cramping or a change in vaginal discharge, but many other conditions can cause these symptoms. Any amount of vaginal bleeding in the second or third trimester should be evaluated immediately; but some women spot occasionally after intercourse, and certain vaginal infections can cause spotting. A gush of fluid may indicate rupture of membranes, but often it is normal vaginal discharge or bladder incontinence related to fetal movement. Urinary tract infections can both cause and mimic preterm labor. Medical conditions such as appendicitis, cholecystitis, and even gastroenteritis can trigger preterm labor.

Women who show symptoms of preterm labor are more likely to have an increase in symptoms if they engage in sexual activity (including breast stimulation and any activity that produces orgasm); long-distance travel in cars, trains, or buses; carrying heavy objects; prolonged standing; and strenuous physical activity. The preterm delivery rate in heavy smokers (more than half a pack a day) is one in five pregnancies, or more than twice the rate of nonsmokers.

If you suspect preterm labor, transport the woman on her left side and be vigilant for sudden delivery. Premature infants of low birth weight have lower perinatal morbidity and mortality rates when they are delivered at a tertiary-care center. Birth may be delayed if the mother is instructed to pant and blow rather than push. Many women in preterm labor do not feel contractions and may deliver unexpectedly. If preterm delivery does occur, choose a side-lying maternal position whenever possible because this reduces pressure on the fetal head. Premature infants are more likely to suffer brain hemorrhage during birth, and every measure must be taken to make birth gentle and easy. Coach the mother to push without holding her breath, and encourage her to push with short grunts, expelling air from her nose or mouth with each effort.

The EMS provider should employ full resuscitation if there are any signs of life at delivery. BLS resuscitation can be employed to assure the family and patient that all efforts were attempted, even if you are not sure whether the infant is viable. Do not attempt if the fetus is decomposing or is severely malformed (e.g., heart on outside of body, open skull with missing cerebrum). Premature infants should be transported to a hospital with a neonatal intensive care unit if possible, but do not lengthen transport time more than a few minutes to reach one. Premature babies are often born vigorous and then quickly develop problems such as dyspnea and hypothermia. (See chapter 9.)

Threats to Mother and Fetus 117

Carbon Monoxide Poisoning

Many kinds of accidental or environmental poisoning are possible; but in the industrialized world, carbon monoxide (CO) is the leading cause of poison-related mortality and morbidity. CO is an odorless, colorless gas formed by the incomplete combustion of organic compounds. CO toxicity may occur when exhaust systems malfunction, when ventilation is obstructed, or when equipment designed for the outdoors is used in confined areas. Possible sources include gas water heaters, kerosene space heaters, charcoal grills, propane stoves, and propane-fueled forklifts. House fires may generate high amounts of CO where it occurs in the presence of other toxins such as cyanide, complicating diagnosis and treatment. Deliberate exposure to CO is a common mechanism of suicide. Fumes from some spray paints, solvents, degreasers, and paint removers are converted to CO in the liver.

Carbon monoxide binds with adult hemoglobin with an affinity 200–250 times greater than that of oxygen, and fetal hemoglobin has an even stronger attraction. CO combines with the hemoglobin to form **carboxyhemoglobin (COHb)**. COHb levels are an unreliable indicator of severity of intoxication or prognosis for mother or fetus. Fetal COHb levels can be as much as 10–15% higher than those of the mother, and the fetus can suffer severe damage even if maternal symptoms are moderate. Carbon monoxide is an **abortifacient** and a teratogen. Exposure can result in immediate or delayed pregnancy loss, physical malformations, and neurological impairment. Risk is greater when the patient is exposed to CO for an hour or more or is in an enclosed space during exposure.

The nervous system and heart are very susceptible to damage from CO poisoning, but other organs are also affected. Because the hemoglobin is saturated with CO, it cannot pick up oxygen, and the patient becomes hypoxic at the cellular level. Intracellular uptake of carbon monoxide may also be a mechanism for injury. Hypoxia alone would not explain why many patients develop neurological and psychiatric abnormalities up to 40 days after exposure. Long-term effects range from subtle cognitive deficits to incapacitating movement disorders.

Symptoms and signs of CO poisoning may include headache, dizziness, nausea, flu-like symptoms, malaise, exertional dyspnea, chest pain, ventricular dysrhythmias, disorientation, lethargy, hallucinations, agitation, lack of coordination, abdominal pain, syncope, seizure, and coma. Cherry-red skin color is rare; most CO poisoning victims are pale and cyanotic. Neonates are at great risk because their hemoglobin picks up and holds CO more readily than does adult hemoglobin. Small infants may present with only vomiting and may show symptoms before the rest of the family do. Patients who present with these symptoms

carboxyhemoglobin (COHb)
A compound formed when carbon monoxide combines with hemoglobin in the blood.

abortifacient
A substance or device that causes abortion.

should be questioned about the use of gas- or oil-fueled appliances and the presence of similar symptoms in other household members, in pets, or in neighbors.

Emergency treatment of the pregnant woman with CO poisoning is identical to the treatment of a nonpregnant woman. Priorities include stabilization of airway, breathing, circulation, removal from the toxic environment, application of 100% oxygen, cardiac monitoring, and rapid transport. Intubate if there has been a thermal airway injury or if the patient cannot reliably maintain her own airway. Seizures should be treated with diazepam as would be seizures from other causes. Pulse oximetry is inaccurate in the presence of COHb and will read as normal in even the seriously compromised patient. The prehospital responder should draw a blood sample on scene, if possible, to document levels of COHb before treatment is initiated.

The pregnant patient with a high COHb level or serious symptoms may require treatment with hyperbaric oxygen at a regional facility. Hyperbaric oxygen accelerates the clearance of CO from the body, correcting hypoxia and preventing central nervous system damage.

ON TARGET The prehospital provider should not use a pulse oximeter on the patient with CO poisoning. Hemoglobin saturated with CO will produce a false normal reading.

Substance Abuse

In the United States, about 6% of pregnant women report using illicit drugs while pregnant. Most drug abusers use more than one substance concurrently. Substance abuse during pregnancy can have adverse long-term and short-term effects on the fetus. Substance abuse can be found in all age, ethnic, and socioeconomic groups. The EMS provider should remain alert for indications that a patient has been abusing drugs and consider complications that may result.

Cocaine and Crack

Whereas cocaine is water soluble and administered orally, intravenously, or nasally, crack is smoked. A 1993 study suggested that as many as 10% of pregnant women use cocaine, more in urban areas. Cocaine is a potent stimulant, elevating pulse, constricting vessels, and elevating blood pressure while giving a feeling of euphoria. The resulting hypertension can cause placental abruption, maternal brain hemorrhage, heart and lung disorders, rapid delivery, preterm delivery, spontaneous abortion, or sudden death. The infant can also suffer cerebral infarcts and hemorrhage, malformations, behavioral abnormalities, low birth weight, SIDS, and withdrawal symptoms.

Opiates

Opiates, including illegal drugs such as heroin and legal prescription narcotics, affect the central nervous system and cause changes in mood, pain tolerance, sensations, and alertness. Opiates are physically addictive, and the user requires progressively higher doses to reach the desired effect. Heroin use in pregnancy increases the likelihood of stillbirth, prematurity, neonatal death, IUGR, and behavioral disturbances. The neonate of a woman who has high blood levels of opiates at the time of delivery may be lethargic at birth and suffer respiratory depression.

fetal alcohol syndrome

A set of congenital anomalies (e.g., small head, slow growth, mental retardation, hyperactivity) caused by excessive consumption of alcohol during pregnancy.

Alcohol

Alcohol use during pregnancy is strongly associated with fetal abnormalities. One-third of pregnant women who consume six or more drinks a day give birth to children with **fetal alcohol syndrome**, the leading preventable cause of mental retardation in the United States. Lesser amounts of alcohol may have milder physical, cognitive, or behavioral effects, including central nervous system dysfunction, facial abnormalities, and growth problems. Alcohol abuse causes bleeding in the first trimester, infection, and abruption. No amount of alcohol has been proven safe for pregnant women.

The acutely intoxicated pregnant woman should be managed no differently than any other person in that condition, with emphasis on ABCs and preventing injury. Position on left side for transport and have suction ready in case of vomiting if she has difficulty clearing her airway.

The alcohol-dependent pregnant woman may have withdrawal seizures as early as 12–48 hours after her last drink.

Amphetamines

Amphetamines encompass a large family of stimulants, including speed, meth, ecstasy, and the designer drugs. Amphetamines cause the vessels feeding the uterus and placenta to spasm, reducing oxygen and nutrient flow to the fetus, and sometimes causing abruption, preterm labor, intrauterine growth restriction, and stillbirth. Abnormalities such as cleft lip, microcephaly, and cardiac defects have been attributed to these drugs, as have behavioral and cognitive problems. These drugs curb maternal appetite, sometimes causing maternal and fetal malnutrition. A woman on amphetamines will appear energetic, if not hyperactive, and may sometimes suffer paranoid delusions or hallucinations. She is at risk for hypertension and tachycardia. Withdrawal brings lethargy and deep depression.

Tobacco

Tobacco causes vasoconstriction and reduces blood flow to the placenta. In addition, smoke from cigarettes, cigars, and pipes contains many toxic substances, such as carbon monoxide and formaldehyde. Smoking sharply increases the risk of abruption, low birth weight, prematurity, spontaneous abortion, and stillbirth. The infant mortality rate of smokers is 60% greater than that of nonsmokers. If the mother smokes more than a pack a day, the risk increases an additional 35%.

Summary

The pregnant patient offers a wide range of challenges to the prehospital health care provider. Pregnancy not only complicates but also is complicated by many conditions, from the obvious (such as trauma) to the obscure (such as hypoglycemia). Many of these conditions are, or can quickly become, life threatening to mother or fetus. In general:

- With a few noteworthy exceptions, the pregnant patient should be treated as any other patient.
- Treating the mother first is the best means of ensuring the survival of mother *and* fetus.

1. What three mechanisms are responsible for most of the trauma suffered by pregnant women?

2. How does pregnancy work against successful resuscitation of the woman in cardiac arrest?

3. What factors increase the risk of thromboembolism?

4. Does asthma worsen or improve in pregnancy? How would the EMS provider treat the pregnant woman with asthma exacerbation?

5. What are some possible signs of preterm labor? What other disorders cause or mimic preterm labor?

CHAPTER 5

The Woman in Labor

Objectives

By the end of this chapter you should be able to

- Recognize the signs of impending labor
- Understand the stages of labor
- Differentiate between false labor and labor
- Understand the methods of labor induction
- Take a history and assess a woman in labor
- Manage a precipitous delivery

CASE Study

Responding to a call for "possible labor," Kim and Edward rolled the ambulance up the long driveway of a farmhouse remote from the nearest hospital. Grabbing an OB kit, equipment kit, and oxygen bag just in case, they headed up the walk. A nervous woman met them on the front porch.

Speaking rapidly, Amanda told them that this was her second baby and that her first delivery had been very quick and intense. With her last labor, she left home as soon as her contractions began and was fully dilated by the time she arrived at the hospital. After 15 minutes of pushing, she delivered a healthy 9-lb boy. Her midwife expected the second baby to arrive even faster.

Now she was 38 weeks pregnant with another boy, estimated fetal weight of 7 lb by sonogram several days earlier. At that time her midwife assessed her cervix as 3–4 cm dilated, soft and very thin, and the fetal head was very low in the pelvis. "Do you think you're in labor?" Kim asked, confused because Amanda showed no signs of pain, puttering around with abundant nervous energy and appearing utterly unlike the classic picture of a woman in labor.

"I don't know," Amanda replied. "I'm having contractions 4 minutes apart, have been for about 2 hours or so. They don't hurt, but they didn't last time, either. And I am having a lot of pressure down there and some pink discharge. I really don't know what to do! I don't want to go in for a false alarm, but I'm scared that we're going to have the baby in the car if we drive in ourselves."

"It's usually better to go in for a false alarm than to take chances," Edward explained. "We can certainly take you into the hospital for evaluation." Amanda sighed in relief and affirmed that she would feel much safer with an ambulance transport.

"I just have to grab my bag," Amanda said as she vanished down the hall.

As she returned she stopped, cringed, and a tremendous gush of clear fluid cascaded down her legs. She rushed to the bathroom, sat on the toilet, and groaned. Amanda was suddenly lost in her bodily sensations, oblivious to the ambulance crew. It appeared that she was having hard contractions one on top of the next.

"Kim, toss some towels on her bed and open the OB kit," Edward said. "We need to check for crowning. I think she's going fast." Amanda was now making guttural grunts. Edward tried to coax Amanda to the bed. Amanda whimpered unintelligibly and moaned again, involuntarily pushing. Edward and Kim lifted Amanda from the toilet and carried her to the bed, where they visualized her vulva. No fetal parts were crowning, but there was a moderate quantity of mucusy red blood at her introitus.

Amanda moaned as another contraction peaked, and she pushed mindlessly. Another push, and a hairy scalp showed, compressed into folds by the pressure of birth, then withdrew and disappeared. With the next push, Edward used a gloved hand to apply a 4 in. × 4 in. gauze to Amanda's perineum as it bulged. He spread his fingers over the emerging head and applied careful counterpressure.

"Gentle pushes, Amanda," he said. "Very gently, breathe your baby out slowly." This time the head crowned fully, then emerged. Edward asked Amanda to stop pushing and began to feel around the neck for the cord. Amanda suddenly pushed forcefully and the baby shot out, slipping between Edward's hands and landing safely on the bed a few inches from Amanda. Edward picked him up, placed him on his mother's abdomen, and began to dry and stimulate him with a towel. The infant was purple but flung up his arms in a Moro reflex and opened his eyes. Edward sucked mucus from his airway with a bulb syringe. Moments later, the baby began crying heartily, and his lips and body turned a reassuring pink.

Questions

1. What features of Amanda's history suggested that her delivery would be quick and easy?
2. Describe how the EMS provider should assess rupture of the amniotic membranes.
3. If Edward had been unable to move Amanda off the toilet before delivery, how would he have managed the birth?
4. What concerns would Kim and Edward have about the third stage of labor?

Introduction

Labor is often a protracted, physically demanding process, taxing the physical and emotional resources of the woman. Conversely, birth can occur unexpectedly with barely any warning, sometimes in awkward or unusual settings. Changes that herald approaching parturition may occur days and weeks prior to the event. Prehospital providers must consider all possible contingencies when assessing the laboring woman, and provide comfort measures and interventions that safeguard the well-being of mother and fetus.

KEY TERMS

active labor, p. 131	crowning, p. 132	meconium, p. 128
amniotomy, p. 137	effacement, p. 126	nitrazine® paper, p. 127
cephalopelvic disproportion, p. 138	grand multipara, p. 132	vernix caseosa, p. 127
	malpresentation, p. 132	prostaglandin, p. 125

Mechanism and Stages of Labor

prostaglandin
A hormonelike substance that may affect metabolism, blood pressure, smooth-muscle activity, or nerve transmission.

Labor is the process by which uterine contractions cause progressive cervical change that results in the expulsion of the fetus, placenta, and membranes. Researchers continue to gain insight into the physiology of labor and attribute a complex interplay of genetic programming, maternal and fetal hormones, **prostaglandins**, psychological influences, and mechanical stimuli.

Like any other muscular contraction, a uterine contraction is produced by the shortening of muscle fibers. Unlike other physiological muscular contractions, uterine contractions of labor are painful. With each contraction, the muscles of the upper uterine segment shorten and pull upward on the passive lower uterine segment and cervix, causing them to thin and open over the baby's head (much like pulling on a turtleneck sweater) as the upper segment contracts and retracts. These muscle fibers do not return to their original length between contractions; the upper part of the uterus becomes thicker over the course of labor, while the lower uterine segment thins. Unlike the toning Braxton Hicks contractions of pregnancy (see chapter 1), labor contractions progressively thin and open the cervix.

Signs of Impending Labor

Changes that herald labor may occur hours, days, weeks, or even months before labor begins. Sometime during the third trimester, the fetal presenting part descends into the pelvis. The cervix remains long, thick, and closed throughout pregnancy, sealed with a plug of dense mucus that inhibits the ascent of bacteria into the uterus. Before labor commences, the cervix usually effaces, dilates, and softens, and the mucus plug may be expelled—although this process may not begin until labor with some individuals. **Effacement** describes the thinning of the cervix, expressed in percentages. Many women are more than 80% effaced and 3 or more centimeters dilated for weeks before labor commences.

effacement
Shortening and thinning of the cervix in preparation for birth, expressed in percentages. A cervix that is 100% effaced is paper thin.

Lightening
Weeks before labor, the presenting part of the fetus may move down and enter the pelvis, informally described as the baby "dropping." See Figure 5-1. The expectant mother may find that she can breathe easier and feels "lighter" because the fetus is no longer beneath her ribs compressing her diaphragm. The trade-off is that the descent of the fetus puts additional pressure on her bladder, and she may urinate frequently or even experience urinary incontinence. Lightening often increases pressure on pelvic nerves and veins, causing leg and back pain and increased pedal edema.

Rupture of Membranes
Rupture of membranes (ROM) precedes labor in only 12% of births. An intact amniotic sac cushions both the presenting part and the umbilical cord during labor, and in most women it does not spontaneously rupture until the second stage. Sometimes the amnion does not rupture at all, and the baby is born "in the caul," traditionally considered a harbinger of good luck. (In this case the EMS provider need only tear the membrane and remove it from the baby's face before the first breath.)

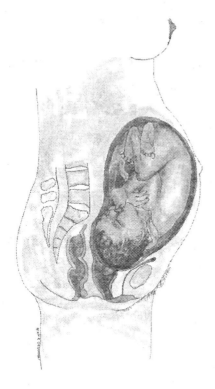

FIGURE 5-1
Lightening.

Lightening is the term for when the baby moves into the pelvis in preparation for delivery, also known as the baby "dropping." This movement can happen during labor or many weeks before.

Illustration by Bonnie U. Gruenberg

In most cases of ROM at term, labor begins spontaneously within 24 hours of rupture. Infection, however, becomes a concern once there is an open passage between the uterus and the outside world, and most hospitals induce labor within 24 hours after a woman ruptures membranes at or near term.

Rupture of membranes can occur as a gush of a quart or more of warm fluid or as a small leak that the woman experiences as persistent dampness. If membranes rupture while the patient is on the toilet, the EMS provider may notice bits of **vernix caseosa** (which resembles globs of moisturizing cream) and fetal hair in the water.

Vaginal drainage on undergarments or sanitary pads should be evaluated for color and scent. Amniotic fluid should be clear and almost odorless, or have a vague bleachlike odor. Fluid that is thin and yellow or smells like urine may *be* urine. A watery vaginal discharge can also mimic rupture of membranes.

The patient's physician or midwife diagnoses ROM by sterile speculum exam, which will reveal pooling of fluid in the vagina and perhaps seepage through the cervix. Amniotic fluid also turns **nitrazine® paper** deep blue and dries in a distinctive ferning pattern on a microscope slide. If these tests are equivocal, an amniotic fluid index (AFI) can be measured sonographically to quantify the volume

vernix caseosa
A white, greasy, tenacious substance secreted by fetal sebaceous glands that adheres to the body hair and protects delicate fetal skin *in utero.*

nitrazine® paper
Paper impregnated with phenaphthazine, an indicator dye, used to determine the pH of solutions by its change in color.

of fluid present in the uterus. A low AFI may indicate ruptured membranes.

Any patient who reports rupture of membranes should be evaluated by her provider at the office or hospital. ROM carries the risk of cord prolapse, which can reduce or stop blood flow to the fetus. Prolapse is more likely if the fetus is not in a vertex (head down and flexed) position. Fetal heart rate or presence of fetal movement should always be assessed as soon as possible after ROM to assess fetal well-being.

The potential for infection may become greater with every hour a patient's membranes are ruptured, especially if she carries the group B strep bacteria in her vaginal flora or has placed anything in her vagina. Chorioamnionitis is indicated by fever, uterine tenderness, malaise, elevated maternal or fetal heart rate, and foul-smelling yellowish vaginal drainage (see chapter 3).

meconium

The tarry blackish-green substance excreted in a baby's first bowel movement, which ideally occurs shortly after birth, but may occur *in utero*.

If the fetus has passed **meconium** (moved its bowels *in utero*), the amniotic fluid will appear pale greenish or tan; thick meconium may resemble pea soup. Dense, black, tarry meconium issuing from the vagina often indicates a breech presentation. Meconium can denote fetal distress and poses a risk of airway compromise in the newborn (see chapter 9).

Mucus Plug

The mucus plug is a glob of mucus that seals the cervix during pregnancy. It is gelatinous and blood streaked, much like thick nasal mucus. When the cervix loosens near term, the mucus plug may dislodge. Mucus-plug passage may herald the onset of labor, or it may occur weeks before labor commences. Often the woman has an increase in vaginal discharge after the mucus plug has dislodged, which serves to deter microorganisms from ascending into the uterus.

Bloody Show

During labor, progressive cervical stretching ruptures capillaries, causing pink or reddish, mucus-laced vaginal discharge—"bloody show." It tends to increase in volume when labor is progressing rapidly and at the end of first-stage labor. (Frank vaginal bleeding may indicate a more serious condition, such as abruption or placenta previa.) Bloody show can also follow a vigorous cervical exam by the patient's obstetrical provider.

Recognizing Labor

False Labor

The contractions of false labor are irregular, spasmodic, and often sharp, and do not progressively dilate the cervix. Braxton Hicks contractions

Table 5-1   Differences between True and False Labor

True Labor	False Labor
Pain at regular intervals	Irregular contractions
Intervals gradually shorten	No change in pattern over time
Duration and severity increase	
Pain starts in the back and moves to the front	Pain felt mostly in front
Walking increases intensity	No change with walking—or change in activity may stop contractions altogether
Bloody show often present	No bloody show
Cervix effaced and dilated	No change in cervix or fetal descent
Presenting part descends	

grow stronger and more frequent toward the end of pregnancy, sometimes occurring in a pattern that mimics labor. Prolonged standing, physical exertion, dehydration, and emotional stress may make the uterus irritable and initiate runs of contractions that can be very painful. These contractions can begin weeks before the onset of labor, sometimes last for days, and cause sleeplessness and frustration for many pregnant women.

Whereas in true labor, contractions generally grow closer, more regular, and longer in duration, the contractions of false labor usually remain irregular. See Table 5-1. Other times, these contractions may be regular and mimic labor, only to disappear if the woman changes activity or increases her fluid intake. Sometimes a woman will present with the pelvic and back pain of a urinary tract infection coupled with painful runs of contractions, making it difficult to determine whether she is truly in labor.

True Labor

The EMS provider should time contractions from the beginning of one to the beginning of the next and also note the duration of an average contraction. In most cases, labor contractions settle and grow longer, stronger, and more frequent over time, eventually occurring every 2–3 minutes and lasting 60–90 seconds. Most commonly, the woman experiences the pain of labor contractions as a spasm that starts in the lower back, curls around her hips, and knots above the pubic bone.

Labor is not always clear-cut or obvious, and even obstetrical professionals cannot always diagnose labor in the first minutes of patient contact. Labor involves progressive cervical change, but it is never appropriate for an EMS professional to perform a vaginal examination.

Prehospital providers must infer a woman's progress in labor through external physical and behavioral cues, but these can vary greatly and may be unreliable indicators of the woman's true status. The patient who reports that she is in agony may actually be in very early labor, and the calm and apparently comfortable patient may be in advanced labor.

As always, it is helpful to generalize, but remember that human reproductive processes are inherently variable. Sometimes a woman's contractions *never* become closer than 5 minutes apart or become completely regular.

PEARLS Palpate contractions at the uterine fundus, where the greatest muscular contraction takes place, rather than the suprapubic area, where the mother usually feels most of her pain.

Stages of Labor

ON TARGET The savvy prehospital provider realizes that human reproductive processes are inherently variable.

Labor occurs in three stages:

- First-stage labor (the dilation phase) is from onset of dilation to complete (10 cm) dilation of the cervix.
- Second-stage labor (the expulsion phase) begins with complete dilation and ends with the birth of the baby.
- Third-stage labor (expulsion of the remaining products of conception) lasts from the birth of the infant to the expulsion of the placenta and membranes.

Some clinicians refer to a fourth stage of labor (the hemostasis phase) continuing from the delivery of the placenta until the woman is hemodynamically stable, 1–4 hours after delivery.

First-Stage Labor

Prodromal (Latent) Labor

The latent phase of labor is from onset to about 3–4 cm dilation. True labor usually begins slowly and subtly, especially with a primipara. The cervix progressively effaces and dilates, and contractions become more regular, more intense, longer, and more frequent. Women in latent-phase labor can usually converse throughout the duration of their contractions and are typically upbeat and excited about labor.

Some women are significantly effaced and dilated for weeks before labor begins, and may progress rapidly when membranes rupture with the onset of regular contractions. Progress from a closed cervix to 3–4 cm dilation is often slow, especially for primiparas. It can be frustrating for a woman to endure more than 6–8 hours of painful, closely spaced contractions only to find that she is 3 cm dilated—yet this is typical of first labors. The latent phase can last up to 14 hours for a multipara (average 5.3 hours) and 20 hours for a primipara. Labor may be preceded by days of false labor, making the time of onset unclear. Some multiparas (and, rarely, primiparas) have painless latent phases or bypass the prodromal stage entirely; they may labor intensely and deliver rapidly.

Active Labor

active labor
First-stage labor, between about 3–4 and 10 cm dilation, characterized by frequent, strong contractions 60–90 seconds in duration.

First-stage labor between about 3–4 and 10 cm dilation is termed **active labor.** It is characterized by increased frequency, longer duration, and greater intensity of contractions. By the end of the active phase of labor, contractions are usually 2–3 minutes apart and last 60–90 seconds. A woman in active labor often abandons her social veneer and develops a distracted, turned-inward quality as she focuses entirely on coping with contractions. She may grow discouraged, irritable, or frightened. A primigravida usually progresses at about 1 cm per hour; a multipara typically dilates faster. It is not uncommon for a multiparous patient to progress from 6 cm dilation to delivery of the infant in less than an hour. A woman who has ingested cocaine may also have a rapid labor and delivery.

Transition

Near the end of first-stage labor, between about 8 cm and complete dilation, the woman enters a phase of labor termed transition, the deceleration phase between first-stage (dilation) labor and second-stage (expulsion) labor. This is the most intense phase of labor, and the woman may lose confidence in her ability to cope. She may become anxious, irritable, or restless. She may fall asleep in the brief intervals between contractions, may appear exhausted or frustrated, and may resist following directions. Her skin is often diaphoretic, and the caretaker may note shaking legs, chattering teeth, belching, vomiting, grunting, and involuntary pushing efforts. Bloody show may increase, and her membranes may rupture at this point. As she approaches complete dilation, she may experience increasing rectal pressure and a strong need to bear down.

Second-Stage Labor

After her cervix has dilated fully, the expulsion stage begins. Second-stage contractions occur on average about every 2–3 minutes and are

crowning
Emergence of
widest part of the
fetal head from the
vagina. In com-
mon usage this
term can mean any
fetal presenting
part distending the
vaginal opening.

usually accompanied by a strong urge to push caused by the pressure of
the fetal head low in the pelvis. Some women have little urge to push,
and others may be so frightened and overwhelmed by the stretching,
burning, and pressure that they resist pushing. The woman will feel
significant rectal pressure as the baby presses on nerves that usually
signal the need to defecate. As the head descends and begins to stretch
the tissues of the pelvic floor, the birth attendant will first observe
bulging of the perineum, then the presenting part of the fetus itself.
When the vaginal opening encircles the fetal head, the fetus is said to be
crowning.

Third-Stage Labor

Third-stage labor lasts from the birth of the infant to the expulsion of the
placenta and membranes. The woman is at her greatest risk for hemorrhage during and immediately after third stage.

Factors Affecting Length of Labor

The average woman delivering her first baby will experience approximately 12 hours of labor. A woman who has delivered before has an
average labor length of 6–8 hours. The average primigravida will push
for an hour, but a multipara usually pushes for 20 minutes or less. In
general, first labors are long, slow, and difficult, and subsequent labors
are faster and easier. The size of the fetus is sometimes a significant
consideration; a woman who has delivered a 6-lb baby rapidly may
struggle to give birth if her next infant weighs 10 lb and has wide
shoulders.

grand multipara
A woman who has
given birth many
times, usually
more than five.

Grand multiparas often have easy, fast births, but overall they do
have a higher rate of **malpresentations** because of lax abdominal tone.
After the fourth delivery, dysfunctional contraction patterns are more
likely to occur, and her progress through active labor may be slow.

malpresentation
Abnormal position
of the fetus that
may make vaginal
delivery difficult or
impossible.

Back Labor

A woman with back labor will experience most of her labor pain in the
sacral area. This pain can be severe and often persists between contractions. Back labor may indicate that the fetus is in an occiput posterior
position—spine toward the mother's spine and skull pressing against her
sacrum as the head descends. When the fetus is in the occiput posterior
position, all stages of labor may be prolonged unless the fetus rotates.
(see Malpresentations and Cephalopelvic Disproportion, chapter 7.)

The Four *P*s

It is helpful to consider the four *P*s of childbirth: the passage, the passenger, the powers, and the psyche. Successful delivery depends on the relationships among these four variables.

Passage

The woman's birth passage comprises the bony pelvis and the overlying soft tissues. The female pelvis is designed for childbearing, but some pelvic shapes and sizes are more conducive to an easy delivery. An observer cannot infer the suitability of a woman's pelvis from the curve of her hips—it is the internal dimensions that determine whether a baby of a particular size will fit. A petite 5-ft woman with a favorable pelvis may have no trouble delivering a large infant. A broad-hipped 6-ft woman may be unable to deliver a much smaller baby if her internal pelvic dimensions are narrow. The resistance of the cervix and pelvic-floor muscles can also influence the progress of labor, and maternal position can affect the ability of the pelvis to expand.

Passenger

The size and position of the fetus has great influence over the course of labor and delivery. See Figure 5-2. If he is too large in relation to the mother's pelvis, adopts a transverse position, or extends his head so that

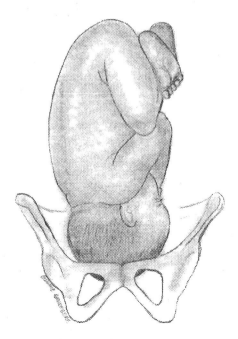

FIGURE 5-2
Occipito-Anterior.
Occipito-anterior is the optimal fetal positioning for delivery.
Illustration by Bonnie U. Gruenberg

the widest part enters the pelvis, vaginal birth may become more complicated or prevented entirely (see Malpresentations and Cephalopelvic Disproportion, chapter 7). Even an appropriately sized, properly positioned fetus may not fit the pelvis if he tilts his head or positions his arm alongside his ear.

Fetal position is a result not only of uterine shape and available space but also of the mother's position and movements and the fetus's own activities. The fetus is not a passive passenger—fetal position is voluntary to some extent. In the same way a newborn can wriggle across his crib and wedge himself in a corner, a fetus helps to determine his birth position with crawling and stepping reflexes. Fetuses have even been known to crown slowly, then suddenly withdraw until the head is no longer visible, rotate 90°, then descend again to deliver easily. A stillborn infant by contrast is utterly passive and is more likely to deliver as a brow or face presentation because of his tactile unresponsiveness and lack of tone.

Powers

This refers to the power generated by uterine contractions. Strong, long, frequent, well-coordinated contractions hasten delivery. If the uterus does not contract hard enough or frequently enough, vaginal birth will not occur. Maternal position influences the powers of labor. Supine positioning decreases the strength of contractions but increases frequency; left lateral increases strength and decreases frequency. Ambulation can increase the intensity and frequency of contractions.

Psyche

The expectant mother's psychological state—self-concept, attitude, confidence, level of preparation, experience of pain, coping ability, and social support—can affect the course of her labor and her reaction to it. Women with unresolved fears are more likely to have longer labors, more fetal distress, and more obstetrical interventions at the hospital. Emotional dystocia refers to dysfunctional labor caused by emotional distress and the accompanying production of catecholamines, or "fight or flight" hormones. Excess catecholamines can cause inefficient contractions and reduce fetal oxygenation. A woman experiencing emotional dystocia may harbor deep fears related to previous difficult births or the prospect of motherhood. She may have suffered previous traumatic experiences, such as physical or sexual abuse. She may be dealing with cultural factors such as profound modesty or language barriers limiting her understanding. Contractions commonly become weaker and widely spaced on the way to the hospital and for the first hour following admission, presumably due to anxiety associated with an unfamiliar environment.

Maternal Response to Labor

Childbirth is in most cases a natural process, but it is as physically demanding as participating in an athletic event. It draws on the woman's deepest physical and psychological resources. It can be a triumphant, loving, and empowering experience or a terrifying and agonizing one, depending on her physical circumstances and emotional state. A woman may have an easy, virtually painless delivery with one child and a tense, excruciating delivery with another. Cultural expectations and the personal meaning a woman ascribes to the pain alter her perceptions of it. Childbirth education has been shown to reduce fear and increase coping ability.

An observer cannot ascertain the amount of pain the woman feels by observing her reaction. Accept that her pain is whatever she says it is. A quiet woman may be experiencing *more* pain than her demonstrative counterpart. There is no correct way to respond to labor, and the moans and cries of a vocal woman are neither better nor worse than stoic silence.

Vital Signs

It is important to measure blood pressure between contractions, because readings increase an average of 10–20 mmHg systolic and 5–10 mmHg diastolic during contractions. Pain and fear can elevate blood pressure, but preeclampsia must always be considered a possible source of hypertension. The patient's pulse rate can also climb markedly during contractions.

In most EMS systems, fetal heart tones are not routinely monitored. A fetal heart rate, however, can give valuable information about the status of the unborn child. If fetal heart tones are auscultated during first-stage labor, they should be obtained along with maternal vital signs every 30 minutes for low-risk women and every 15 minutes for high-risk women. If a woman is in crisis, vital signs and fetal heart rate should be evaluated every 5 minutes. If the EMS provider notes significant increase or decrease in the fetal heart rate, position the mother in whatever position yields the best fetal heart rate, administer oxygen, and run an intravenous infusion of isotonic crystalloid intravenous solution at a rate of 200–300 ml an hour (or as local protocol dictates).

Bladder Function

Women in labor may feel the need to urinate often, and it is essential that they do so because a full bladder can obstruct delivery and contribute to postpartum hemorrhage. Prolonged pressure on the bladder can result in difficulty urinating after delivery. Sometimes a full bladder will produce a telltale bulge just above the pubic bone. If the patient voids scant quantities of dark, concentrated urine, consider dehydration or preeclampsia and treat accordingly.

Gastrointestinal Changes

Gastric motility and digestive efficiency are greatly reduced in labor. Many physicians restrict a woman in labor to clear liquids or nothing by mouth to reduce the chance of aspiration if she requires general anesthesia for an unexpected complication. Midwives, on the other hand, tend to encourage their clients to consume small amounts of light foods such as soup or yogurt for energy in labor, and research has shown this practice to be safe and beneficial. Maintaining hydration and adequate blood-sugar levels staves off exhaustion, which leads to complications, such as inadequate uterine contractions, and does not increase the risk of harm from aspiration. EMS professionals, however, should not allow the woman anything other than sips of water in labor and nothing at all by mouth if she is a high-risk patient.

Fluids and Electrolytes

It is common for a woman to become diaphoretic during labor, especially during transition and second stage. Hyperventilation and slightly elevated body temperature also increase insensible fluid loss. Urinary output increases during labor, perhaps because greater cardiac output during labor increases blood flow to the kidneys. If the woman has not maintained adequate fluid intake or vomits frequently during labor, she may become dehydrated. Intravenous normal saline or lactated Ringer's should be initiated as appropriate.

Induction of Labor

If the doctor or midwife deems that immediate delivery is in the mother and/or baby's best interest, labor may be artificially induced. This may be a multiday process and may result in a cesarean section if the procedure causes fetal distress or does not produce adequate labor. For successful induction, the woman must have a ripe cervix and adequate contractions. If the cervix is thin, soft, and significantly dilated, an intravenous pitocin

amniotomy
Deliberate rupture
of the amniotic
membranes.

drip should start contractions. Sometimes **amniotomy**, or artificial rupture of the amniotic membranes, is also performed. A woman with a long, thick, closed cervix will require cervical ripening before starting pitocin.

At the end of pregnancy, some obstetrical providers will "strip membranes" in the office (sweep a finger in a circular motion between the cervix and the amniotic membranes) to encourage labor to begin. After having membranes stripped in the office, a woman can expect to cramp and have bloody show for the next day or two. Sometimes the symptoms subside; in other cases they progress to true labor.

Sometimes women attempt to induce labor themselves using herbs or folk remedies. Some of these methods are clearly ineffective, some seem to work, and many are of unknown efficacy. Pennyroyal, red raspberry leaf, and black or blue cohosh, related homeopathics such as cimicifuga and caulophyllum, and evening primrose oil are used by women who wish to start or intensify labor. Castor oil ingestion can cause intense, turbulent labor, painful cramping without labor, or severe diarrhea with potential for dehydration.

Impediments to Labor

Some labors progress at an average or accelerated rate, but others proceed slowly or come to a standstill. Possible causes of slowing or stoppage include

- **Uterine exhaustion.**   Prolonged labor, a large fetus, and malpresentations affect the contractility of the uterine muscle.

- **Overstretching of the uterus.**   A large fetus, multiple gestation, or excess amniotic fluid can overdistend the uterus and interfere with its ability to contract.

- **Anxiety and pain.**   It is common for contractions to grow weaker and widely spaced upon transport to the hospital. Many women experience a period of decelerated labor when removed from the security of home. Women who have been sexually abused may experience flashbacks that reduce their ability to cope with labor. Fears of "splitting apart" at delivery or fears of impending motherhood can slow labor progress.

- **Maternal exhaustion.**   When a woman depletes her energy stores, she may not have the reserves necessary for effective pushing. Persistent vomiting may cause dehydration. Intravenous fluids should be administered as indicated, and vital signs and blood glucose levels should be monitored.

cephalopelvic
disproportion
A condition in
which the size or
position of the fetal
head with respect
to the maternal
pelvis prevents
progress in labor.

- **Malpresentation.** If the presenting part does not exert pressure on the cervix, dilation and descent will be slower. Sometimes a malpresented fetus is unable to deliver vaginally.

- **Cephalopelvic disproportion** (fetus does not fit pelvis). Fetal descent can slow or stop because of **cephalopelvic disproportion.**

- **Maternal position for pushing.** Some maternal positions (especially supine) can slow the descent and expulsion of the fetus.

Comfort Measures

EMS personnel do not have the option of administering pain-relieving medications to the laboring patient, so discomfort must be managed with nonpharmacological methods, such as positioning, massage, and encouragement.

- **Social support.** Relatives and friends are often very important to a woman in labor. Do not separate her from her loved ones unless absolutely necessary. Find ways for them to assist. Consider assigning family members the task of comforting the mother, freeing EMS personnel to attend to the medical concerns at hand. If the patient speaks a language other than that of the EMS crew, and a family member can translate, keep that person with her to serve as interpreter. The patient can give true consent only if she has full understanding, so reliable two-way communication is important.

- **Ambulation.** It is beneficial for a healthy woman in normal early labor to walk to the ambulance under her own power. Walking stimulates labor and helps the baby find an optimal position.

  Do not allow the woman to ambulate in late first-stage labor if she is a multipara, during second-stage labor if she is a primipara, or with rapidly progressive labor. Doing so could result in an unexpected standing or squatting delivery.

  Never allow a woman to walk if she displays signs of a potentially dangerous condition, such as abruption, placenta previa, or preeclampsia. Do not allow a woman in preterm labor to ambulate or she may stimulate unwanted contractions. Further, preterm babies are more likely to be breech and therefore are at increased risk for cord prolapse.

- **Coping strategies.** A caregiver's knowledge of comfort measures can be enormously advantageous to the woman in labor. Childbirth classes help the laboring woman cope with the pain and fear of labor. She may learn breathing techniques and may have her mate or a friend serve as her birthing coach. The EMS professional should audit childbirth classes whenever possible for a review of the birth process and a discussion of useful relaxation and pain-relief strategies.

- **Positioning.** If possible, allow the woman to choose a position of comfort (avoiding the supine position because of the risk of hypotension). If she has no strong preference, default to a left lateral position. Not only does side lying maximize cardiac output, but it also results in stronger, less frequent, more efficient contractions.

- **Back pain.** If the patient is experiencing back pain, a hands-and-knees position can help rotate the baby and take pressure off her back; but it may be difficult or unsafe to maintain in a moving ambulance. If back pain is intractable, try positioning her on her right side for transport, facing the wall. Sit on the bench and massage her sacrum firmly. Try deep massage with thumbs, knuckles, or a firm object such as a tennis ball or small rolled towel. Side lying may also encourage the baby to rotate into a position that puts less pressure on her back.

- **Temperature.** Cold or hot packs applied to the woman's back or lower abdomen effectively reduce pain. Ask the woman which she prefers. On a long transport, alternate hot with cold about every 15 minutes. Women in active labor generate heat, and many like to be fanned during a contraction. A damp washcloth placed on the forehead may also provide comfort.

- **Controlled breathing and relaxation.** Relaxation during and between contractions speeds labor and reduces pain. Distraction techniques, including breath control, can also decrease the perception of pain. Slow, deep abdominal breathing can be taught on the spot. Hold eye contact and breathe with her to the count of four: "In through the nose, out through the mouth. In . . . two . . . three . . . four . . . out . . . two . . . three . . . four." Inhalation and exhalation should take about 5 seconds each. Gaining control of her breathing pattern is especially important if the woman tends to hyperventilate. Another useful method is to encourage the woman to "pretend she is asleep," breathing deeply and becoming limp and relaxed. Some EMS professionals incorporate visualization techniques, such as encouraging her to imagine herself relaxing on a beach or some other place that gives her peace. Some women benefit greatly from these techniques; others ignore and resist coaching.

Effleurage is a distraction technique of tracing light circles with the fingertips over the woman's abdomen during a contraction. In theory it confuses the transmission of pain impulses and reduces the perception of discomfort, providing both psychological and physiological relief. The patient can quickly learn to do this herself.

If the woman is receptive to touch, watch her body for signs of tensing and encourage her to relax to your touch. For example, as you lay your hand on a tight shoulder, tell her, "Loosen your shoulder. Feel the tension melt away under my hand." A woman may find this comforting during early active labor, and then abruptly reject any touch during transition.

* **Leg cramps.** Leg cramps are common in pregnancy, especially in labor. Pregnant women are at increased risk for thrombophlebitis, so avoid massaging the calf. Instead, straighten the leg and firmly dorsiflex the foot (bring the top of the foot toward the shin) to stretch the calf muscle. Hold the position until she expresses relief.

* **Cleanliness.** A woman with ruptured membranes will continue to leak fluid until the baby is delivered. Place a sanitary pad or folded towels between her legs to absorb the fluid. Ensure that she stays clean and dry by changing underpads as they become saturated. If she is perspiring, she may also appreciate having perspiration sponged from her neck and face.

Evaluation of Labor

Taking a History and Assessing a Patient in Labor

In general, expect a rapid delivery in a multigravida who reports a history of rapid deliveries and a slower pace in a primigravida. It is important to gather information rapidly when encountering a woman in labor. Many of the techniques discussed in chapter 2 apply.

* **Age.** If the woman is under 16 years of age, she is at higher risk for preeclampsia, anemia, and malnutrition. Women older than 35 years of age are at higher risk for numerous complications, including hypertension, gestational diabetes, preterm delivery, multiple gestation, and chromosomal anomalies in the fetus.

* **Gravida/para.** In general, primigravidas have longer labors, and multigravidas have shorter labors. Multigravidas who have had more than 4–5 pregnancies have increased risk of prolonged labors, placental abruption, placenta previa, and postpartum hemorrhage. Not all patients are forthright with their histories, and they may not disclose that there have been prior births or abortions.

* **Previous deliveries.** Some obstetrical problems, such as postpartum hemorrhage or precipitous delivery, tend to recur. It is useful to be forewarned.

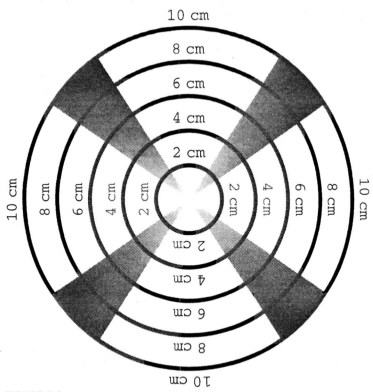

FIGURE 5-3
Cervical Dilation Chart.
Cervical dilation occurs when the tissue of the cervix opens. The cervix progressively thins and opens around the baby's head until no part of it obstructs the baby's exit, usually at 10 cm of dilation.

- **Condition of cervix.** It is helpful to ask whether her provider checked her cervix in the office and what the findings were. See the cervix dilation chart in Figure 5-3. A woman who had a cervix that was long, firm, and closed yesterday is less likely to deliver precipitously today than one with a cervix that was 4 cm, thin, and soft. Most women can accurately relay what a provider has told them about their cervixes.

- **Prior cesarean.** A woman who has delivered by cesarean section may be at increased risk for uterine rupture, especially if she has a classical (vertical) incision into her uterus. Some clinicians allow a woman with a previous cesarean to deliver vaginally if she meets certain criteria. Determine why she had the cesarean. If it was performed for contracted pelvis or excessive fetal size, the condition may repeat, and vaginal birth may not be possible. A condition such as cord prolapse is unlikely to recur. Vaginal delivery after cesarean in the field is likely to proceed identically to any other vaginal birth. If she has never labored before or delivered vaginally, her labor pattern may be more like that of a nulliparous woman. Consider the possibility that her uterus may rupture in labor, and that there may be difficulties with placental expulsion after the birth.

* **Gestational age.** An infant's chances for survival are greatest if he is born at term, that is, between 37 and 42 completed weeks of gestation. An infant born before 37 weeks may be immature and face life-threatening complications. An infant born after 42 weeks may be postmature.

* **Last oral intake.** It is important to establish the woman's nutritional and hydration status and whether she has been vomiting. If she requires anesthesia at the hospital, her provider will want to know what and when she last ate.

* **Bladder status.** Ascertain whether the patient has been voiding regularly and whether the quantity was sufficient. A full bladder can obstruct labor.

* **Medical and obstetrical history** (see chapter 2).

* **Provider's name and hospital of choice.**

* **Maternal vital signs and fetal well-being.** Evaluate baseline vital signs and take serial readings as indicated, including fetal heart rate. Also ask the mother whether the fetus is moving normally.

Differentiate between False Labor and True Labor

* **Assess contractions.** Consider time of onset, frequency and duration, pain pattern, and intensity. The contraction is most effectively palpated at the fundus. When palpated, a mild contraction will feel like a slightly flexed biceps muscle, a moderate contraction like a tightly contracted biceps, and a strong contraction as hard as the back of the hand. Contraction strength may be difficult to assess in a woman with a thick abdominal adipose layer.

* **Presence of bloody show.** Bloody show tends to increase near the end of first stage.

* **Rupture of membranes.** The prehospital provider should assess whether the woman's water has broken and, if so, when it ruptured and whether the vaginal drainage has any odor or color. Has the baby been moving normally since the time of rupture?

Stay and Deliver or Transport?

The decision to stay and deliver the infant on scene or transport the patient to the hospital is not always easy or clear-cut. The woman and her obstetrical provider may strongly prefer that the delivery take place in the hospital or birth center as planned; but in most cases an EMS professional can successfully deliver a healthy baby in the field. Your primary task is to control the scene dynamics, ensure that both mother and infant are stabilized, watch for complications that require assistance, and let nature take its course. Every effort should be made to get to the hospital before delivery, but most deliveries will proceed normally if they occur out of the hospital.

High-risk pregnancy and delivery are a different matter. The woman with complications should deliver in a hospital, and field delivery can reduce the likelihood of survival for the infant and possibly the mother. Preterm delivery, severe preeclampsia, multiple gestation, maternal bleeding disorders, and breech delivery are only a few high-risk situations best managed in a hospital setting. The decision to transport a patient is ultimately based on the best judgment of the EMS provider and the medical control physician, who must weigh several considerations, including

- **Expected length of labor.** A primigravida is more likely to have a long, slow labor and a multigravida a shorter, faster one; but not every woman delivers as expected. A multipara may deliver unexpectedly with two pushes, or she may push for over an hour.

- **Stage of labor.** The woman's stage of labor may be hard to determine. She may appear in extreme discomfort and seem to be in advanced labor at only 2 cm of dilation or may remain stoic or even smiling as she approaches complete dilation. Are her contractions firm to palpation? How far apart are they?

- **Urge to push.** A strong urge to push is the hallmark of second-stage labor, but in some cases the woman may feel the urge for hours before she is completely dilated. Other women feel no urge to push until the baby reaches the pelvic floor. Remember that the average primigravida pushes for nearly an hour before delivering, and a 2-hour pushing stage is still considered normal.

- **Rectal pressure and bulging.** Rectal pressure, a result of the fetus pressing on nerves that usually signal the urge to defecate, can be a sign that birth is imminent. She may pass feces as the fetus descends. Before crowning occurs, the perineum bulges, and the anus everts.

- **Mother's judgment.** If a woman says, "I am having the baby—NOW!" believe her!

- **Rupture of membranes.**   Membranes often rupture at the end of the first stage of labor or as the mother begins to push. Frequently when membranes rupture spontaneously in a multiparous patient in advanced labor, the baby rapidly follows.

- **Crowning.**   The term refers to the vagina stretching around the widest part of the fetal head, moments before birth, but in common usage it can mean any glimpse of fetal presenting part at the vaginal opening.
   The time between crowning and delivery is usually short, but may vary. With a multiparous patient, so little time may elapse between perineal bulging, glimpsing a hint of fetal scalp, and delivery of the infant, the attendant may barely have time to glove. With a primiparous woman, the head may show more than 30 minutes before delivery. Small or preterm babies may be expelled rapidly, but very large infants may take longer to emerge.

- **Distance to the hospital.**   Location is an important consideration. If the patient is likely to deliver en route, she may be better off where she is.

- **Complications.**   If you must deliver high-risk pregnancies in the field, call for backup—extra hands are helpful if both mother and baby need close attention. Sometimes a birth can be delayed if the mother breathes or pants rather than pushes, other times the pushing urge is involuntary and undeniable.

Precipitous Delivery

With a precipitous delivery, a single push can bring the baby to the perineum, and a second push can propel the entire baby into the world. In this case there is little time for grace or finesse. The priority is to ensure that the infant does not slip out of the birth attendant's hands and fall. Precipitous deliveries may occur unexpectedly in a standing position, and if a birth attendant is not present to catch the infant, it may land on the floor and suffer skull fracture or other damage.
   Many precipitous deliveries at home or in public places occur into the toilet, when the woman mistakes the rectal pressure of impending delivery for a need to move her bowels. If the EMS provider attends a woman who is in the process of delivering on the toilet, the safest procedure is to move her to the floor and deliver the infant there. If the woman will not leave the toilet and the baby is emerging, the EMS provider can encourage the woman to move forward and sit on the edge of the seat for delivery, allowing the toilet to serve as a kind of birthing chair as the attendant catches the baby. More commonly, the baby is

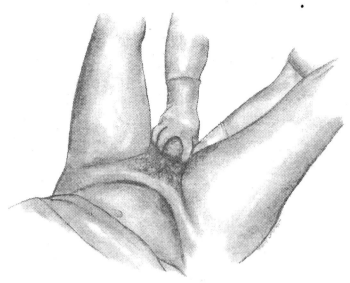

FIGURE 5-4
Precipitous Delivery.
The head emerges while the birth attendant applies gentle counterpressure with a palm or the underside of the fingers.
Illustration by Bonnie U. Gruenberg

born into the toilet before anyone realizes what is happening. In this case, lift the baby out, warm him, and attend to resuscitation if indicated. In most cases the baby will be vigorous, but hypothermia and aspiration of toilet water are considerations.

Most precipitous deliveries are easy and uneventful, although rapid delivery often bruises the baby and causes lacerations to the mother's perineum. The fetus is less likely to deliver explosively if you position the mother on her side and ask her to breathe rather than actively push. Hold gentle counterpressure on the fetal head without holding the baby back (see Figures 5-4 and 5-5). Some women are so overwhelmed by sensation that they ignore coaching, push forcefully, and rapidly expel the baby. Allow the baby to deliver directly onto the bed between her legs (Figure 5-6), or catch him as he emerges, guiding him upward in an arc that places him on his mother's abdomen (Figure 5-7). The placenta usually delivers soon after the birth, but the risk of hemorrhage is increased following a precipitous delivery.

If the woman appears to be delivering in a standing position, throw a pillow or blanket on the floor beneath her to provide a cushion if the baby falls. It can be difficult for a birth attendant to get a secure grip on the baby and when a woman delivers standing, and a fall could snap the cord or cause injury to the infant.

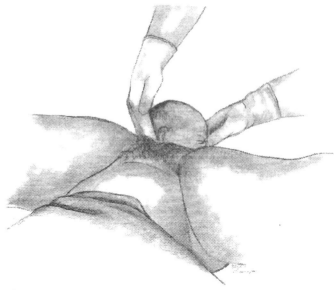

FIGURE 5-5
Precipitous Delivery I.
After the head is out, ask the mother to stop pushing while you check
for the presence of the cord around the neck (see chapter 6).
Illustration by Bonnie U. Gruenberg

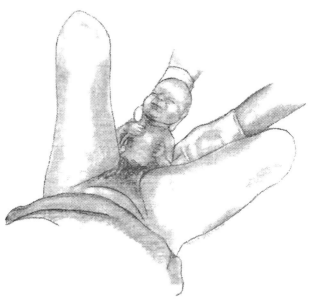

FIGURE 5-6
Precipitous Delivery II.
The birth attendant may choose to rotate the baby to face his
mother after he emerges.
Illustration by Bonnie U. Gruenberg

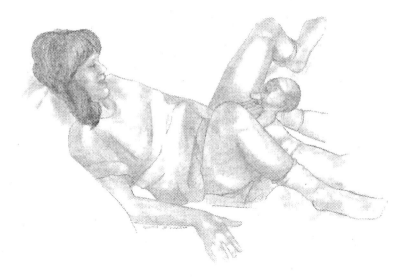

FIGURE 5-7
Precipitous Delivery III.
Lift the baby and place him on his mother's abdomen.
Illustration by Bonnie U. Gruenberg

Summary

The signs of labor and its stages may be clear or confusing, and the responses of women to the process differ greatly and can change suddenly. Prehospital providers must form their impressions from the patient's physical and behavioral clues alone, without the benefit of sonograms, speculums, or digital vaginal exams. Sharp assessment skills and a working knowledge of the physiology of labor allow the EMS responder to evaluate the parturient woman, increase her comfort and confidence, and promote optimal outcomes.

REVIEW QUESTIONS

1. Describe maternal changes that may herald the imminent onset of labor.

2. Define the "Four Ps" of childbirth and discuss how they relate to successful delivery.

3. Discuss factors that would influence your decision to stay and deliver on scene or initiate transport.

4. What comfort measures might the prehospital provider use with a laboring patient?

5. How can the EMS provider distinguish between labor and false labor?

Normal Delivery
Management

Objectives

By the end of this chapter you should be able to

- Safely attend a normal delivery

- Reduce a tight nuchal cord

- Manage a normal third-stage labor

- Manage the immediate care of a normal neonate

- Reduce the risk of perineal lacerations

CASE
Study

shoulder dystocia
A bone-on-bone obstruction in which the fetal shoulder is caught behind the maternal pubic bone, preventing delivery.

"One more little push and her head will be out," Chris told Natalyia, who bore down. The baby's wet, blond head emerged into the paramedic's gentle hands as he knelt in the back of the minivan. Chris swiftly checked for a nuchal cord. The Doppler had identified deep decelerations in fetal heart rate with contractions, with slow recovery. Chris suspected cord compression.

His suspicions were correct. Around the baby's neck he felt an unusually thin, tight umbilical cord and attempted to reduce it by hooking his finger beneath it and gently easing it over the baby's head. Suddenly, the cord snapped.

Chris immediately placed his hands on the baby's head and asked Natalyia to push with all her strength. Praying that he would not encounter a **shoulder dystocia**, he guided the baby's head down until he saw the anterior shoulder, and then up until the baby's body slipped into his hands. The cord was extremely short and had been tight around the neck. It had been stretched thinner with every push. That explained the decelerations Chris had auscultated. The newborn had no tone at all, pale color, no respirations.

Questions

1. What crucial procedure should Chris perform next?
2. What resuscitation measures will this baby need?
3. What maternal or fetal conditions could cause a thin, weak cord that would be susceptible to breakage?
4. What third-stage problems might Chris encounter?

Introduction

Childbirth has a unique standing in the field of emergency medical services. Virtually every other situation that prompts an ambulance call involves a deviation from a normal process. Childbirth is a normal process, but laboring patients benefit from the expertise of trained professionals who can intervene when complications develop. Unlike other emergencies, in which active intervention is warranted and expected, attending normal childbirth involves watchful waiting and gentle assistance.

KEY TERMS

acrocyanosis, p. 166

closed-glottis pushing, p. 159

engagement, p. 155

intrapartum, p. 155

introitus, p. 163

lithotomy position, p. 152

nuchal cord, p. 162

shoulder dystocia, p. 149

vertex presentation, p. 155

Equipment and Setting

The prehospital provider cannot always choose the setting for an emergency delivery and may have to improvise equipment. Knowledge, confidence, and a patient-centered attitude are the EMS responder's most valuable attributes in any situation. Necessary medical care always takes priority over patient comfort or preference, but emergencies can usually be managed with concern, consideration, and compassion.

Thoughtful gestures build trust and cooperation. Respect the woman's modesty at all times and drape her with sheets as appropriate. An underpad should be placed below the woman and changed as needed to keep her dry and comfortable.

Even in an emergency situation, the EMS crew can usually find a private setting for delivery, out of the elements and away from crowds. A bedroom is ideal. The back of an ambulance provides less room to maneuver, but better access to equipment.

If possible, choose a warm room for delivery, heated to at least 74–76°F. Close windows and doors to reduce drafts, which contribute to convective heat loss in the neonate. Hypothermia is a significant threat to all newborns.

Keep oxygen readily available in case of maternal or fetal hypoxia or the need for infant resuscitation. Administering oxygen to the laboring woman is unnecessary unless she is having a problem (bleeding, hypertension, decelerated fetal heart rate, malpresentation, etc.). Cardiac monitoring is unnecessary unless she is hemodynamically unstable or presents with metabolic abnormalities, a history of cardiac disease, chest trauma, or other indications for monitoring.

If everything remains normal, the woman probably does not need intravenous access, but life-threatening complications such as postpartum hemorrhage can arise unexpectedly. Therefore, it is prudent to initiate an intravenous line of lactated Ringer's or normal saline if time permits.

Within easy reach, organize the bulb syringe, a supply of 4 in. × 4 in. gauze sponges, disposable towels, infant hat, cord clamps, scalpel or scissors, placental container, and medications for hemorrhage such as oxytocin and methergine (if protocols permit). Have your newborn resuscitation kit (endotracheal tubes, pediatric epinephrine doses, oxygen, suction, etc.) available in case of a depressed baby.

Many prepackaged OB kits do not include baby blankets. Flannel bath blankets are ideal for newborns, but towels will suffice. If time permits, prewarm them by wrapping them around chemical hot packs. If the delivery is at home, the mother probably has blankets or linens that she can contribute—the more, the better. You will need enough to dry the baby immediately to prevent chilling, then to wrap him in dry blankets. The mother may feel chilled after delivery and require blankets as well.

If protocols indicate, use a Doppler or stethoscope actively during the birth, monitoring the fetal heart rate every 5 minutes and listening through and after contractions. As the baby moves through the pelvis, heart sounds will move lower in the mother's abdomen. The fetal heart-rate may decrease to about 100 when she pushes, then recover to the normal range between contractions.

Universal precautions are essential at a birth. Body fluids of many kinds are abundant at delivery and may harbor disease organisms. Amniotic fluid and blood may gush, splash, and spurt unpredictably. Gloves, gown, and a mask with a vision shield or goggles offer appropriate protection. The provider who will actually deliver the infant should don sterile gloves; other providers may remain nonsterile. If possible, scrub hands and arms before gloving.

Blood and fluid can ruin a mattress—a potential hardship for patients with limited resources. If time permits, ask a family member to spread newspapers or some other barrrier over the mattress as you assist the patient to the bedroom. A vinyl shower curtain or tablecloth makes a good waterproof layer and is readily available in many households. Place a sheet and underpad on top of these for the woman's comfort.

As in any emergency, the EMS professional should not only *remain* calm but also *project* calm. A composed, confident demeanor can bring order out of the chaos of an emergency scene.

Maternal Positioning

Squatting

For thousands of years and in most cultures, women have traditionally given birth in the squatting position. The pelvic outlet of a squatting woman can increase in diameter more than 28%, and gravity augments maternal pushing. This position is often impractical in the field, however. Many women find squatting difficult and awkward and require assistance to maintain it. Squatting is contraindicated for women with severe varicosities of the legs because it can reduce venous flow from the lower extremities. Perineal swelling and laceration may be increased in this position. Further, squatting may make it difficult for the inexperienced birth attendant to support the perineum and control the delivery of the head.

Supine (Dorsal, Lithotomy)

lithotomy position
Lying on the back with the legs apart or elevated.

The supine position is an adaptation of the **lithotomy position** popular in delivery rooms for most of this century. The lithotomy position, supine with the legs elevated in stirrups, was developed by physicians 200 years ago to provide them better visibility and greater control of the delivery process through interventions such as episiotomy and use of forceps. The dorsal position resembles the lithotomy position, but without stirrups. Sometimes the hips are elevated on a towel to allow better visualization of the perineum.

A woman's cardiac output is lowest in the supine position; in some women blood pressure can decrease by 30%. Consequently, fetal hypoxia may develop more rapidly in this position. The uterus may impinge on the diaphragm, causing the woman to experience shortness of breath. The vagina angles upward, so she is pushing against gravity. Dorsal positioning limits the degree that the pelvis can expand to accommodate the baby's head. Radiological studies show that pelvic measurements are least favorable for delivery in this position. Perineal lacerations are more likely. Supine positions can lengthen the second stage of labor and increase the incidence of fetal heart-rate abnormalities and fetal hypoxia. The supine and lithotomy positions are sometimes useful in a hospital setting when the obstetrical provider wishes to use specific interventions to hasten birth, but in the field dorsal positions are best avoided.

Semi-Sitting

Semi-sitting at a 45°–60° angle is a good compromise between supine and squatting that works very well in the field. Upright postures use gravity and abdominal muscles to advantage, allow the mother to view the birth, improve cardiac output over supine positioning, and permit the birth attendant full access to the perineum. Semi-sitting also makes it convenient for the provider to place the newborn on the maternal abdomen or chest after the birth.

Left Lateral Recumbent

Left lateral recumbent is an excellent position to use for field deliveries. Help the woman lie on her left side with her left leg extended and her right leg bent and drawn up toward her abdomen, or with both knees bent. The woman can support her own leg by grasping the knee and pulling it toward her shoulder when she pushes, or an assistant can provide leg support if the woman is inflexible or resistant to direction.

Lateral recumbent positioning maximizes cardiac output and can help to normalize the blood pressure of hypertensive patients. It reduces the risk of aspiration in the patient with an altered mental status. It can improve placental perfusion and thereby improve the condition of a distressed fetus. It may also slow precipitous deliveries and reduces the risk of shoulder dystocia. Left lateral position can encourage rotation of an occiput posterior fetus, especially if one leg is lifted. Most women find this position comfortable, and it minimizes tearing of the perineum. The birth attendant can easily control delivery of the head and has a good view of the perineum as the baby crowns.

Hands-and-Knees

Midwives often encourage hands-and-knees positioning position for birth. Hands-and-knees may reduce back pain and encourage rotation of the occipto-posterior fetus, and it can improve placental and umbilical blood flow in case of fetal distress. In field births, hands-and-knees can be especially helpful in case of shoulder dystocia (see chapter 7).

Delivery in this position may be awkward for the inexperienced attendant. When the baby is born, the baby is usually placed on the bed behind the mother, and he cannot be moved to the maternal abdomen until the woman rolls over—an awkward maneuver before the cord is cut. The mother may also tire of holding this position.

In general:

* Forward-leaning positions and asymmetrical positions (one leg elevated) tend to reduce back pain and encourage fetal rotation.

* Dorsal positions decrease cardiac output, increase back pain, and result in more frequent, more painful contractions that are less effective in expelling the fetus, but increase visualization for the birth attendant.

* Upright birth positions (sitting, squatting, birth stools) shorten the second stage and improve fetal heart-rate patterns over dorsal positions. Upright positions also result in less discomfort, easier pushing, and a more normal delivery, but studies suggest that they cause almost as much perineal trauma as dorsal positions.

* Except in many industrialized Western countries, almost all women give birth in an upright position such as standing, sitting, or squatting.

* Whatever position the patient delivers in, flexion is desirable. Encourage the woman to curl around her baby as she pushes and flex her chin toward her chest. Encourage her to relax her legs and bottom as she pushes.

* When positioning the woman, allow at least 2 ft of space below the woman's vulva for working on the baby and delivering the placenta as indicated.

PEARLS No matter how inconvenient delivery may be in a given situation, it is never appropriate to hold a woman's legs together to attempt to delay the birth. To do so may cause fetal hypoxia.

Mechanism of Second-Stage Labor (Cardinal Movements)

intrapartum
A noun or adjective pertaining to the period of pregnancy from the onset of labor through the expulsion of the placenta.

In the field, **intrapartum** complications can appear without warning and may not reflect anything previously encountered in textbooks or in life. It is important that the EMS professional understand the basic mechanism of normal labor to better address deviations from normal as they occur.

Optimally (and in the vast majority of cases) the fetus will enter the world in a **vertex presentation** (head down and flexed). The vertex baby may present either occiput anterior or occiput posterior. Occiput anterior position is the most favorable for easy birth—head down, back toward the mother's abdomen, chin flexed to chest, presenting the smallest diameters of his head to the pelvic corridor. Occiput posterior places the back of the fetal head at the maternal sacrum, causing back pain and slowing the progress of labor. After the cervix is fully dilated, the fetus must rotate while negotiating a maze of bony maternal projections and stretching the musculature of the pelvic floor. Occiput anterior vertex delivery occurs through predictable alterations in fetal position.

vertex presentation
A fetal presentation in which the top of the head enters the pelvis first.

engagement
Passage of the widest diameter of the fetal presenting part through the pelvis.

- **Engagement.** Engagement occurs when the widest part of the head enters the pelvic inlet, the first bony obstacle to be negotiated.

- **Descent.** The head enters the pelvis in a transverse position to conform to the shape of the pelvic inlet.

- **Flexion.** As the fetal head descends, it encounters resistance from the muscles of the pelvic floor, which increases flexion. Flexion allows the smallest diameter of the head to move though the pelvis. (If the head is not flexed, a wider portion of fetal skull must negotiate the pelvic passage.)

- **Internal rotation.** The midpelvis is widest from front to back, so the fetus rotates to face his mother's sacrum. Only the head makes this turn—the shoulders remain oblique (diagonally positioned). See Figure 6-1.

- **Extension.** The back of the head reaches the pubic bone and pivots beneath it. Then the head extends to follow the direction of the vagina and its supporting muscles. At this point, the birth attendant observes perineal bulging, crowning, and then the birth of the head, facing the mother's anus. See Figures 6-2, 6-3, and 6-4.

(Continued on page 158)

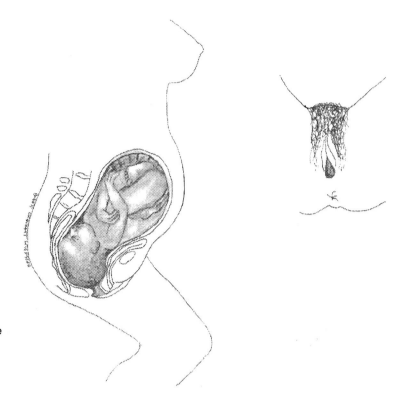

FIGURE 6-1
Internal Rotation.
The fetal head faces
the maternal sacrum.
The birth attendant
may see gaping of the
vagina and a dark
hollow within.
Illustration by Bonnie U.
Gruenberg

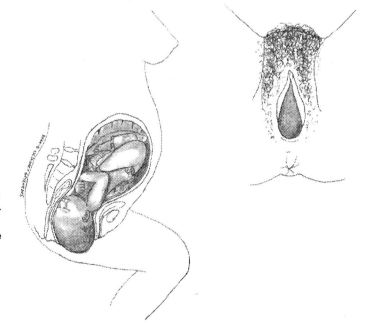

FIGURE 6-2
Extension.
The fetal head reaches
the pelvic floor and be-
gins to extend. The
birth attendant can see
the fetal scalp with
each push, but it re-
cedes between push-
ing efforts.
Illustration by Bonnie U.
Gruenberg

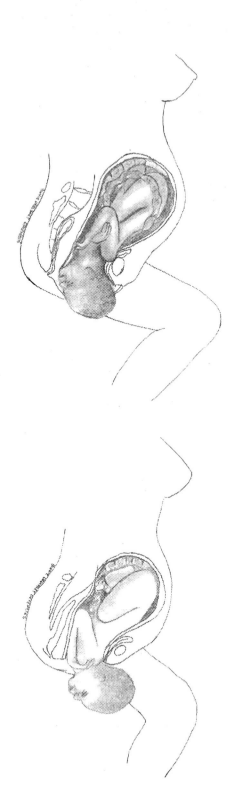

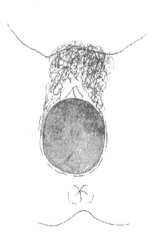

FIGURE 6-3
Full Crowning.
The vagina encircles the
widest part of the fetal
head. Birth is imminent.
Illustration by Bonnie U.
Gruenberg

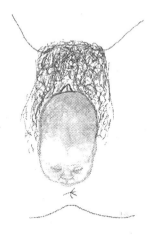

FIGURE 6-4
Birth of Head.
The head emerges
facing the maternal
perineum.
Illustration by Bonnie U.
Gruenberg

Normal Delivery Management   157

- **Restitution.** When the baby's head is born, it faces the anus while his shoulders remain positioned diagonally inside the pelvis. As soon as the head is free, the baby's neck turns to the right or the left to re-align with the shoulders. See Figure 6-5.

- **External rotation.** Now the head turns farther to the side as the shoulders rotate internally to the anteroposterior diameter. See Figure 6-6.

- **Expulsion.** The anterior shoulder slides under the pubic bone and is born by lateral flexion. The posterior shoulder is born next, and the body should follow quickly.

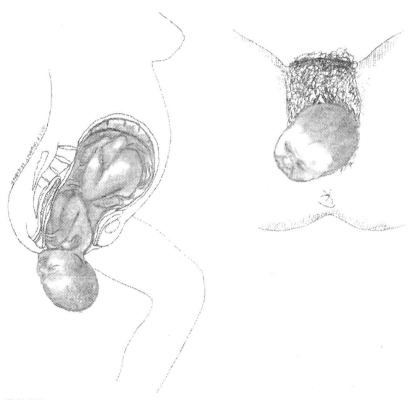

FIGURE 6-5
Restitution.
The head turns to the side to realign with the shoulders.
Illustration by Bonnie U. Gruenberg

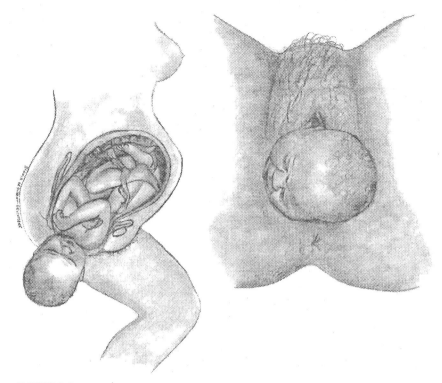

FIGURE 6-6
External Rotation.
The head turns farther to the side.
Illustration by Bonnie U. Gruenberg

Pushing Techniques

Closed-Glottis Coached Pushing (Valsalva Pushing)

closed-glottis pushing
Pushing the infant down and out while holding the breath; Valsalva pushing.

Many professionals teach laboring/women to push with a closed glottis. The woman is taught to take a deep breath, hold it, and bear down to the count of 10, whereupon she expels her breath, takes another breath, holds it, then pushes again, until the contraction subsides. This **closed-glottis pushing,** or Valsalva pushing, was once thought to shorten the second stage of labor by increasing the effectiveness of maternal pushing.

Recent research suggests that closed-glottis pushing does not shorten second-stage labor and might actually lengthen it. Forced exhalation against a closed glottis increases intrathoracic pressure, reducing venous return and diminishing cardiac output. Lower cardiac output reduces maternal blood pressure and placental blood flow, which may cause fetal hypoxia and acidosis. Valsalva pushing also results in an increased incidence of perineal tears and maternal exhaustion. It can be effective, however, in moving the baby past bony obstacles that may slow delivery. It is also helpful if the woman does not have a strong pushing urge or says that she does not know how to push.

Open-Glottis ("Natural") Pushing

A woman who has not taken childbirth classes and has not otherwise been "taught" to push will instinctively give a series of short, open-glottis pushes lasting 6 seconds or less. Open-glottis pushing is a series of short pushes that alternates brief breath holding and exhalation, or pushing with no breath holding at all, only small grunts similar to that used for defecation.

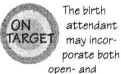 The birth attendant may incorporate both open- and closed-glottis pushing as the labor proceeds.

Research shows that open-glottis pushing does not decrease the pushing effort and may shorten the second stage. Maternal and fetal vital signs remain more stable with open-glottis pushes, and the woman is less likely to become exhausted by pushing efforts. This style of pushing is less likely to cause cervical swelling or trauma if begun before cervical dilation is complete. Open-glottis pushing is especially useful in the field, where EMS providers are unable to determine cervical dilation.

Normal Delivery

As the baby descends, certain clues herald imminent delivery. The woman often utters low-pitched grunts in second-stage labor. As the baby compresses rectal nerves, she may complain that she needs to move her bowels. She may push involuntarily with contractions.

As the fetal head reaches the pelvic floor, maternal tissues bulge, and the labia part to reveal the fetal scalp. The pressure of the head on the pelvic floor often triggers a powerful pushing urge. Typically the head appears with contractions, only to retreat between pushes. With the primigravida, 30 minutes or more may elapse between the first glimpse of scalp and delivery of the infant. Most multiparous women deliver within a few pushes after the head becomes visible, but progress is highly variable.

As the head begins to distend the perineum, the woman may expel feces. Do not contaminate your sterile gloves. Have your partner remove feces with tissues or 4 in. × 4 in. gauze to avoid contamination of the birth area, or cover the feces with a dressing or towel.

The woman may also involuntarily urinate with pushing efforts. Cover her urethral opening with a towel to avoid spraying. Urination is beneficial, because a distended bladder can obstruct birth and cause postpartum hemorrhage.

Palpate contractions for intensity and duration. Check maternal vital signs every 15 minutes during the pushing stage of labor—every 5 minutes if the patient is unstable. If protocols require, auscultate fetal heart tones every 5 minutes, listening during and after a contraction. It is common and often benign for fetal heart tones to dip briefly during a contraction as a vagal response to pressure on the descending head, but many serious complications also present with decreased fetal heart rate. If the heart rate drops below 90, transport with the mother on oxygen with IV access in left lateral position to an appropriate facility.

The woman may instinctively tense as the head reaches the perineum. It may feel to her as if she were splitting apart, burning, stretching impossibly, or having an enormous bowel movement. Encourage her to let go, to open. Encouraging her to touch the emerging head with her hand may help her make a vital connection with the infant, stop resisting, and surrender to the process.

Allow the head to emerge slowly to reduce the risk of tearing in the mother and reduce the risk of neonatal intracranial bleeding from abrupt pressure changes. As the head stretches and thins the perineum, encourage small, gentle, open-glottis pushes. Be patient. You may support the perineum by applying the palm of your dominant hand to the area between the vagina and anus, thumb and forefinger curved in a C-shape around the vaginal opening. You may opt to hold a 4 in. × 4 in. gauze between your hand and the perineum to reduce rectal contamination. The finger pads of your other hand should apply gentle counterpressure to the bones of the emerging fetal head to slow delivery and encourage flexion.

ON TARGET Apply gentle counter-pressure as the head crowns, but never hold the head back forcibly.

As the head begins to emerge, coach the mother to stop pushing. This may be difficult for her. Encourage her to "breathe the baby out" or to pant. If the baby is in occiput anterior position, the head will emerge facing the mother's anus. It usually rotates a quarter-turn to the right or left, then rotates further so that it faces directly left or right. If the amniotic sac is intact, tear it away from the baby's face before the first breath. If there has been meconium in the fluid (see chapter 10), vigorously suction the mouth first, then the nose.

Research suggests that if there is no meconium in the fluid, suctioning on the perineum has little value. Mechanical compression of the chest during delivery squeezes fluid from the baby's lungs and oropharynx, effectively reducing fluid in the airways. Aggressive suctioning can also cause bradycardia and tissue trauma in the infant. Irritation of nasal mucous membranes sometimes causes swelling and increased production of mucus in the hours following birth, resulting in rebound nasal congestion. Some protocols still recommend bulb suctioning upon delivery of the head regardless of the condition of the fluid. As always, the EMS provider should follow local protocols.

If you choose to bulb suction while the head is on the perineum, squeeze the air out of the bulb, insert the tip, and release. Squirt the aspirated fluids out of the bulb, compress, and repeat. Suction quickly, then look for a nuchal cord.

Nuchal Cord

nuchal cord
An umbilical cord wrapped around the fetal neck.

The umbilical cord is wrapped or draped around the neck (**nuchal cord**) in about 25% of all deliveries and may be looped four or more times. Slide your finger along the baby's neck and shoulder to check for the presence of a cord, which will feel firm, knobby, and pulsating. Check thoroughly but quickly. Your fingers may slide *beneath* the cord to find bare neck, and you may erroneously conclude that there is no nuchal cord. Most nuchal cords easily reduce if the birth attendant gently grasps the cord in a hooking motion and slips it over the head. If this does not work, attempt to loosen the cord and slip it down over the shoulders.

If the cord is tight and will not reduce, you may clamp the cord in two places, cut between the clamps, then unwind the cord from the neck. The provider must do this quickly, before the next contraction. Remind the mother to keep panting or blowing instead of pushing, but do not be surprised if she is unable to restrain herself and pushes anyway.

 If a tight nuchal cord must be cut, it is safest to use sterile bandage or umbilical scissors.

Unfortunately, most OB kits come with only a scalpel for cord cutting, and it can be very dangerous to work with a sharp, unprotected blade so close to a baby's face and neck and a woman's genitals. This dilemma can be circumvented by stocking sterile umbilical or bandage scissors with the OB kit to use in the event of a tight nuchal cord. If you must cut with a blade, direct the edge away from the infant.

Remember that if you must sever the cord before the baby is out, you will cut off his only supply of oxygen. It is imperative to deliver the baby quickly after the cord is cut and stimulate him to breathe on his own as soon as possible. If shoulder dystocia occurs and delivery is delayed (see chapter 7), the baby may be in serious trouble.

The other option for delivering a child with a tight nuchal cord is to employ the "somersault maneuver." This is sometimes the only safe option if the infant is slipping into your hands faster than you can cut and unwind the cord. To perform the somersault, flex the baby's head toward the mother's thigh and hold it there while the body slips out. In this way, the baby's neck does not move more than an inch or so from the

introitus
The entrance
to the vagina,
between the labia
minora.

mother's **introitus,** and the cord does not tighten excessively. Once the body is out, it is simple task to unwind the cord from the neck. The somersault is easier to understand and learn with practice on obstetrical mannequins, and the EMS provider is encouraged to rehearse the procedure before using it in the field.

After delivery, leave the baby between the mother's legs at the level of the introitus and allow the cord blood to transfuse back into the infant. Babies with tight nuchal cords are often born hypovolemic, pale, and stunned. The EMS provider can start resuscitation from this position, stimulating and warming the child, giving blowby oxygen or assisting respiration while allowing the child to benefit from a minute or more of volume infusion and oxygenation from the intact and pulsing cord. Resuscitation should never be delayed to let the cord stop pulsing. If it will benefit the infant to sever the cord immediately and take him elsewhere for resuscitation, do it.

Delivering the Body

Some babies will grimace, open their eyes, and attempt to cry as soon as the head is delivered. Some will just lie passively, and others will clench their jaws, making it difficult to insert the bulb syringe.

It is important to remember that while the baby's head is on the outside, the shoulders may still be held by the bony pelvis. *Never pull or twist a baby's head!* It is easy to apply excessive pressure, and damage to the delicate nerves in the baby's neck may be permanent.

Place your palms on either side of the infant's head, taking care not to cover his face with your fingers. With the next contraction, ask the woman to push gently, then carefully guide the head down (toward maternal posterior) to encourage the anterior shoulder to slide beneath the pubic bone. See Figure 6-7. When you see the shoulder, gently raise the

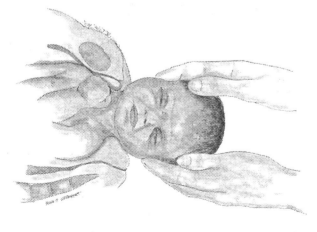

FIGURE 6-7
Guiding Head for Anterior Shoulder.
Guide the baby's head gently down until
you see the anterior shoulder.
Illustration by Bonnie U. Gruenberg

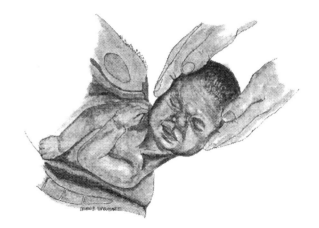

FIGURE 6-8
Guiding Head for Posterior Shoulder.
After the anterior shoulder emerges, gently guide the head and body up and out of the vagina.
Illustration by Bonnie U. Gruenberg

head up (toward maternal anterior), and the posterior shoulder will slip out, often with the rest of the body. See Figure 6-8. Forceful traction is never appropriate. The mother's pushing delivers the shoulders; gentle guidance is all that is required from the birth attendant. See Figure 6-9.

The baby will be extremely slippery and may slide from your grasp if you are not prepared. Delivery on a bed or stretcher makes delivery safer, and you can allow the baby to be born directly upon the bed without fear of dropping him. Otherwise, as the posterior shoulder is born, allow one hand to support the infant, your thumb and forefinger gently circling the base of the neck, following the infant's body with your other hand as it is expelled, and catching one or both legs or feet as they emerge. Your partner should note the time of birth.

The baby should be placed immediately on the mother's abdomen, skin to skin, head lower than the body to allow fluids to drain from the respiratory tract. Most babies will start crying within 15 seconds after delivery, stimulated mostly by cold, touch, and the release of pressure. The cord is still pulsing and supplying oxygen to the baby during this time. Unless the infant requires extensive resuscitation, most assessments and interventions can be accomplished with the infant on the mother's abdomen. Skin contact enhances maternal bonding, comforts the infant, and helps keep him warm. The infant may remain skin to skin with the mother en route to the hospital unless either becomes unstable.

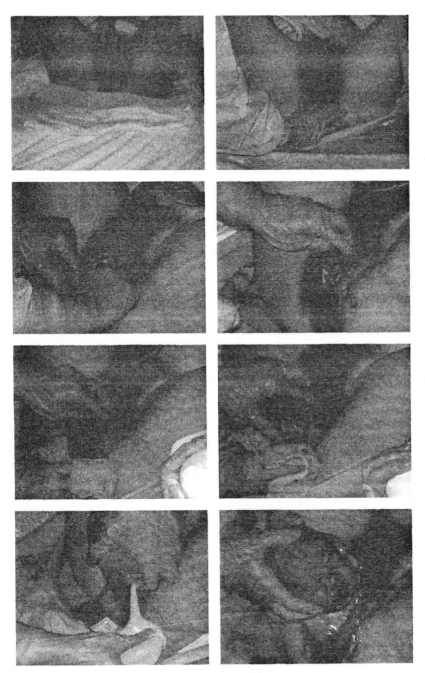

FIGURE 6-9
A Birth Sequence.
Most births require little more than gentle assistance and supportive care.

Immediate Care of the Normal Newborn

First ask yourself, *Is this a normal newborn?* Sweep your eyes over the baby as you dry him and look for obvious abnormalities. Observe him for indications that he will need assistance. It is reassuring if he cries, expels mucus, wriggles, and pulls his limbs tightly against his body.

Dry him rapidly, because chilling will compromise even a vigorous baby. Discard the wet towels and wrap dry, warmed blankets around the infant, keeping him skin to skin with his mother and thus using her body heat as a warming table. Cover his head with a baby cap or fold of blanket—the greatest heat loss occurs through the head, especially in babies with sparse hair. If he does not begin to breathe right away, stroke his back up and down, flick his feet with thumb and forefinger, and run your thumbs up and down the soles of his feet. Babies find these actions extremely irritating, and most will respond to the stimulation (see Neonatal Resuscitation, chapter 10).

ON TARGET *Childbirth is a natural process. Most babies delivered outside the hospital are born healthy, even if no provider is present.*

Newborn Management Priorities

○ Establish a clear airway. Position the head lower than the body for drainage, wipe fluid from the face, and suction if the baby sounds gurgly or shows excess fluid at the mouth or nose. Some agencies use a DeLee suction trap attached to a suction source to clear the airway. Use caution. Suctioning can cause bradycardia and trauma to the mucus membranes.

○ Maintain warmth. Heat loss can lead to hypothermia, hypoglycemia, and respiratory distress.

○ Place the baby on the maternal abdomen and keep him there at least until the cord is clamped. It may be appropriate to keep him there until you arrive at the hospital.

○ Monitor the infant's condition and stimulate or resuscitate as necessary.

○ Monitor maternal condition and watch for hemorrhage or shock.

○ Clamp and cut the cord after pulsations cease.

○ Assign Apgar scores.

acrocyanosis
Blue coloration of the extremities of a neonate that may persist for the first week.

The baby will usually appear purplish at birth because oxygen is less abundant *in utero*. After a few lungfuls of air, the baby should become pink and vigorous. Blue hands and feet (**acrocyanosis**) are a normal finding within the first few hours of life.

Drying and bulb suctioning the baby will stimulate crying and movement. Newborns should breathe at a rate of 30–60 per minute; but in the first 2 hours following birth, respirations of 70 are considered normal. Irregular respirations are a normal finding, sometimes with pauses lasting 5–12 seconds followed by a burst of rapid respirations. A 12-second pause may be considered normal if the infant's oxygen saturation remains normal, there is no change in skin color, and bradycardia does not occur. Crackles (rales) are common immediately after birth.

retraction
Pulling in of the flesh above and below the sternum, between the ribs, and around the neck when a newborn breathes, a sign of respiratory distress.

Retractions, nasal flaring, expiratory grunting with respirations, and audible gurgling are all signs that the infant may be experiencing respiratory distress. Cyanosis around the mouth (circumoral cyanosis) or trunk (central cyanosis) indicates that the baby is not oxygenating well and needs assistance.

Heart rate can easily be determined by auscultation or by palpating the junction of the umbilical cord and the abdomen. Neonatal hearts continue to beat at the fetal rate of 120–160, although immediately after birth the rate may rise to 180.

While assessing the infant, keep an eye on the mother. Remain alert for signs of placental separation or postpartum hemorrhage. If the mother needs your full attention, ensure that your partner remains focused on care of the infant. Sometimes babies who are vigorous at delivery become apneic soon after if mucus obstructs the airway or if there are underlying abnormalities.

Cutting the Umbilical Cord

Recent research indicates that the practice of delaying cord clamping until pulsations cease poses no significant risks, and the practice confers significant health benefits on preterm and full-term babies. The American Academy of Pediatrics and the World Health Organization endorse delayed cord clamping to reduce neonatal anemia and improve the flow of red blood cells to the brain, lungs, extremities, and intestines. It may also protect against persistent pulmonary hypertension of the newborn (see chapter 10).

Early cord clamping can reduce the amount of blood the newborn receives at birth by more than 50%. As long as the cord pulses, oxygen exchange continues between infant and mother as it did *in utero,* helping the newborn make the transition to extrauterine life. Once the cord is cut, the baby loses this maternal assistance. Most of the placental blood volume is transfused within 3 minutes after delivery.

Meanwhile, the initial steps of resuscitation can be accomplished just as easily with the baby on the mother's abdomen. Unless the infant requires intubation, ventilation, or chest compression, leave him on the mother's abdomen with the cord intact until cord pulsations have stopped. Although pulsations may persist for some time close to the baby, they stop first near the mother's vulva. When pulsations stop in any part of the cord, it can be cut without interrupting oxygen exchange.

You may let the mother decide who is to cut the cord. Cutting the baby free may be very meaningful to the father or others significant in her life.

Within 5–7 minutes of birth, vessels spasm in the umbilical cord, so it is not necessary to cut the cord before transport. It may be preferable to leave the baby attached to the placenta if, for example, the woman delivered some time ago, and both baby and placenta are wrapped in soiled laundry on a filthy floor. Cutting a dirty cord may introduce bacteria into the baby's system, so it is acceptable to transport the baby with the placenta.

In most cases the birth attendant will sever the umbilical cord. This is done by placing two clamps on the cord about 2 in. apart, 6 in. from the infant's abdomen, and cutting between them. Clean string ties or umbilical narrow tape, at least 15 cm in length, can also be used, tied tightly in two places. If the cord is not clamped before cutting, the infant may hemorrhage. If you have only one clamp, attach it 6 in. from the infant and cut the cord on the placental side. Blood lost from the placental end of the cord is fetal in origin, *not maternal,* and should not be considered in the maternal blood loss estimation. It is acceptable to use one clamp and allow the placental end to drain into a pan until the placenta is ready to deliver. This procedure is dangerous only if there is an undiagnosed twin *in utero.*

After applying the first clamp, some clinicians squeeze the cord flat and strip the blood from an inch or two of cord before applying the second clamp. This prevents blood from spurting upon cutting the cord, in accordance with universal precautions.

If the delivery occurs distant from equipment or supplies, cord clamps can be improvised. Select a fairly wide and flexible substitute. Clean shoelaces are acceptable, as is gauze bandage, knotted tightly around the cord in the same fashion as clamps. Narrow ties such as wire or dental floss can cut into or through the cord and allow hemorrhage to occur, defeating the purpose of clamping. Monitor the infant's cord stump, and add another clamp immediately if a clamp loosens.

ON TARGET Blood lost from the placental end of the cord drains from the placenta. It is fetal in origin, *not maternal.*

Apgar Scores

Apgar scoring is a method of evaluating a baby's initial response to the extrauterine world. Dr. Virginia Apgar developed it in the 1950s, and each of the five criteria scored conveniently corresponds with a letter in her last name (see Table 6-1). The baby earns 0–2 points on each of five criteria:

Appearance (skin color)
Pulse rate
Grimace (reaction to stimulus, usually the bulb suction)
Activity (muscle tone)
Respiratory effort

Table 6-1   Apgar Scores

	0	1	2
Appearance (skin color)	Body blue or pale	Body pink, extremities blue	Pink all over
Pulse rate	Absent	Under 100 bpm	Over 100 bpm
Grimace (reaction to bulb suction in mouth)	No response	Grimace	Cough, sneeze, cry
Activity (muscle tone)	Limp	Some flexion of extremities	Active movement
Respiratory	Apnea	Slow and irregular	Strong cry

The Apgar score simply evaluates how quickly and effectively the baby transitions to life on the outside and whether resuscitation is needed. It cannot predict health. Babies with severe anomalies can have excellent Apgars, and babies with poor Apgars may ultimately do very well.

The birth attendant should assign Apgar scores at 1 and 5 minutes of age. Infant care or resuscitation should not be interrupted for scoring, however. Rather, take a good look at the infant as you work and note whether he is crying or apneic, floppy or tightly flexed, pink or blue. Heart rate is easily obtained by touching the umbilical cord or listening to the chest (see Neonatal Resuscitation, chapter 10). A healthy term newborn should score between 7 and 10 at both 1 and 5 minutes of age.

Once mother and infant are stable, the infant may be encouraged to breastfeed. Nursing triggers the mother's pituitary to release oxytocin, a hormone that contracts the uterus and may help reduce bleeding. Even mothers who have chosen not to breastfeed may opt to put the baby to breast if you explain that it is a natural, healthy way to minimize her blood loss.

Ideally, the healthy infant will be transported skin to skin with his mother. This placement keeps him warm and helps to stabilize his vital signs. Observe mother and infant closely en route.

Placenta Delivery

The third stage of labor consists of separation and expulsion of the placenta. Contractions begin 3–5 minutes after delivery of the infant, but may not be painful. Normally the placenta will be expelled within 5–20 minutes of delivery of the infant. Afterward, the uterus contracts to minimize blood loss. In a multiparous woman, the uterus may have difficulty remaining contracted, and the woman may experience severe afterpains as the uterus tightens, relaxes, and tightens again.

After the baby is expelled, the uterus contracts, and the placenta shears off the uterine wall. Signs of placental detachment:

- A sudden trickle or small gush of blood. Often there is little or no bleeding before the placenta separates.
- The part of the umbilical cord protruding from the vagina lengthens.
- The uterus, as felt through the abdominal wall, contracts into a globular, grapefruit-like mass and rises in the abdomen.

Expulsion can occur by the Shultz mechanism (shiny, membranous fetal side first) or Duncan mechanism (meaty, bloody maternal side first).

Interference with this normal process causes more problems than it solves.

- *Do not pull on the umbilical cord!* The cord may snap off in your hand, necessitating manual removal of the placenta at the hospital. Incomplete separation may cause hemorrhage. Pulling on the cord may also cause the uterus to invert, resulting in massive, life-threatening hemorrhage.
- Do not try to deliver the placenta unless you are sure that it has separated.
- Always deliver the placenta with a contraction, using the mother's pushing effort to expel it.

ON TARGET Mismanagement of the third stage of labor can result in severe maternal hemorrhage.

During the minutes after delivery, the EMS provider should remain vigilant for maternal hemorrhage and signs of placental separation. Without massaging or stimulating the uterus, the crew member not responsible for the baby should place one hand on the abdomen to feel for the fundus to change shape and position, signaling placental detachment. It is not necessary to delay transport to wait for the placenta.

In some cases, the placenta does not deliver at all. There are many reasons for this occurence, and sometimes lack of separation or partial separation can cause infection or severe hemorrhage. In rare cases, the placenta has actually grown into or through the uterine muscle and can be removed only surgically.

The safest way for an EMS provider to deliver the placenta is to let the mother expel it. Observe her for signs of placental separation, then help her into an upright position, such as squatting. When she says that she feels a contraction, ask her to push. It is helpful to have your partner brace the uterus by placing the edge of a hand above the pubic bone and pressing inward. The placenta should slide out, and you can assist by gently guiding the cord outward.

Sometimes the amniotic membranes trail the placenta. These are very fragile and can break off inside the mother, creating the potential for infection. As the placenta emerges, catch it in both hands and deliver it slowly, or allow it to slide gently into a basin positioned at the level of the vagina. Sometimes you can close a 4 in. × 4 in. gauze around any trailing membranes and gently tease them out by rocking them side to side while you or your partner supports the placenta to prevent tension on the membranes. It is also possible to hold the placenta in two hands and turn it over repeatedly, so that the membranes become ropelike and less likely to tear as they emerge. This maneuver can be difficult for the inexperienced. If you observe tearing and retention of membranes, make note of this condition and inform hospital personnel.

After the placenta is out, immediately place your hand on the uterus through the abdominal wall. It should feel hard and grapefruit-like, no higher than the umbilicus. The uterus maintains hemostasis by remaining firmly contracted and midline. If the uterus feels "boggy" (soft and doughy), massage it vigorously between your two hands until it is firm. Always support the lower part of the uterus with your hand when massaging the fundus. The fundus should be checked frequently and massaged if boggy in the hours following birth. You can teach the woman to do this herself, freeing your hands for other tasks, but monitor her closely.

Bleeding should be minimal. Watch slow trickle bleeding carefully because blood loss can add up over time. If you find the uterus firm, but displaced above the umbilicus and to the right, the woman probably needs to empty her bladder. The uterus can be difficult to palpate in an obese woman.

Examining Placenta and Membranes

Emergency obstetrical kits come with a bag for the placenta. Before sealing the bag, look carefully at the placenta. It weighs an average of about 1.5 lb, approximately one-sixth the weight of the newborn. Small babies usually have small placentas, and large babies have large ones, though diabetes can cause the placenta to grow large and edematous. See Figure 6-10.

The side of the placenta that was attached to the mother will appear dark-red and meaty, similar to a piece of liver in color, but segmented into lobules. The opposite side of the placenta, the fetal side, is slick and shiny, with a treelike pattern of blood vessels branching from the umbilical cord insertion. Two layers of membrane can be observed, the chorion and the amnion, adhering to each other to form the sac that encased the fetus and amniotic fluid.

ON TARGET Check the placenta carefully for missing pieces that may remain inside the mother.

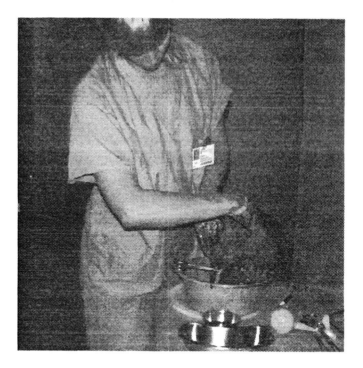

FIGURE 6-13

Examination of Placenta.
Carefully examine the placenta for
missing pieces that may have been
retained in the uterus. A fragmented
placenta can cause hemorrhage.
Photo by Phyllis Block

Note how many vessels are present in the umbilical cord. It should have three: two small arteries and a larger vein. A two-vessel cord can indicate anomalies in the infant and should be reported to the hospital.

Sometimes a piece of the placenta is left in the uterus, preventing adequate contraction and creating the potential for hemorrhage (see Postpartum Hemorrhage, chapter 7). Look at the pattern of blood vessels on the placenta and membranes. Are there any places where blood vessels end abruptly at a torn edge? A rough area can indicate torn tissue. Let the hospital know if you suspect retained placental fragments. Hospital personnel will want to inspect the placenta themselves and may wish to send it to pathology for evaluation.

Torn Umbilical Cord

The umbilical cord is elastic and will stretch as the fetus descends or when the birth attendant removes a snug cord from the neck during birth. Uncommonly, the umbilical cord may tear or break during delivery. The human umbilical cord can bear a load of 4–24 lb (the average breaking strength is 10–14 lb). A weak cord may break under minimal stress. The cord is most likely to break if it is thin and unhealthy or abnormal, as in cases of malnutrition, maternal smoking or hypertension, intrauterine growth restriction, oligohydramnios, or genetic anomalies. Causes of a short cord include chromosomal anomalies, genetic predisposition, and decreased fetal activity.

Often the first indication of a torn cord is unexpected, abundant bleeding. It may be difficult to localize the source of the bleeding, because a tiny surface tear can spray in all directions. A cord hemorrhage can result in a hypovolemic baby. Do not waste time looking for the source if you suspect the cord has torn. Simply clamp the cord immediately between the baby and the likely site of the tear.

The cord may snap when the birth attendant tries to reduce a thin, tight nuchal cord, resulting in fetal hemorrhage while the body is yet unborn. If so, have the mother push forcefully and deliver the baby immediately, then clamp the baby's end of the cord to prevent further blood loss. Resuscitate the infant as necessary and consider that fluid volume replacement may be necessary if the blood loss is significant. Bleeding from the maternal end of the cord is insignificant; it is simply draining from the placenta. Use caution in the third stage when the umbilical cord is weak. Minimal traction on the cord may cause breakage, potentially causing third-stage hemorrhage and necessitating manual removal of the placenta. Placental abnormalities may also exist.

Perineal Lacerations

The vagina is designed to stretch to accommodate passage of a term baby. Sometimes, however, minor or extensive trauma occurs.

Perineal trauma is classed by degree:

- **First degree.** Involving perineal skin only. This may be seen as minor abrasions or split skin on the vagina, perineum, or labia.
- **Second degree.** Involving muscle and skin.
- **Third degree.** Partial or complete disruption of the anal sphincter.
- **Fourth degree.** Involving complete disruption of the external and internal anal sphincter.

A third- or fourth-degree laceration, even when carefully repaired by a physician, leaves the woman with a 30–40% risk of long-term incontinence of flatus or feces.

Episiotomy is an incision into the perineum sometimes cut by the physician or midwife at the time of crowning to enlarge the vaginal opening. Episiotomies are cut either mediolaterally, across the grain of several layers of muscle, or midline, with the grain—risking extension of the cut toward the anus. From the turn of the last century through the 1970s, episiotomy was routinely practiced on nearly all American women during delivery, with the intention of preventing fetal intracranial hemorrhage and benefiting the long-term integrity of the pelvic floor.

Recent research, however, has revealed that episiotomies create more problems than they solve in the vast majority of cases and should not be performed routinely. Although a surgical cut is neater and easier to repair than a laceration, it is also likely to continue tearing along the path of the incision, creating a third- or fourth-degree laceration that might not otherwise occur. Studies show that women who underwent episiotomy experienced significantly more anal incontinence, even without extension, than did women who delivered over an intact perineum *or* women who tore spontaneously. Women with a prior episiotomy are also like to suffer separation of the scar during subsequent births, especially if their healing capacity is impaired by diabetes, smoking, or poor nutrition.

Progressive clinicians no longer reflexively reach for the scissors, but carefully deliver babies over intact perineums using techniques that minimize the likelihood of tearing. The EMS provider, for whom episiotomy is not an option, can also take steps to minimize perineal trauma.

Studies have attempted to determine whether a woman is less likely to tear if the birth attendant supports the perineum or allows birth to proceed without touching the mother. Results of the two approaches proved comparable, but supporting the perineum does reduce the amount of vulvar pain experienced for up to 10 days after delivery.

Sometimes perineal trauma is beyond the control of the birth attendant. Heavy smokers, drug addicts, and women with poor diets or chronic illnesses may have fragile tissues that tear rather than stretch. Babies born with a hand at the neck frequently drag an elbow upon delivery, causing a deep tear, and large or poorly positioned babies can cause vaginal trauma. Some women are unable to control the pushing urge and expel their babies so rapidly that tissues do not have time to stretch. Primiparous women are more likely to suffer lacerations than are women who have borne previous infants. A woman with a trichomonas vaginal infection may have swollen, congested vaginal tissues that lacerate easily, and genital warts tend to make the tissue more friable. Scar tissue from a prior deep tear or episiotomy may rupture if a woman's babies are closely spaced or if infection or poor nutrition prevented proper healing.

The EMS professional attending a delivery can recognize patients who are at higher risk for perineal laceration and take steps to prevent it.

- Side-lying positioning decreases the likelihood of laceration by allowing the baby to emerge slowly and gently. Consider this for primiparous patients and others at high risk for tearing.

- Slow crowning reduces lacerations. As the head distends the perineum, discourage forceful pushing and allow the baby to emerge gradually. As long as the vital signs of both mother and fetus are reassuring, take the time to let the mother stretch. Vigorous closed-glottis pushing results in more perineal trauma than spontaneous pushing with an involuntary, open-glottis technique.

- Control the emergence of the head by keeping gentle counterpressure on the infant's head as it emerges.

- The sensation of crowning is terrifying to many women. If the patient can relax her bottom and tolerate the stretching rather than tensing against the pain or forcefully expelling the infant, she is more likely to deliver without tearing. Reassure her that she will feel burning and stretching and may feel as if she is going to split apart, but these are normal and expected sensations.

Lacerations can bleed significantly after delivery, but bleeding often stops on its own. The perineum is the most likely structure to tear in childbirth, but anterior tears into the labia, urethra, and even clitoris can occur. These structures are vascular and rich with nerve endings; injuries to these areas are extremely painful and may bleed profusely.

 PEARLS Do not attempt to stop vaginal bleeding by packing the vagina.

Excessive bleeding after delivery usually originates from the uterus and is only occasionally related to perineal trauma. Always ensure that the uterus is well contracted before attending to lacerations. The EMS provider can apply direct pressure to any obvious external injuries until bleeding diminishes or stops. Usually, the birth attendant need only apply a perineal pad and instruct the woman to press her thighs together. Ice packs applied to the perineum effectively staunch bleeding and are very soothing to painful torn tissues. A woman may also lacerate her upper vaginal wall or cervix, and the EMS provider can only conjecture that this is the case by observing excessive bleeding with a well-contracted uterus. Any woman who is bleeding excessively should be rapidly transported to a hospital with intravenous fluids infusing rapidly and oxygen in place.

Your record should include the following information:

- Position of the infant at birth
- Presence of nuchal cord
- Time of birth
- Apgar scores
- Sex of infant
- Initial management of infant
- Time of placenta delivery
- Appearance and intactness of placenta
- Any observed tearing of perineum
- Mother and infant's condition
- Estimated blood loss

Summary

Childbirth is essentially a natural process. The birth is more likely to remain normal if the birth attendant refrains from needless interference and simply provides watchful, patient, supportive care. The role of the prehospital provider is to gently support the delivery process while anticipating problems and intervening quickly when complications arise.

REVIEW QUESTIONS

1. Compare and contrast the following maternal positions for delivery—supine, semi-sitting, lateral recumbent, squatting, and hands and knees.

2. You have just delivered the infant's head and feel a snug loop of cord around the neck. What should you do?

3. What techniques can a prehospital provider use to decrease the likelihood of perineal lacerations during delivery?

4. What are the signs that the placenta is ready to deliver?

5. Describe how to clamp and cut the umbilical cord.

Maternal and Fetal
Complications of
Labor and Delivery

Objectives

By the end of this chapter you should be able to

- *Treat the woman who is experiencing postpartum hemorrhage*

- *Recognize and treat the patient with amniotic fluid embolism*

- *Recognize dysfunctional patterns of uterine contraction*

- *Transport the patient with fetal heart-rate decelerations*

- *Assist delivery of the infant in breech presentation*

- *Manage the delivery of twins*

- *Resolve shoulder dystocia*

CASE
Study____

Hannah had apparently been pushing for some time when Sonia and Javier arrived. Her last two deliveries had been uneventful and resulted in healthy 9-lb babies. Her friend had lent her a book that advocated unattended deliveries, and Hannah thought it would be a very spiritual experience to give birth without medical intervention and just her husband there for support. Hannah secretly planned not to call her physician when labor began.

But when she had pushed for 2 hours and still no scalp was showing, her concerned husband called for an ambulance. The crew arrived to find Hannah squatting with determination in a steaming shower, pushing with her contractions. Sonia talked her out of the shower, and Hannah somewhat reluctantly allowed the paramedic to examine her genitals. A moderate amount of scalp had finally begun to part her labia when she pushed.

Hannah was 10 days post dates, and a sonogram the week before indicated a fetal weight of $9\frac{1}{2}$ lb. Sonia positioned Hannah carefully while Javier set up equipment for neonatal resuscitation.

Hannah pushed forcefully, and gradually the head crowned. It emerged slowly to the chin, then retracted tightly against the perineum—turtle sign. The head was slow to restitute to the side. When Sonia checked around the neck for a nuchal cord, her fingers were a tight fit. The baby's head began to turn dark purple. It was a shoulder dystocia.

Questions

1. What is shoulder dystocia and what are its risk factors?
2. What is the procedure for resolving a shoulder dystocia in the field?
3. What are the risks to Hannah's baby during and after a shoulder dystocia?
4. What are the risks to Hannah during and after a shoulder dystocia?

Introduction

The vast majority of deliveries proceed without complication and result in a healthy mother and a healthy infant. Emergencies can occur with unexpected suddenness, however. Every EMS provider should periodically review the management of obstetrical emergencies so that in the event of a problem, the plan is clear and actions are reflexive.

KEY TERMS

asphyxia, p. 183

asynclitism, p. 188

atony, uterine, p. 180

congenital, p. 188

dehiscence, p. 183

dizygotic, p. 204

monozygotic, p. 203

occiput posterior (OP), p. 189

Maternal Complications

Third-Stage Hemorrhage

After delivery, the placenta shears away from the uterine wall and is expelled, allowing the contraction of uterine muscles to control bleeding by closing off the open ends of blood vessels. A trickle or gush of blood normally signals that the placenta is ready to deliver. Ordinarily, all the attendant need do is deliver the placenta, then massage the uterus. See Figure 7-1. Sometimes the placenta will come out easily if the mother is helped to a squatting position and encouraged to push.

Sometimes, however, part of the placenta adheres while the rest of it detaches. Blood courses from the exposed vessels underlying the detached area, but the placenta still *in utero* prevents the uterus from clamping down. This blood loss can be rapidly life threatening. If the placenta does not come out, the EMS provider must act quickly.

• Prepare for rapid transport. Some of cases of third-stage hemorrhage can be resolved only in the operating room, so it is essential to take the patient to a hospital with the capacity for immediate surgery.

• Firmly massage the uterus. Normally, uterine massage is not performed until after delivery of the placenta, but it becomes necessary in the case of hemorrhage from a partially detached placenta. You may guide the placenta out by bracing the contracted uterus above the pubic bone with one hand and gently guiding the cord downward as the mother pushes. You will get a better grip on the cord if you grasp it with a clamp or 4 in. × 4 in. gauze.

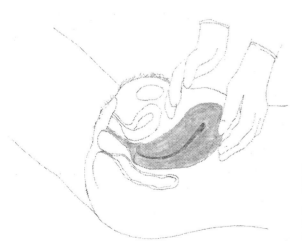

FIGURE 7-1
Fundal Massage.
To control postpartum bleeding, the birth attendant should massage the fundus until it contracts.
Illustration by Bonnie U. Gruenberg

Caution! If you use too much traction the cord will tear off, or a life-threatening uterine prolapse may result. Cord traction will *not* deliver a placenta that is still adherent to the uterus. Never use cord traction if the uterus is not firmly and obviously contracted. Always guard the uterus with a hand above the pubic bone when employing cord traction. Although hemorrhage is bad, uterine inversion is worse and can be caused by the birth attendant.

● If you do not have intravenous access, have another crew member start two large-bore IVs of lactated Ringer's or normal saline while you massage the uterus. Draw blood, if local protocols allow, to expedite laboratory studies at the hospital.

● Administer high-flow oxygen and position the woman for shock.

● Transport rapidly.

 Do not use excessive traction when attempting to deliver the placenta. The cord may snap off in your hand, or the uterus may invert, either of which may contribute to uncontrollable hemorrhage.

Postpartum Hemorrhage

About 4% of women suffer postpartum hemorrhage, defined as blood loss of greater than 500 cc. Postpartum hemorrhage is a major cause of maternal mortality and can progress rapidly. Excessive bleeding most commonly develops by 30 to 60 minutes after the birth of the infant, but may occur as late as 8 or more weeks after delivery.

The most common causes of postpartum hemorrhage are uterine atony; vaginal, perineal, or cervical lacerations; retained or fragmented placenta; and maternal blood-clotting abnormalities. Risk factors include an overstretched or overworked uterus, as with a long, difficult labor; a rapid, intense labor; multiple gestation; polyhydramnios; a large baby; preterm delivery; a history of preeclampsia; prior postpartum hemorrhage; previous cesarean delivery; nulliparity; and grand multiparity. The risk of hemorrhage is also increased after a long third stage. It rises significantly if the time between the birth of the baby and the birth of the placenta exceeds 30 minutes.

If the perineum is intact and hemostasis is achieved quickly after the placenta delivers, blood loss for a typical birth is often 300 cc or less. Estimated blood loss should not include any blood that flows out of the placenta from the cut end of the umbilical cord. Placental blood is fetal in origin and is distinct from maternal blood loss.

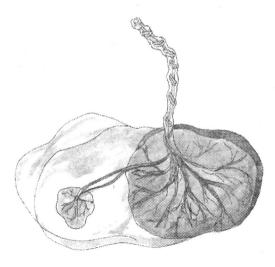

FIGURE 7-2
Succenturiate Lobe.
A succenturiate lobe may remain in the uterus after
the rest of the placenta has delivered, causing
hemorrhage.
Illustration by Bonnie U. Gruenberg

Retained Placental Fragments

Hemorrhage may occur if part of the placenta is left in the uterus after the completion of third-stage labor. Typically, the woman will achieve adequate hemostasis immediately following the delivery, but begin to hemorrhage hours, days, or weeks later. The EMS professional should carefully examine the placenta for missing fragments that might have remained inside the uterus. At the hospital, retained segments can be surgically removed.

A succenturiate lobe is a satellite placenta that is occasionally attached to a primary placenta by blood vessels and membranes. In this situation, the placenta may deliver and leave the succenturiate lobe inside and attached, so that the uterus cannot clamp down effectively to control bleeding. See Figure 7-2. Blood clots can also fill a uterus and thwart contraction.

Atony

atony, uterine
Loss of uterine
muscular tone,
which may impede
the progress of
labor or cause
postpartum hem-
orrhage.

When excessive bleeding follows the delivery of the placenta, the most common cause is uterine **atony** (failure to contract). In a normal delivery, bleeding is minimized by firm contraction of the empty uterus, which effectively constricts the blood vessels that moments before fed the placenta. If the uterus does not contract, the blood vessels remain open, and blood flows freely.

If bleeding continues in a steady flow after delivery of the placenta, or if a heavy gush occurs and does not stop, act quickly. Grasp the uterus through the abdominal wall with your two hands and knead it firmly. The fundus should be palpable roughly at the level of the umbilicus and ideally should feel rigid. In the case of uterine atony, the uterus will feel boggy (soft and doughy). It is essential that you stimulate it vigorously enough to cause a contraction. This will be extremely painful to the woman. Warn her that what you are about to do will hurt, and explain its necessity as you work.

If bleeding does not slow immediately,

- Have a crew member establish at least one large-bore intravenous line and rapidly infuse lactated Ringer's or normal saline.

- If local protocols allow, administer 10 units of pitocin intramuscularly or 10–20 units diluted in 1,000 cc of lactated Ringer's or normal saline (or both IM and IV pitocin if protocols permit). If the uterus does not respond, follow with 0.2 mg of intramuscular methergine if the patient has no history of hypertension.

- Treat for shock. Administer high-flow oxygen. Cardiac monitoring is indicated if the patient is seriously hemorrhaging. Monitor vital signs closely. Transport rapidly to the nearest appropriate facility. Continue to vigorously massage her uterus en route.

A distended bladder can cause or worsen postpartum hemorrhage. If your laboring patient has risk factors for postpartum hemorrhage, establish intravenous access, and draw blood if protocols permit. In some systems the EMS provider may be required to insert a Foley catheter.

PEARLS Methergine is contraindicated in patients with preeclampsia or high blood pressure, or with a history of either condition.

Retained Placenta

Typically the placenta delivers within 5–15 minutes, although a third stage of up to 30 minutes is not uncommon. Delay in placental separation is more likely to occur with premature infants.

Do not wait for placenta delivery to begin transport. If the placenta is slow to emerge, try putting the infant to the mother's breast en route to the hospital. Breastfeeding causes the release of oxytocin, which triggers contractions, promoting placental separation and reducing the likelihood of hemorrhage. Often a placenta that appears retained is really positioned in the cervical os, ready to be delivered, but blocking the flow of blood that heralds separation. In this case, helping the mother into an upright or squatting position encourages delivery. Try waiting for a contraction, then help her into an upright position over a bedpan and ask her to urinate. While waiting for the placenta, monitor the woman's vital signs and bleeding.

ON TARGET
The prehospital provider should not wait for placenta delivery to begin transport.

If the placenta remains attached, manual removal may be necessary upon arrival at the hospital. In some cases, the placenta has grown into the uterine wall (placenta accreta), into the uterine muscle (placenta increta), or entirely through the uterine wall (placenta percreta). The last-named condition is rare, and it is more likely to occur in a uterus scarred by prior cesarean section or other surgery. Treatment of a retained placenta should include transport, establishing intravenous access, monitoring vital signs closely, and treating for shock if hemorrhage occurs.

Uterine Rupture

dehiscence
Splitting open or rupture of a surgical wound or scar.

Uterine rupture is rare, but serious, carrying a 5% mortality rate for the mother and 50% for the fetus. Uterine rupture can be as minor as the partial separation of an old scar (**dehiscence**) or involve disruption of the entire thickness of the uterine wall, sometimes extruding the fetus into the abdominal cavity. Thirteen percent of uterine ruptures occur outside the hospital. Prediction and recognition of the condition in the field are crucial to maternal and fetal well-being.

Any woman who has a scarred uterus is at risk for uterine rupture. Previous cesarean section with a "classical" (vertical) uterine incision confers the highest risk. In about one-third of cases of classical scar rupture, the rupture occurs before labor begins. Sometimes a woman will have a horizontal scar across her abdomen and a vertical one on the uterus, so taking a history becomes important—but the woman does not always know which technique was used. Horizontal cesarean incision scars rupture, too, but less commonly and usually with less severe consequences. Other uterine surgeries, such as removal of large fibroid tumors or repair of a Müllerian defect, also increase the risk of uterine rupture. Malpresentations can also lead to uterine rupture—especially in a woman who has had many pregnancies, which may have left her lower uterine segment especially thin. Blunt trauma or cocaine use can also precipitate uterine rupture.

Uterine rupture can present subtly or dramatically, and it is not always easy to diagnose. Ominous changes in the fetal heart-rate pattern may herald uterine rupture. These include decelerations immediately following contractions, an abrupt, persistent decrease in rate, or loss of heart tones altogether. Suspect rupture when the woman experiences a sudden change in the character of pain, usually at the peak of a contraction. She may feel the sensation of "something tearing inside." Sometimes uterine rupture is preceded by increased abdominal tenderness or unusual patterns of pain radiation. Sometimes, though, pain is minimal.

Contractions often continue after uterine rupture. The woman may bleed vaginally in small or great quantities. Free blood in the peritoneal cavity can cause chest or shoulder pain, creating a presentation that resembles pulmonary embolism. The fetus may be palpated in a different position, and it may suddenly become easy to palpate if it has been expelled from the uterine cavity into the abdomen. The fetus may kick violently upon rupture, then fall still.

Frequently the mother subsides into shock. Her pulse becomes rapid and thready, her skin is pale and moist, and her blood pressure may plummet. She may vomit or faint. The only treatment is emergency surgery to deliver the infant.

The woman with suspected uterine rupture should be treated similarly to any patient in hypovolemic shock. Position her on her left side with the stretcher flat, establish two large-bore intravenous lines of lactated Ringer's or normal saline, administer high-flow oxygen by mask, and transport rapidly to the nearest facility with the capacity for immediate surgery.

 The woman with suspected uterine rupture should be treated like any patient in hypovolemic shock.

Uterine Prolapse (Uterine Inversion)

A uterine inversion occurs when the entire uterus turns inside out and protrudes through the cervical os (incomplete), into the vagina (complete), or beyond the vulva (prolapsed). Spontaneous occurrence is very rare—uterine inversion is usually due to mismanagement of the third stage of labor. Most typically, this situation is caused by excessive traction on the umbilical cord or pulling out the placenta before the uterus has contracted. Prolapse is most likely to occur with multiparous women because the musculature and ligaments anchoring the uterus tend to be lax.

 Uterine inversion may not be obvious to the EMS provider. Except in cases of prolapse (protrusion beyond the vulva), the inverted uterus is invisible from the outside.

The result is usually shock with life-threatening hemorrhage. If the uterus protrudes from the vagina, diagnosis is obvious. But because EMS personnel do not perform vaginal exams, they may not detect a uterine inversion that they cannot see. If inversion is suspected, transport rapidly to the nearest facility.

Treat for shock with two large-bore IVs of lactated Ringer's or normal saline running wide. Saline-soaked sterile gauze should be applied to any part of the uterus protruding from the vagina. If the placenta is adherent to the inverted uterus, do not remove it, or uncontrollable hemorrhage may ensue.

Amniotic Fluid Embolism

Amniotic fluid embolism (AFE) is a rare complication that can occur during or immediately after delivery. It warrants mention in this text because it is one of the most common causes of maternal death. Occasionally a small amount of amniotic fluid enters the maternal circulation, triggering what may be either an anaphylactic reaction or pulmonary embolism from fetal skin, hair, and vernix contained in the fluid. The woman with this condition will present with sudden shock or even cardiac arrest, often accompanied by DIC. Treat as you would hypovolemic shock or DIC, but bear in mind that there is no evidence that any treatment improves prognosis in true cases of AFE.

Chorioamnionitis

Chorioamnionitis, infection of the fetal membranes, is potentially life threatening to both mother and fetus. Intact amniotic membranes protect the sterile environment of the uterus from microorganisms. Once the membranes rupture, there is the potential for infection, which becomes more likely if membranes have been ruptured more than 24 hours. Chorioamnionitis also occurs sometimes with intact membranes.

Chorioamnionitis is characterized by maternal fever and tachycardia, fetal tachycardia (which often precedes maternal symptoms), tender uterus, and foul-smelling amniotic fluid. The infant may have poor Apgar scores or may be born vigorous and suddenly decline 10–25 minutes after delivery. Newborn hypothermia is also common. Treatment for chorioamnionitis includes

- Rapid transport to hospital
- Hydration with intravenous fluids (lactated Ringer's or saline) and protection from hypothermia

- Frequent vital signs
- Preparation for newborn resuscitation

If possible, save the placenta in a sterile container or bag because it will be sent to pathology at the hospital.

Uterine Dysfunction

Expulsion of the fetus requires strong contractions with a normal gradient, in which the strongest muscular contraction occurs in the fundus and the weakest in the lower uterine segment. Variations of uterine activity can impede or halt the progress of labor. The EMS provider should be aware of their existence.

Hypotonic Contractions

Hypotonic contractions are usually infrequent, short, and mild. They are characterized by a normal gradient, but they are weak overall. The mother is usually comfortable, but may contract for many hours without making much progress. Prolonged uterine activity puts her at risk for postpartum hemorrhage and possible infection if her membranes have ruptured. In the hospital, pitocin is often used to augment these weak contractions.

Hypertonic Contractions

In hypertonic uterine dysfunction, the uterus contracts erratically. Some isolated sections contract harder than others, and the greatest muscular contraction occurs in the middle section instead of the fundus. Hypertonic contractions are very painful and difficult and do not dilate the cervix effectively. Hypertonic contractions are more likely to occur during the latent phase of labor and are seen most frequently in primigravidas. A woman in early labor who seems to be in great pain may very well be coping with hypertonic contractions. The mother may become exhausted or discouraged, and the fetus may become stressed if the contractions compromise placental blood flow. Obstetrical providers often treat hypertonic contractions by administering narcotics or barbiturates to allow the woman to rest. Often she will awaken with an effective contraction pattern.

Fetal Complications

Fetal Heart-Rate Abnormalities

A normal fetal heart rate is an indicator of fetal well-being. Unfortunately, it can be very difficult to auscultate a fetal heart rate in the best of circumstances. Many ambulances do not carry a Doppler, and a stethoscope or fetoscope is frequently useful only if the patient is in her third trimester, the fetal back faces the maternal abdomen, and there is not much maternal fat shielding the uterus. Clearly it is important not to waste time searching for a fetal heartbeat in an emergency situation, but auscultation of the fetal heart can provide valuable information on fetal well-being and sometimes dictate the course of care. A detailed description of fetal monitoring is beyond the scope of this book, but a basic understanding of fetal assessment can be valuable in the field.

The normal fetal heart rate ranges from 120 to 160. With maturation of the nervous system later in gestation, the rate tends to rise during wakefulness and REM sleep, and drop during quiet sleep. It is easy to confuse the fetal and maternal heartbeats, especially if the latter is rapid because of medication or labor pain, or the fetus is in distress. Use of a pulse oximeter on the maternal finger will differentiate between fetal and maternal rates.

A fetal heart rate that shows persistent decelerations, or dips in rate, may denote either poor placental perfusion or umbilical cord compression. Cord compression can occur if there is decreased amniotic fluid or if the cord is wedged between fetal or maternal body parts. A cord wound tightly around the fetal neck or body may cause slowing of the heart rate, especially during delivery. Changing the mother's position from one side to the other or placing her in the knee-chest position (cheek, chest, and knees on the stretcher, rump in the air) often shifts the fetus and improves the fetal heart rate. Intravenous fluids can improve maternal hydration and sometimes increase amniotic fluid volume, potentially taking pressure off a compressed cord.

If you note periodic or sustained decelerations in the fetal heart rate,

- Transport quickly if birth is not imminent.
- Call for backup and prepare for resuscitation if delivery occurs.
- Administer high-flow oxygen by mask.
- Begin intravenous hydration.
- Change maternal positioning and transport in whatever position best improves fetal heart rate.

Malpresentations and Cephalopelvic Disproportion

For birth to occur, the fetus must pass through his mother's pelvis. Cephalopelvic disproportion (CPD) is the term used when the fetal head is unable to make the passage. CPD is not limited to large babies. A small baby with his head in an extended or tilted position can fail to descend into the pelvis. A woman whose pelvis is narrowed by prior pelvic fracture or **congenital** defect may be unable to deliver even a well-positioned baby.

congenital
Present at birth or during uterine development, as a result of either hereditary or environmental influences.

True malpresentations are uncommon. Approximately 95% of the time, the fetus presents vertex—head down with chin flexed to the chest. This posture efficiently presents the smallest diameter of the baby's head to the pelvis, simplifying the birth process. Any deviation from this position can make labor slow and difficult, or even prevent vaginal birth. Premature infants are more likely to adopt unusual birth positions, because they are small in relation to amniotic fluid volume and can easily change position. The EMS provider who is attending the birth should be aware of potential variations in presentation, some of which are challenging to manage or even life threatening to mother and infant.

Cephalic Malpresentations

The fetus who presents head-down, but with his head extended to some extent (deflexed), or a fetus with his head tilted to the side instead of in alignment with the shoulders (**asynclitism**) faces a more difficult birth, because he presents a wider diameter of his head to the pelvis.

asynclitism
Tilting of the fetal head at an oblique angle.

Face Presentation   The face presentation (in which the face is the first fetal part to enter the pelvis) is the most extreme example of deflexion. See Figure 7-3. The fetus often may assume this attitude during labor, so even a woman who has had a recent ultrasound can be unaware that her fetus is delivering face first. The first sign of a face delivery in the field is usually the crowning of nose, eyes, and mouth. The face is usually swollen and bruised from dilating the cervix, especially if membranes have been ruptured for hours. The chin will be facing the pubic bone (a chin facing the sacrum is not deliverable vaginally and will not progress to crowning). The head is born by flexion, externally rotates, and the shoulders move into the usual position for delivery. The rest of the delivery proceeds as usual.

As many as 60% of infants delivered in face presentations have some sort of deformity that encourages this position. Babies with anencephaly and microcephaly (both malformations including small heads) often present face first, as do babies with goiters and tumors of the neck.

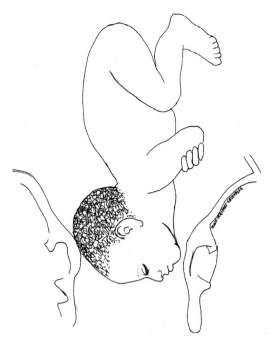

FIGURE 7-3
Face Presentation.
In an attitude of extreme deflexion, this fetus hyperextends
his neck and presents face first.
Illustration by Bonnie U. Gruenberg

Facial swelling from the pressures of birth may create airway problems
for the newborn. Commonly, the baby will continue to hold the hyperextended posture for days after birth.

**occiput posterior
(OP)**
A fetal position in
which the occiput
of the fetal skull is
directed toward
the mother's
sacrum.

Occiput Posterior   The **occiput posterior** (OP) fetus lies with his
back toward his mother's spine. See Figure 7-4. Occiput posterior babies
are somewhat deflexed because the head drops back into the hollow of
the maternal sacrum. Every contraction pushes his skull into the
sacrum, often causing painful "back labor." During labor, the baby can
be encouraged to turn by positioning the mother on her side or hands
and knees. The mother usually appreciates pressure, hot packs, or cold
packs applied to her lower back. Often the fetus rotates to occiput anterior before delivery, but if not, the child is born facing the ceiling. If the
child should deliver in an OP position, perineal or periurethral tearing
is more likely. The head is born by flexion first, then extension. The
head externally rotates as the shoulders move into the usual anterior-
posterior position.

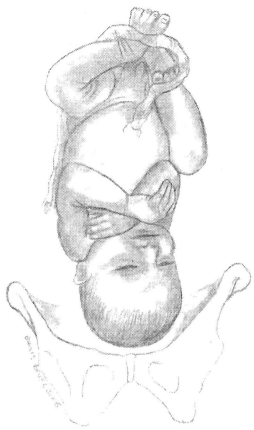

FIGURE 7-4
Occiput Posterior.
A fetus in the right occiput posterior position (ROP).
Illustration by Bonnie U. Gruenberg

Noncephalic Malpresentations

Shoulder or Transverse Presentation   Some babies lie obliquely across the uterus, a position that cannot be delivered vaginally. This situation will sometimes present to the EMS provider as an arm hanging out of the vagina or a prolapsed cord. See Figure 7-5. This is a life-threatening situation for the fetus. Rapid transport to the hospital is essential, ideally with the mother in the knee-chest position, on oxygen, and receiving IV crystalloid solution. (See treatment for prolapsed cord later in this chapter.)

Breech   Breech presentation, or buttocks or feet at the cervix, is the most common of the noncephalic malpresentations, occurring in 3–4% of labors at term. Breech positioning is more common with

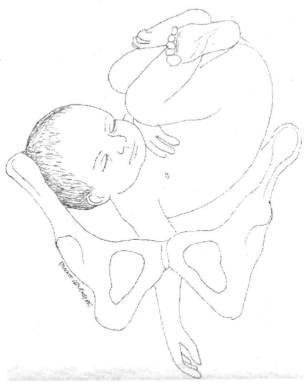

FIGURE 7-5
Shoulder Presentation.
A shoulder presentation is not deliverable vaginally, and an
immediate cesarean section is indicated.
Illustration by Bonnie U. Gruenberg

premature delivery because many babies do not assume a head-down
position until well into the third trimester. Breech is also more likely
with grand multiparity, polyhydramnios or oligohydramnios, certain
fetal anomalies, uterine abnormalities or fibroid tumors, multiple gestation, or previous breech.

Breech positions are further classified as

- **Frank breech.** The fetal buttocks enter the pelvis, with hips
flexed, legs extended, and the feet by the baby's head. The extended
legs make it difficult for the baby to somersault to vertex, and often he
remains stuck in the frank breech position. Frank breech accounts for
about half of all breech presentations and is most favorable for a vaginal delivery. See Figure 7-6.

- **Complete breech.** With complete breech, the fetus is squatting or
sitting cross-legged on the cervix.

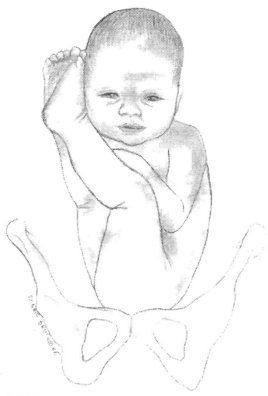

FIGURE 7-6
Frank Breech.
The sacrum of the frank breech fetus is the part that
presents to the maternal pelvis.
Illustration by Bonnie U. Gruenberg

  ● **Footling breech.**   One or both hips and knees are extended and
one or both feet are presenting. A variation of this is the kneeling
breech. See Figure 7-7.

 PEARLS Frank breech is the most common of breech presentations and
is most favorable for a vaginal delivery.

    Vaginal breech deliveries carry a perinatal risk of death three to five
times that of nonbreech deliveries. (Some of these deaths are due to
anomalies or prematurity that predisposed the baby to the breech positioning.) Vertex delivery places the largest part of the baby first and
allows the head to mold over time, presenting the smallest possible

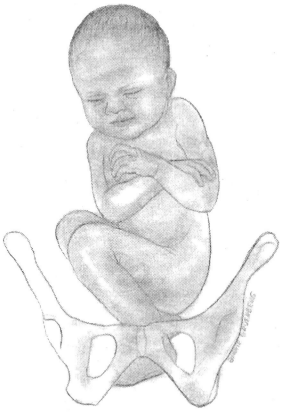

FIGURE 7-7
Footling Breech.
The footling breech enters the maternal pelvis feet first,
increasing the likelihood that the umbilical cord will prolapse
around the presenting part.
Illustration by Bonnie U. Gruenberg

asphyxia
Extreme hypoxia
with increased
carbon dioxide in
the blood, leading
to coma or death.

diameter to the pelvis and conforming to its shape. In a breech delivery, the body is born first, followed by the larger shoulders, and then the largest and most solid part, the head, without the benefit of molding. If the head is unable to fit the pelvis, this fact may not become apparent until the body is born. The cord may prolapse around the infant's legs when the water breaks or may become pinched between the pelvis and the fetal head causing **asphyxia.**

The child may suffer birth trauma, especially if the birth attendant tugs on the body in an effort to free it. Sometimes the cervix will open wide enough to allow the smaller diameter of the legs or body to slip though, but leave the head entrapped. Sometimes the partially empty uterus will contract and release the placenta, cutting off the baby's oxygen supply before it is completely born, while it is unable to breathe for itself.

Maternal and Fetal Complications of Labor and Delivery 193

Yet sometimes the infant will emerge uneventfully, so fast that the responder scarcely has time to prepare for the birth. It is impossible to know until events unfold whether a breech delivery will proceed easily or become obstructed. Some midwives and physicians will attempt vaginal breech delivery in controlled circumstances, but most opt for cesarean section if attempts to turn the baby before labor fail. The EMS provider has no such option and must cope with the situation as it occurs.

Managing the Breech Delivery   The diagnosis of breech presentation is often far from obvious. Sometimes the mother reports that the fetus was breech at the last office visit. Experienced hands might palpate a large hard head in the fundus that can be balloted between the fingers of two hands. Even experienced obstetrical providers occasionally mistake a hard sacrum for a head when feeling the abdomen or even when examining the vagina for the presenting part. Some breech deliveries do not become apparent until crowning occurs, when the birth attendant is startled to see protruding feet or bottom.

Every effort should be made to allow the breech birth to take place in the hospital. If the EMS provider positions a woman on her side and encourages her to avoid pushing and to breathe through contractions, birth may be delayed long enough for transport. When delivery is imminent, the responder must cope with a field delivery.

British midwife Margaret Myles is famous for her admonition "Hands off the breech!" There is much to be said for allowing the breech infant to deliver with minimal handling. A hands-off approach encourages the fetus to maintain a position of flexion during the birth, simplifying delivery. The sensation of being grasped can stimulate the emerging baby, causing his hands and arms to fly up in a Moro "startle" reflex. This can extend the neck and present larger diameters of the head to the pelvis, or even wedge an arm up alongside the head. Temptation is great to "help" the baby deliver by pulling on whatever parts emerge. This can cause serious injury to the infant, including organ damage and limb fractures.

This text will detail how to deliver the frank breech. Other breech presentations follow a similar course if delivery proceeds normally. Any basic life support crew handling a breech delivery should call for advanced life support backup. The infant is more likely to be premature, have physical anomalies, suffer trauma, and require resuscitation.

The frank breech usually delivers with one hip toward the pubic bone and the other toward the mother's sacrum, his back to either the right or left. See Figure 7-8. First the anterior hip delivers, then the posterior hip with lateral flexion, the body emerging to the umbilicus. Encourage the mother to push *hard* with contractions. External rotation should occur until the baby's back faces up, and you should gently guide the infant to a backup position if he does not naturally

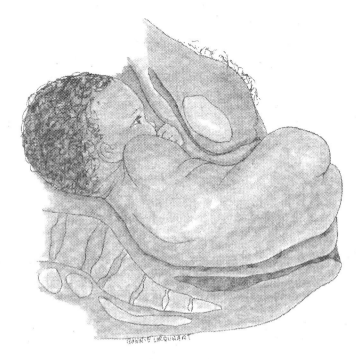

FIGURE 7-8
The Buttocks Emerge.
The frank breech fetus usually delivers with one hip toward the pubic bone and the other toward the mother's sacrum, his back to either the right or left.
Illustration by Bonnie U. Gruenberg

achieve that on his own. When the umbilicus is seen, if the cord appears to be pulled taut, the birth attendant may gently pull a few inches of umbilical cord down to create slack for delivery. This is the crucial point of the delivery. At this stage, the head has entered the pelvis, and the cord is probably compressed between the pelvic bones and the baby's head. To reduce the risk of asphyxia, the head should be born within 5 minutes.

Eventually, the feet should spring free as the body descends. See Figure 7-9. The birth attendant should wrap the emerging infant in a warm towel or blanket. See Figure 7-10. Cool air may cause hypothermia and can stimulate breathing efforts with the head still unborn. If the trunk is slow to emerge, gentle downward traction may be applied by placing both hands on the fetal pelvis, thumbs on the sacroiliac regions, fingers on the iliac crests and applying gentle downward traction at a 45° angle. Grasp the infant *only* over the bony pelvis—to grasp the infant at any other point may cause serious injury. Maternal pushing is the force that delivers the infant—do not attempt to pull the baby out. The arms should deliver spontaneously. If the arms are caught and seem to be impeding delivery, you may gently free them by sweeping them over the chest and out.

Delivery of the head is the most hazardous part of the breech delivery. Gently lift the fetal body upward, but the angle should be no more than parallel to the floor to avoid injuring the neck through

ON TARGET Maternal pushing is the force that delivers the breech infant—do not attempt to pull the baby out.

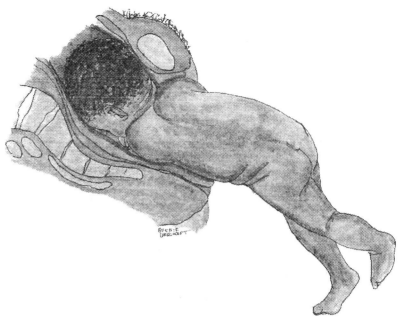

FIGURE 7-9
The Legs Spring Free.
First the anterior hip delivers, then the posterior hip with lateral flexion, the body emerging to the umbilicus. Eventually, the feet should spring free as the body descends.
Illustration by Bonnie U. Gruenberg

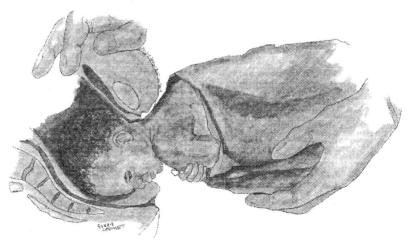

FIGURE 7-10
Wrap a Blanket around the Baby.
The birth attendant should wrap the emerging infant in a warm towel or blanket. Grasp the infant *only* over the bony pelvis—to grasp the infant at any other point may cause serious injury. Maternal pushing is the force that delivers the infant.
Illustration by Bonnie U. Gruenberg

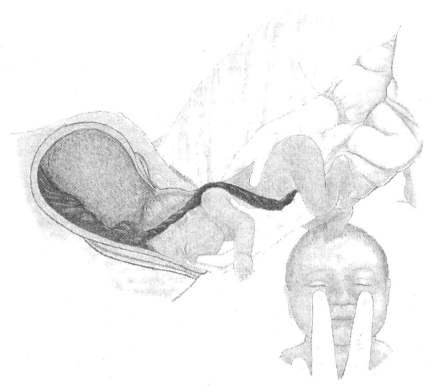

FIGURE 7-11
Placement of the Fingers to Maintain Airway in a Breech Birth.
If the head does not deliver, the birth attendant must make an airway for the baby.

hyperextension. An assistant can apply pressure directly behind the maternal pubic bone (*not* fundal pressure!) to keep the fetal head flexed and aid delivery. In most cases, the head will spontaneously deliver.

If the head does not deliver, minutes count if the baby is to have any chance of survival. Rapid transport is critical. Immediately insert your hand into the vagina and make an airway for the baby by keeping the maternal tissue away from his face. See Figure 7-11. Thread oxygen tubing into the space you have created and supply blowby oxygen at a rate of 6–8 L/min. If the umbilical cord is still pulsing, keep it warm and moist and avoid handling it. If the circulation between mother and fetus remains intact, the child has a vastly improved chance for survival. Ensure the fetal body remains wrapped in dry warm towels or blankets to preserve heat. Establish intravenous access in the mother with a large-bore catheter and a crystalloid solution, and put her on high-flow oxygen. Have the mother continue to push hard with contractions, while you lift the fetal body parallel to the floor and have an assistant apply suprapubic pressure.

Be on guard for maternal hemorrhage. After the fetal body delivers, the uterus might clamp down and attempt to expel the placenta. With the head and placenta still retained in the mother's body, the uterus might not be able to control its own bleeding, and hemorrhage may ensue. If she begins to bleed heavily, intravenous fluid bolus in indicated, along with the high-flow oxygen and rapid transport that should already be underway.

Compound Presentation

Compound presentation occurs when a hand presents alongside the head, enlarging diameters and complicating the delivery. If you recognize this problem, gently pinch the fetal fingers, and very often he will pull the hand back and out of the way. Be prepared for extensive maternal lacerations if the child delivers with the hand alongside the head. See Figure 7-12.

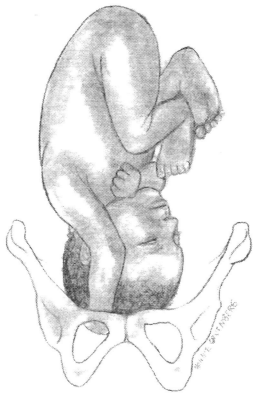

FIGURE 7-12
Compound Presentation
A compound presentation occurs when the arm lies alongside the fetal head, a situation that may obstruct delivery.
Illustration by Bonnie U. Gruenberg

Shoulder Dystocia

Shoulder dystocia is one of the most frequently occurring complications of labor and delivery and can be life threatening for the baby. Shoulder dystocia occurs after delivery of the head, when the anterior fetal shoulder becomes impacted against the maternal symphysis pubis and the width of the fetal shoulders is wider than the maternal pelvic inlet.

Although a very large baby is more likely to encounter shoulder dystocia at delivery, about half off all cases occur with average-sized fetuses. Risk for shoulder dystocia is increased with gestational diabetes, prior shoulder dystocia, postterm pregnancy, short maternal stature, and abnormal pelvic structure.

Uterine atony and subsequent hemorrhage are common following shoulder dystocia. Shoulder dystocia can result in maternal tissue trauma, including an increased risk of vaginal, third-degree, or fourth-degree tears.

The most serious risk that shoulder dystocia poses to the fetus is hypoxia that may result in neurological damage or death. This risk increases if there is a significant delay in delivery of the fetus. The fetus may also suffer brachial plexus palsies, which cause nerve damage and paralysis in the baby's arm that usually resolves within the first year of life, but may be permanent. Fractures of the fetal clavicle or humerus may occur.

Because shoulder dystocia can occur with any headfirst delivery, the EMS provider should consider this possibility with any birth and rehearse the steps of management on the way to any potential delivery.

Shoulder dystocia may be preceded by a long, slow crowning of the infant's head. When the head emerges, external rotation is slow to occur or does not occur at all. The fetal head appears to pull back against the perineum (this is known as "turtle sign"). When you check for the nuchal cord, you feel the head is tightly applied to the perineum and your fingers have difficulty reaching the neck. The fetal head begins to turn purple, then black. When you attempt to deliver the body, all you feel is resistance. *Do not pull on the baby's head!* True shoulder dystocia is a bone-on-bone impaction, and attempting to effect delivery by pulling and tugging will only injure the infant's neck. Keep in mind that with every minute delivery is delayed, the fetal pH drops precipitously. Call for backup immediately.

The first step in resolving a shoulder dystocia is to straighten the pelvic angles and increase the diameter of the pelvic inlet by changing the mother's position. If she is on a bed or stretcher, create space beneath the mother's bottom. Bring her hips to the edge of the bed or slide a cushion or bedpan under her bottom. Have her grasp her knees and pull her thighs back onto or alongside her abdomen, as if she were trying to put her knees in her armpits. Her shoulders are flat on the bed. This is called McRobert's maneuver. This position effects delivery by flattening

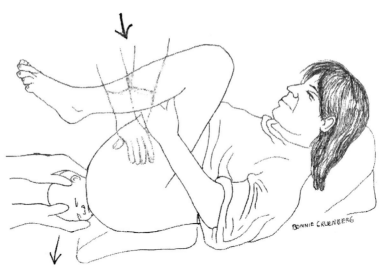

FIGURE 7-13
McRobert's Maneuver.
In the event of shoulder dystocia, place the mother in McRobert's position and apply suprapubic pressure. Have the mother bear down forcefully while you gently, but firmly guide the head downward.
Illustration by Bonnie U. Gruenberg

the sacral promontory, shifting the pubis, and pushing the posterior shoulder into the hollow of the sacrum, creating more room for the anterior shoulder to move under the pubic bone. Assistants, if present, can help her bring her legs back.

When the woman is in McRobert's position, an assistant should stand on the side of the baby's back (the side that the baby's emerging head faces away from) and apply deep pressure straight down just above the mother's pubic bone, similar to the pressure applied in a CPR compression. See Figure 7-13. This serves to adduct the anterior shoulder and reduce the diameter of the shoulder girdle, allowing it to move beneath the pubic symphysis. The assistant should use a steady pressure at first while you attempt to deliver the infant, and then if unsuccessful, should apply pressure in a rocking motion. Never use fundal pressure.

While the mother is on her back with legs pulled close and the assistant is providing suprapubic pressure, have the mother push with focused effort. Most women will marshal extra reserves of strength and courage when they know their baby is in trouble. Guide the head downward with gentle pressure, taking care not to stress the neck. It is easier to guide the head downward if there is space beneath the mother's bottom. If you are delivering over the side of a bed, be prepared for a sudden release of resistance if your maneuvers are successful—followed by a slick infant slipping into your grasp. Placing pillows on the floor

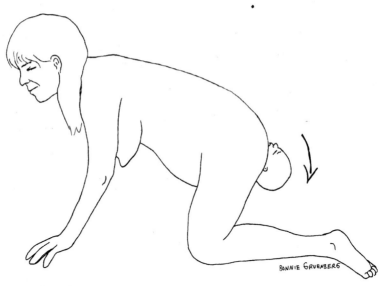

FIGURE 7-14
Gaskin Maneuver.
If McRobert's position fails to resolve shoulder dystocia, turn the mother on
hands and knees. Guide the fetal head downward to release the posterior
shoulder, then upward to complete the birth.
Illustration by Bonnie U. Gruenberg

beneath the woman provides a safer landing zone for the baby if he
should slip though your hands and fall.

In most cases, these two maneuvers will resolve the shoulder dystocia.
If they do not, immediately flip the woman to her hands and knees (not
knee-chest). Grasp the fetal head and gently guide it downward, attempting to deliver the posterior shoulder (which is now uppermost). This is the
Gaskin maneuver, which will resolve most shoulder dystocias by changing
the angles of the pelvis and enlarging the pelvic diameter. The act of turning from supine to hands and knees often shifts the fetal position to allow
for delivery. See Figure 7-14.

If none of these maneuvers are successful, rapid transport to the
nearest facility is in order. Transport the mother in either the hands-and-
knees or McRobert's position, and continue repeating the maneuvers
described here en route. Initiate high-flow oxygen for the mother, and
start a large-bore intravenous line of crystalloid solution.

If delivery is accomplished, the infant may be stunned or hypoxic
and may require resuscitation. Observe the baby carefully to assess
whether he is moving his limbs and if there is bruising or any other
evidence of trauma present. Document your findings carefully.

The mother is very likely to hemorrhage after a shoulder dystocia,
usually immediately after delivery of the placenta. Treat as with any
postpartum hemorrhage.

Umbilical Cord Prolapse

Umbilical cord prolapse involves a cord that lies beside or below the presenting part. This is most likely to occur with the fetal head high in the pelvis, or with polyhydramnios, multiple gestation, or fetal presentation other than vertex. Cord prolapse can be immediately life threatening to the fetus. See Figure 7-15. If the cord becomes compressed or if the vessels within it begin to spasm, his oxygen supply is cut off.

When encountering a cord prolapse, the first step is to place the mother in a knee-chest position immediately or lay her on her back with several pillows elevating her hips. Knee-chest is probably better for sustaining a good fetal heart rate, but may be hard to maintain in a moving ambulance. See Figure 7-16. Immediately don sterile gloves and insert your entire hand (if possible) into the woman's vagina. Find the

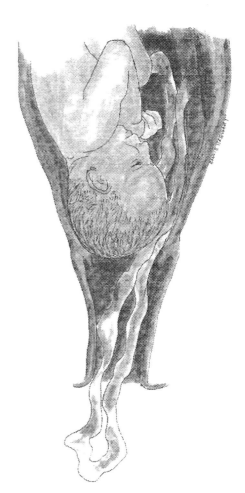

FIGURE 7-15
Prolapsed Cord.
Umbilical cord prolapse carries the risk of life-threatening hypoxia or anoxia for the fetus. Treatment is immediate cesarean section.
Illustration by Bonnie U. Gruenberg

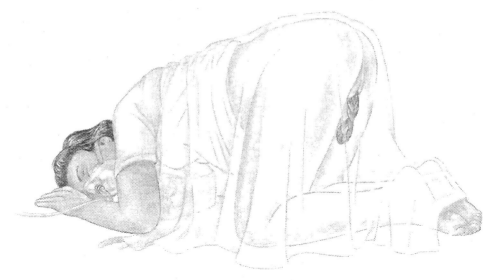

FIGURE 7-16
Patient Positioning for Prolapsed Cord.
Positioning the patient with umbilical cord prolapse.

presenting part of the fetus and push it upward, off the cord. The cervix might be only partially dilated, so this is not always easy to manage. Uterine contractions will be forcing the baby down toward you at regular intervals, but your task is to hold the fetus back and prevent compression of the cord. Once your hand is in the vagina, it will remain there until the baby is delivered by cesarean section at the hospital. You will probably remain under the drapes between the woman's legs during the surgery until the baby is delivered.

A pulsing cord is reassuring if you feel it against your hand, but do NOT compress the cord to check the pulse. It is important to avoid spasm of the cord vessels. If part of the cord protrudes outside of the vagina, keep it moist and warm with saline and plastic wrap.

Immediate transport is crucial. The woman should be placed on high-flow oxygen by mask, and intravenous access should be achieved, but ideally this should all be accomplished en route. The fetus might only have minutes of adequate blood supply remaining, and his best chance for survival lies in immediate rapid transport and immediate cesarean section upon arrival at the hospital.

monozygotic
Derived, like twins or other multiples, from a single fertilized egg; identical.

Multiple Gestation

Twin conceptions occur though one of two mechanisms. Identical, or **monozygotic** twins, arise when a single fertilized ovum divides into two

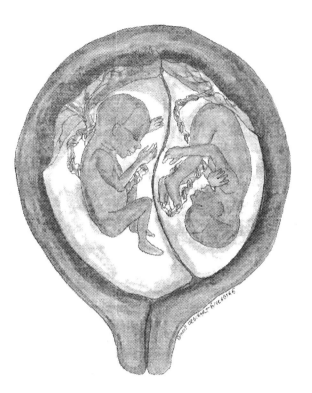

FIGURE 7-17
Twins at 12 Weeks.
These 12-week-gestation fraternal twins are in separate amniotic sacs and have separate placentas.
Illustration by Bonnie U. Gruenberg

dizygotic
Derived, like twins or other multiples, from two separately fertilized eggs; fraternal.

separate clusters of cells that give rise to two separate individuals that share identical genes. They are always of the same sex. Fraternal, or **dizygotic** twins, originate from separate ova and sperm that happen to be fertilized at about the same time. Genetically, they are as closely related as any other siblings. They can be of different sexes, they can even have different fathers, and they may be conceived more than a week apart. See Figure 7-17.

The rate of occurrence for identical twins remains fairly stable at about 1 in 225 births, unchanged by variables such as race, maternal age, and parity. The tendency to bear fraternal twins is hereditary, and these births occur naturally at a rate of about 1 set of twins per 86 births. The rate of twin births in the United States has risen 35% since 1990, and the rate of twins and higher-order multiples also have shown significant increase. Modern treatments for infertility have increased the incidence of twins, triplets, quadruplets, and higher-order pregnancies. African American women are more likely to conceive fraternal twins, as are women of all races between the ages of 35 and 40. The advent of ultrasonography has allowed us to observe pregnancies from soon after conception and has revealed twin conceptions occur far more frequently than previously suspected—loss of one twin while the second is carried to term is not an uncommon occurrence.

Higher-order pregnancies tax both mother and babies, and carry a higher incidence of complications. Fifty-four percent of twins and 93% of all triplets and higher-order multiples are delivered preterm. Preeclampsia, maternal anemia, gestational diabetes, placental abnormalities, fetal growth restriction, malpresentations, abruption, cord prolapse, fetal death, and maternal hemorrhage are all more likely with multiple gestations. The risk of congenital anomalies and developmental defects are doubled for each twin and more than doubled for monozygotic twins and higher-order multiples.

Potential intrapartum complications include malpresentations (especially breech), cord prolapse abruption, dysfunctional labor, and postpartum hemorrhage. The problems encountered with a breech delivery may be inherent because more than half of multiple births involve at least one breech, and there is the possibility that the first twin may lock heads with the second during delivery, making vaginal birth impossible.

Identical twins can grow in separate amniotic sacs or, more rarely, share a sac. The latter situation is potentially risky to the twins, because of the likelihood of cord entanglement. Identical twins may also share placental blood vessels that can lead to growth discordance—one twin is engorged with a superabundance of blood, the other is wasted and anemic from insufficient circulation. In this case both infants are usually very ill at birth. Sometimes one twin will die *in utero*, and the pregnancy continues with one living fetus. There have also been cases in which one twin will be miscarried, and the second continues to term.

At delivery, the majority (43%) of twins present with both babies vertex, which is also the presentation most favorable for vaginal delivery. In the hospital, many obstetricians choose vaginal delivery over cesarean section when both twins are vertex. Even under the most favorable circumstances, vaginal twin delivery can be complicated by abruption of the second placenta after delivery of the first twin, cord prolapse, and hemorrhage before, during, or following the delivery of the second twin.

The twin with the presenting part closest to the cervix is termed twin A. Thirty-eight percent present with twin A vertex and twin B nonvertex, whereas 19% present with twin A nonvertex and twin B either vertex or nonvertex. In a hospital situation, cesarean delivery is the method of choice if the first twin is nonvertex.

The EMS provider who encounters a twin delivery in the field is forced to cope with the situation as it presents. Often the babies are premature and malpresented, and may have birth defects. The mother may have had no prenatal care and may be entirely unaware that she is carrying twins.

If twin delivery is imminent and you must deliver in the field, get help, preferably advanced life support. Both babies may need resuscitation, and the mother may hemorrhage. If the infants are obviously not the same size (discordant growth), both are extremely likely to

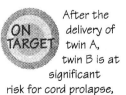

After the delivery of twin A, twin B is at significant risk for cord prolapse, placental abruption, or malpresentation.

develop respiratory distress, intracranial hemorrhage, seizures, and other complications.

Deliver the twins as you would individual infants, being especially gentle with delicate premature babies. Usually the second twin will deliver within 15–20 minutes of the first. You will need a set of infant resuscitation equipment for each baby, including cord clamps, baby hats, and endotracheal tubes, suction catheters, oxygen delivery equipment, neonatal resuscitation bags, blankets, and the like. The most critical time follows the delivery of the twin A, when the second is still *in utero*. Once his sibling has vacated the uterus, twin B is at significant risk for cord prolapse, placental abruption, or maneuvering into an undeliverable malpresentation such as transverse. If twin B is larger than twin A, the cervix might not be sufficiently dilated to accommodate the second baby after the birth of the first. In some cases the cervix recluses after the birth of the first twin.

Use caution when cutting the cord. There have been instances in which the cord of the second twin was tight several times around the neck of the first twin, and in cutting it to free twin A, the birth attendant cut off circulation to twin B still *in utero*. Be sure to clamp the cord twice before cutting—if the twins share placental circulation, allowing the cord to drain after cutting might exsanguinate the twin still *in utero*.

Fetal Demise and Stillbirth

Stillbirth is usually defined as fetal death that occurs after 20 weeks of pregnancy. Up to half occur unexpectedly with low-risk mothers. Fourteen percent of fetal deaths take place during the intrapartum period, and 86% happen antepartally. In some situations, the mother is aware that she carries a dead fetus, although she might not be emotionally prepared for the birth. In other situations, stillbirth is an unexpected shock. A woman who has carried a dead fetus *in utero* for more than 2 weeks is at increased risk for DIC and sepsis.

The most common known causes for stillbirth include

- **Placental problems and cord accidents.** These include abruption and placental insufficiency, cord vessel hemorrhage, and cord compression.

- **Congenital anomalies.** Between 5 and 10% of stillborn babies have chromosomal abnormalities, and others have structural malformations that can result from genetic, environmental, or unknown causes.

- **Growth restriction.** Babies who are growth restricted are at increased risk of death both antepartally and intrapartally, and from unknown causes.

- **Infections.** Bacterial infections are an important cause of fetal deaths that occur between 24 and 27 weeks of gestation, often without symptoms in the mother.

A dead fetus has no muscular tone and may present brow or face first. He may demonstrate extreme molding of the head. The skin begins to peel as soon as a day or two after death, and the provider should be extremely careful not to tear the fragile skin during delivery. (Treating the baby with sensitivity and preserving his appearance as well as possible can be very important to grieving parents.)

Most infants who show no signs of life should still receive full resuscitation efforts. Resuscitation may be withheld, however, if the infant is macerated (softened, with sloughing skin) or if there is a lack of vital signs in conjunction with some profound anomaly obviously incompatible with life (such as an open skull with much of the brain missing). In some cases it will be clear that the fetus is too premature for resuscitation efforts. If the delivery is not witnessed, obtain a complete history en route and establish the time frame of the birth. If the infant is clearly dead, follow local protocols for pronouncement of death and transport procedures.

The EMS provider is not a counselor, but compassionate emotional support can be invaluable in helping bereaved parents cope with the loss of a child.

The EMS provider cannot bring a stillborn infant back to life, but compassionate emotional support can be invaluable in helping the bereaved parents through this crisis. Be honest and forthright. Do not avoid conversation because you feel uncomfortable or are afraid of saying the wrong thing, but beware of empty platitudes. It is appropriate simply to say, "I'm sorry for your loss."

Nearly anything you may say with the intent of making them feel better will miss the mark. You cannot make them feel better. Do not tell the parents that you know how they feel. You do not, even if you have lost a child of your own. Do not tell them what they should feel or do. Do not reassure them that they can have another baby or that it is God's plan. If they ask you questions that you cannot answer, such as what are the chances of this happening again, be honest and say that you do not know.

You can, however, let them cry. You can even cry with them. Encourage them to talk if they want to. Attend to their physical needs. If the parents want to hold their baby in the field, let them. Wrap the baby in a blanket and place a cap upon his head, taking care not to tear his fragile skin in the process. At all times handle the stillborn infant as gently and respectfully as if he were alive, supporting the head and cradling the body. Living or not, he is someone's child. Most hospitals will provide grief counseling for the parents to help them cope with their loss. Parents are often encouraged to hold and name the stillborn infant and are given keepsakes such as footprints, photographs, or a lock of hair. Most parents who have suffered losses report deep appreciation for sensitive, caring attention from professionals at the time of their loss.

Summary

Although most births are uneventful, maternal and fetal complications may arise at any time with no warning. The EMS professional should avoid interfering in natural processes, but stand ready to act decisively and swiftly if complications arise.

REVIEW QUESTIONS

1. How should the EMS provider manage uterine atony in the field?

2. List risk factors for breech presentation.

3. You arrive at a restroom to find a multiparous woman involuntarily pushing. Her water broke 30 minutes ago. You check for crowning and see a male infant's swollen, purple bottom presenting. What do you do?

4. Upon examining the perineum of a pregnant woman with rupture of membranes, you see a loop of umbilical cord at the introitus and no signs of imminent delivery. What should you do?

5. Describe field management of a shoulder presentation.

CHAPTER 8

Postpartum Adaptation

Objectives

By the end of this chapter you should be able to

- Distinguish between normal involution and subinvolution

- Manage the patient with postpartum infection

- Recognize the obstetrical patient at risk for thromboembolism

- Understand the degrees of severity of postpartum depression

- Initiate breastfeeding in the healthy mother and infant

CASE Study

Throughout their EMS careers, Latitia and Maki had longed to deliver a baby in the field. They were overjoyed to find their patient actively pushing when they answered a call for "possible delivery." Kayleigh was unafraid of the pain, radiant, and working with her body beautifully. Latitia supported the perineum as the infant's head slowly emerged, and then Kayleigh spontaneously reached down and completed the delivery, bringing her new daughter up onto her own chest.

The infant looked her mother full in the face with an expression of fascination, as if she found the birth experience extremely *interesting*. She didn't cry, but began to breathe immediately and grew very pink, looking around as if she wanted to understand what had just happened to her. Latitia tucked a dry towel around the infant, leaving her skin-to-skin with her mother for warmth, the cord still uncut, while Maki prepared the stretcher for transport. Latitia severed the cord after it had ceased pulsing, then delivered the placenta. After the placenta emerged, blood began to flow rapidly from Kayleigh's vagina, streaming from her body and pooling beneath her hips.

The baby was pink, alert, and stable, so Latitia bundled her in a blanket and handed her to her father. Maki explained what she was about to do, then vigorously massaged Kayleigh's fundus through her abdominal wall. Kayleigh screamed in pain. Her uterus was soft and un-contracted, and blood was flowing so rapidly it was beginning to drip off the bed. Projecting an attitude of utter calm, Maki continued her vigor-ous massage, but the uterus did not respond.

Questions

1. What should Maki and Latitia do next to control Kayleigh's bleeding? (Local protocols allow them to use medication to control postpartum hemorrhage.)
2. What are risk factors for postpartum hemorrhage?
3. What are the most common causes of postpartum hemorrhage?
4. How long after delivery may postpartum hemorrhage occur?

Introduction

Delivery does not end the reproductive experience for a new mother. Recovery from even an uncomplicated pregnancy and birth is not al-ways short or simple. Numerous physical and emotional complications may occur unexpectedly, and the consequences may be serious. Conditions such as preeclampsia and cardiac disease may worsen in the hours imme-diately postpartum. Others, such as hemorrhage, may arise immediately following delivery or several weeks later. The prehospital provider must guard against the relief and sense of anticlimax that understandably follow as dramatic an event as childbirth. Continued vigilance is indicated after any birth, because the potential for postpartum difficulties is significant.

The EMS provider may assume care for a postpartum woman immedi-ately after delivery, or she may call days or weeks later with a postpar-tum complication. Most women who have had normal vaginal deliveries are discharged from the hospital by 2 days postpartum, and most ce-sarean section patients are home within 3 days. Out-of-hospital birthing centers often discharge patients a few hours after delivery. Women who deliver at home with midwives or lay attendants are usually supervised for several hours, then left in the care of family and friends with in-structions to call if problems present.

Physical Changes

puerperium
The time interval
lasting from child-
birth to the return
of normal uterine
size, about 6 weeks.

The postpartum period, or **puerperium,** begins with delivery and continues about 6 weeks. At the end of this phase, the uterus will have returned to its nonpregnant size. If the woman is not breastfeeding, her
hormonal balance has often reestablished itself. Aside from lactation and
changes in skin and weight, by 6 weeks postpartum the woman's body
has essentially returned to its prepregnant state.

Pulse, blood pressure, and temperature are typically slightly elevated after delivery, but normalize to prepregnant levels within a few
days. Urine output and sweating often increase as the woman diureses
excess fluid maintained during pregnancy.

The Uterus after Delivery

Involution is return of the uterus to normal size after childbirth.
Immediately after delivery, the uterus can be palpated through the
abdominal wall, usually at 2 or 3 finger breadths below the umbilicus. By 6–8 hours after delivery, the fundus rises to the level of
the umbilicus. Thereafter, it descends toward the pelvis at a rate of
1 finger breadth per day, becoming nonpalpable by day 10 after delivery. Breastfeeding accelerates this process by stimulating uterine
contractions.

The Fundus and Hemostasis

When the placenta shears off the uterine wall, the uterus contracts into
a hard mass, effectively squeezing shut the open vessels that once perfused the placenta. The most common cause of excessive postpartum
bleeding is uterine atony, or failure to contract.

After delivery, the birth attendant should palpate the fundus of the uterus through the abdominal wall and assess it for firmness.

After delivery, the birth attendant should palpate the fundus of the uterus through the abdominal wall and assess it for firmness. If the woman is fairly thin and the uterus is very hard, it will be easily palpated as a grapefruit-sized mass just below the umbilicus. If the woman is heavy, it may be harder to determine whether the uterus is firm. If she is bleeding heavily and no firm mass is felt, atony may be assumed; sometimes, however, blood will pool within the uterus or vagina, and external bleeding will not be immediately apparent. If no fundus is felt, or if it feels soft and dough-like, brace the uterus with one hand above the pubic bone and firmly massage the abdomen from umbilicus to a few inches above the pubis to trigger uterine contraction. Fundal massage is painful to the woman, so be sure to explain the necessity of the procedure and show concern for her discomfort. Once the fundus feels firm and bleeding is controlled, it is helpful to teach the woman to massage her own fundus periodically to maintain contraction between your assessments. Any time the woman experiences a gush from the vagina, assess bleeding, recheck the fundus, and massage if necessary.

Afterpains

Persistent painful uterine cramping is more likely to occur in the multiparous woman. The primiparous woman's uterus tends to contract evenly. The uterus of the woman who has borne children before tends to contract, relax, and contract again. These **afterpains** can be very uncomfortable for several days after delivery and may be more intense while nursing the baby.

afterpains
Uterine cramps during the first few days after childbirth.

Lochia

As the uterus heals and cleans itself, the woman experiences bleeding referred to as lochia. **Lochia** changes appearance as the uterus clears out the old epithelial cells, blood cells, and fetal substances such as meconium, lanugo, and vernix.

Lochia rubra begins shortly after birth and is a dark-red flow resembling the first day of a heavy menstrual period. Initially, lochia rubra is fairly heavy and very red. Large gushes are to be expected when the recumbent mother stands, and the pooled blood in her vagina rushes out. Similar gushes are experienced when breastfeeding contracts the uterus. As long as the blood flow slows or stops between episodes, it is considered normal. A flow that continues steadily indicates a hemorrhage.

lochia
Liquid discharged from the vagina after childbirth, containing primarily blood, cellular debris, mucus, and fetal substances such as meconium, lanugo, and vernix.

The passage of small clots is normal. Large clots can be acceptable if bleeding stops after they are passed. Often the uterus will relax somewhat, and blood will pool within, then clot. The uterus will cramp painfully in an attempt to expel the clot. Clots may be very large, often the size of a plum or larger. Usually the uterus will contract effectively after passing the clot, and cramps and bleeding will cease.

By the 2nd or 3rd day postpartum, most women experience a lighter, pinkish, serous flow that continues until about day 10. Lochia alba, a whitish or brownish discharge, continues for the next week or two. Lochia should smell meaty and musty, like menses.

Sometimes the woman will report that her bleeding has almost stopped, then suddenly she begins to bleed a moderate red flow that stops on its own. Often this flow is related to the woman's overexerting herself. If questioned, she may report heavy lifting or restarting an exercise program. Consider that red bleeding beyond 4 weeks may be resumption of the woman's menstrual cycles.

Breastfeeding women do not usually menstruate for at least 6 months after delivery, but some begin as early as 5 weeks. Most bottle-feeding women return to normal cycling between 5 and 12 weeks postpartum and may conceive the next baby as early as 5–6 weeks postpartum—remember to consider spontaneous abortion and implantation bleeding as possible causes of postpartum bleeding.

Subinvolution

subinvolution
Failure of the uterus to return to its prepregnant size after delivery, often because of retained placental fragments or infection.

Subinvolution is a failure of the uterus to revert to its normal size after delivery. This failure may be due to infection or retained placental fragments. If lochia rubra continues for more than 2 weeks, the woman may become significantly anemic, evidencing fatigue, pallor, headache, and orthostatic hypotension. Foul-smelling lochia, abdominal tenderness, and a fever may indicate infection.

Uterus Displaced by Full Bladder

If the fundus is palpated in the right upper quadrant, the woman probably has a full bladder. Postpartum women cannot always identify the need to urinate and may be unaware of a distended bladder. Swelling of the vulva following a long pushing stage or extensive tissue trauma can obstruct urination. A full bladder displaces the uterus upward and to the right and can cause bleeding by preventing effective contraction. See Figure 8-1. In this case, help the woman onto a bedpan or have her urinate on a stack of towels or underpads. Steady slow-trickle bleeding is often helped by urinating in an upright posture, which will help to dislodge clots that may be preventing effective uterine contraction. (Any time you position a postpartum woman in an upright position, watch

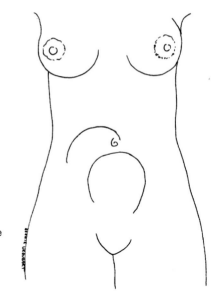

FIGURE 8-1
Uterus Displaced by Full Bladder.
When the fundus is palpable high in the right upper quadrant, the postpartum woman usually needs to empty her bladder.
Illustration by Bonnie U. Gruenberg

for syncope, hypotension, or dizziness. Lay her back down if she becomes hemodynamically unstable.)

Late Postpartum Hemorrhage

EMS professionals may receive calls for postpartum bleeding anytime in the 2 months following delivery. Retained placental fragments may cause bleeding weeks after the birth and can cause life-threatening hemorrhage. Often this bleeding is unexpected, sudden, and copious. Treat as you would manage hemorrhage that immediately follows delivery (see postpartum hemorrhage in Chapter 7).

Large clots with an increase in bleeding could indicate retained placental fragments, which may cause severe hemorrhage. Surgical **dilation and curettage** (D&C) is required for removal of retained placental parts.

If the woman reports soaking a superabsorbency pad in an hour or less for several hours, her bleeding is potentially serious and should be evaluated immediately in the emergency department.

The Vagina and Vulva

The vagina is often bruised and edematous after delivery. Lacerations may occur on the perineum, labia, periurethral area, vagina, or cervix and may extend to the rectum. Shallow abrasions are very common on the inner surface of the labia minora. Persistent tricking of blood after delivery may prove to be from a small but significant torn vessel. If you

dilation and curettage
A surgical procedure in which the cervix is dilated and the lining of the uterus is scraped with a curette, usually performed to obtain tissue samples, to stop abnormal bleeding, to remove placental fragments after childbirth, or as a method of abortion.

localize the source of the bleeding to a laceration, apply a dressing or sanitary pad and hold pressure with an ice pack. *Never pack the vagina.*

Some women have cosmetically pierced labia or clitoral hoods. Stretching during childbirth can create lacerations at the site of these piercings, especially if the jewelry is not removed.

Hematoma

Sometimes the stretching and tearing of the vagina damages blood vessels below the surface, and large painful hematomas can develop in the vagina, vulva, or subperitoneal space. These can develop rapidly and can contain as much as 250–500 cc of blood. Be alert for hypovolemia, because a significant volume of blood can be sequestered within these tissues. Risk factors for hematoma include PIH, first baby, precipitous delivery, vulvar varicosities, or a very large baby. These hematomas may be surgically evacuated or, if small, left to be absorbed on their own. Ice packs may provide some comfort if a hematoma is suspected. The woman may require an indwelling urinary catheter once she gets to the hospital, because the swelling can occlude the urethra and prevent bladder emptying.

Hemorrhoids

Severe hemorrhoids may develop during pregnancy or delivery. Sometimes these anal varicosities become thrombosed (develop blood clots within them) and prompt a call for emergency transport due to extreme pain and the woman's resulting inability to sit in a car. An ice pack can decrease pain and swelling during transport, and a side-lying position is most comfortable.

Postpartum Infections

Postpartum infection occurs in 1–8% of postpartum patients, usually developing in the uterus, breast, urinary tract, or perineal wounds. Women are more likely to develop infections if the immune system is impaired by smoking, diabetes, obesity, stress, anxiety, alcohol or drug abuse, or poor nutrition.

endometritis
Inflammation of the endometrium (the mucous membrane lining the uterus), usually caused by infection.

Endometritis

Endometritis is infection of the uterine lining, most commonly from vaginal or rectal microorganisms that have ascended into the uterus. Risk factors include prolonged rupture of amniotic membranes before delivery, certain vaginal infections, many examinations during labor, cesarean delivery, or invasive procedures such as manual removal of the placenta.

Endometritis can develop anytime during the first 10 days following delivery. It is evidenced by a temperature over 100.4°F, usually 101°–104°F, bloody, foul-smelling discharge, tachycardia, chills, and abdominal tenderness. Milder presentations are also seen, with low-grade fever, persistent bleeding for 6 weeks or more after delivery, a tender uterus that is still palpable in the abdomen weeks after delivery, malaise, and lack of appetite. Infection with group B hemolytic streptococcus may present with scant lochia and without the characteristic foul odor.

Postpartum women can uncommonly develop pelvic cellulitis, a serious infection of the connective tissue of the pelvis. Postpartum peritonitis can also occur, which may evolve into pelvic abscess. Although this condition may be indistinguishable from endometritis to the prehospital provider, the woman will be clearly ill.

Genital Wound Infection

episiotomy
An incision through the vagina, perineum, and underlying muscles to facilitate delivery.

Lacerations and abrasions are common in childbirth, and **episiotomy** is frequently performed by some obstetrical professionals. Childbirth is usually accompanied by defecation and urination and may occur in less-than-clean settings, yet infection of genital wounds is very rare. American women are usually instructed to spray the perineum with a water bottle for days or weeks after delivery to cleanse the healing wounds and provide comfort.

Surprisingly few women suffer infection of perineal wounds. Infection is most likely to occur in the woman whose healing mechanisms are impaired. The woman with a perineal infection will often report severe pain, redness, swelling, and drainage from the wound. Treatment consists of opening and draining the wound, then surgical reapproximation after infection is eliminated.

Cesarean Wound Infection

During cesarean section, the surgeon incises many layers of tissue, including the uterus itself. The infection rate after cesarean delivery is 4–12%, and the woman may not develop symptoms until after discharge from the hospital. As with other wound infections, pain, swelling, redness, oozing, odor, gaping wound edges, and fever may be present.

Postpartum Urinary Tract Infections

Urinary tract infections can occur after childbirth. Because the bladder is often compressed and bruised by the descending fetal head, and because of swelling of pelvic structures, many postpartum women do not recognize the sensation of a full bladder. After childbirth women may delay voiding to avoid irritating raw, sore genitals. Some women are catheterized during or after delivery, a procedure that can introduce infection into the bladder.

cystitis
Inflammation of
the urinary blad-
der, often caused
by infection.

The symptoms of **cystitis**—urinary frequency, urgency, and pain with voiding—typically appear 2 or 3 days postpartum, although they can occur at any time. If it is untreated, bacteria can move from the bladder to the kidney and cause pyelonephritis. Although a kidney infection may also produce these symptoms, its usual signs and symptoms are systemic, including high fever, chills, nausea, and vomiting, with flank pain and costovertebral angle tenderness. Whereas cystitis can usually be treated with oral antibiotics, pyelonephritis usually requires hospitalization and intravenous antibiotics.

Mastitis

mastitis
Inflammation of
the connective tis-
sue in the breast,
usually caused by
bacterial infection.

Mastitis is an infection of the connective tissue within the breast. It can occur anytime during lactation, but usually after the 2nd to 4th week postpartum. The causative microorganisms typically come from the baby's mouth (or the mother's unwashed hands) and move deeper into the breast if the mother's milk is not flowing well. Sometimes the woman has been too busy or ill to feed her baby frequently, and milk distends the breasts. Cracked nipples can allow bacteria easier access to the breast. Fatigue, stress, and poor hygiene may contribute to the development of mastitis.

The woman with a breast infection will be acutely ill. Within a few hours the condition will progress from breast fullness and soreness to systemic fever, vomiting, headache, body aches, and a red, hard area somewhere on the breast. Do not palpate this area—palpation serves no purpose and causes extreme pain. The woman should continue to breastfeed frequently from the affected breast. Infection is less likely to progress to abscess, and symptoms will improve more quickly, if the breast is kept empty. The causative organisms pose no risk to the baby, because they may have come from his mouth to begin with.

Candida albicans
A fungus responsi-
ble for many vagi-
nal yeast infections.

Candida albicans, or yeast, can also cause very painful breast infections, but this condition seldom presents with systemic symptoms. Yeast breast infections are usually bilateral and characterized by shooting pains in the nipple, followed by a broken-glass sensation deep within the breast for hours after a feeding. Certain women are susceptible to yeast infections, and they can be difficult to eradicate, requiring treatment at intervals through the period of lactation.

Prehospital Care of the Postpartum Patient with Infection

The EMS professional who transports a postpartum patient with a suspected systemic infection should start an intravenous line of lactated Ringer's or normal saline, administer a 300–500 cc bolus, then reduce the infusion rate to 125 cc per hour. Sepsis and shock are uncommon but significant complications. Oxygen by nasal cannula at 4 L per minute and cardiac monitoring are in order. For localized infections, treat as vital signs indicate.

Thrombophlebitis

The blood of a pregnant woman clots more readily than that of a non-pregnant woman; pregnancy is a **hypercoagulable state.** Increased ability to clot provides some protection from hemorrhage at delivery but can also contribute to venous thrombosis, the formation of a blood clot in a vein, usually in the lower extremities. If a clot in a deep vessel is dislodged or part of it breaks off, it can travel to the lungs and cause a pulmonary embolism. Embolism is a leading cause of maternal deaths, responsible for about 20% of mortalities.

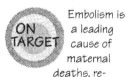

Embolism is a leading cause of maternal deaths, responsible for about 20% of mortalities.

Thromboembolic disease may occur during pregnancy, but it develops more commonly during the postpartum period. Increased levels of clotting factors in the blood, obesity, high parity, anesthesia and surgery, inactivity and prolonged bedrest, hypertension, endometritis, varicosities, and a history of venous thrombosis increase the risk. Thrombus formation may occur in a superficial (surface) or deep vessel. Mild cases may present with local heat, redness, pain, and swelling. Deep-vein thrombosis (DVT) is often more serious and may present with swelling of the distal extremity, fever, and pain. Thromboses can also form in the iliac arteries of the pelvis, causing pain in the lower abdomen. Homan's sign (pain on dorsiflexion of the foot) may or may not be positive with deep-vein thrombosis.

Transport the patient with suspected DVT on oxygen, with the extremity elevated, and with cardiac monitoring. Do not let the patient ambulate. Initiate an IV of lactated Ringer's or normal saline. If the patient is febrile, administer a 300–500 cc bolus, then reduce the infusion rate to 125 cc per hour.

Pulmonary Embolism

Pulmonary embolism (PE) is a common result of deep-vein thrombosis, and the majority of cases are unrecognized clinically. This condition may present during pregnancy or postpartum. Some women with PE present with only vague complaints, and their symptoms may be attributed to normal pregnancy discomforts, or the aches and pains of a woman who has just given birth. Many pregnant women experience apprehension, chest discomfort, and shortness of breath, so it can be difficult to determine whether these symptoms indicate a more serious pathology. Many cases of PE are essentially asymptomatic; only 20% display the classic triad of hemoptysis, pleuritic chest pain, and dyspnea. Pulmonary embolism should be considered in the woman who complains of chest pain, chest-wall tenderness, back pain, shoulder pain, upper abdominal pain, syncope, any new cardiac arrhythmia, tachypnea, dyspnea, tachycardia, or apprehension. Without treatment, approximately one-third of patients who survive an initial PE, whether small or large, die of a future embolic episode.

Pulmonary embolism can be hard to diagnose in the hospital as well, and there are no absolutely definitive tests that can pinpoint the condition with accuracy. Bloodwork is usually normal, as are chest X rays and EKGs. Even the most useful diagnostic modality, the ventilation-perfusion (V/Q) scan, can show false negatives.

Rapid transport is essential for the patient with a suspected pulmonary embolism. Oxygen by nasal cannula at 4 L per minute is suitable for the patient in minor distress; but with dyspnea, high-flow oxygen by mask is indicated. Establish an intravenous line of normal saline at a keep-vein-open rate, and initiate cardiac monitoring. If cardiovascular collapse occurs, resuscitate as appropriate.

Postpartum Thyroiditis

Postpartum thyroiditis is an inflammation of the thyroid gland that occurs in 5–7% of women within the first year following childbirth. This condition is often asymptomatic, but some women present with signs and symptoms of hyperthyroidism for the first few months of the disease, including sensitivity to heat, unexplained weight loss, palpitations, diaphoresis, tremors, irregular menstrual bleeding, and hypertension. During the second phase of this condition, the woman will become hypothyroid, sometimes exhibiting unexplained weight gain, fatigue, sensitivity to cold, amenorrhea, and pale, dry skin. EMS providers should keep in mind that fatigue, depression, and bleeding abnormalities can result from thyroid dysfunction and consider the condition when forming a clinical impression.

Emotional Changes

Postpartum Depression

Psychiatric difficulties of many kinds may arise in the postpartum period. Twelve percent of women experience major depression within the postpartum year, and additional 19% of women experience minor depression. Postpartum depression is often multifactorial, resulting from hormonal, psychological, and lifestyle influences. Levels of the estrogen and progesterone plummet after delivery, and over the next few weeks or months the woman resumes menstrual cycles. These hormonal changes can trigger depression and emotional lability. The persistent fatigue that accompanies caring for a new infant and recovering from the physical stress of giving birth can make the early weeks very challenging. Breast-feeding can be difficult and painful if breast problems develop.

Many women spend their pregnancies imagining themselves becoming the perfect mother and can feel profoundly let down if the daily reality does not match the idealized vision. It can be shattering to a woman's self-image when she learns that parenting is not instinctive, her baby is his own person and will not always conform to her expectations, and perfection is unattainable.

Postpartum depression is more likely when these predictors are present:

- Prenatal depression or anxiety
- Child-care problems or life stress
- Relationship problems or lack of social support
- Poor self-esteem
- Low socioeconomic status
- Unwanted or unplanned pregnancy
- History of psychiatric illness
- Cranky, difficult baby (This is a reciprocal problem—having a depressed mother tends to make the baby more cranky; a cranky baby tends to depress the mother further.)

It is important to address postpartum depression for both the mother's and the baby's sake. Untreated, the woman is at risk for major depression or suicide, and her infant is at risk for abuse and neglect. And a mother's attitude toward her baby strongly influences infant behavior and development.

Postpartum Blues

About 80–85% of women experience postpartum mood instability. This condition is known as the "baby blues," and its primary cause appears to be hormonal fluctuations as the body reverts to its prepregnant state. It is characterized by short periods of emotional lability, often with no identifiable reason. The mother may also feel overwhelmed, anxious, and irritable. Between episodes of this mild depression, the mother feels happier and is able to function normally. The baby blues are usually limited to the first few days postpartum and resolve without intervention, especially when the woman understands that mood swings are to be expected after delivery. Symptoms peak on the 4th or 5th day after delivery and last for several days, but they are generally self-limited and spontaneously resolve within the first 2 postpartum weeks.

Postpartum Major and Minor Depression

Postpartum psychiatric illness was once considered a condition specific to childbearing, but recent research has suggested that it is indistinguishable from major depression that occurs in women at other times. It is characterized by persistent and intense sadness, anxiety, or despair that prevents the woman from performing essential life tasks; tearfulness; inability to enjoy pleasurable activities; insomnia; fatigue; appetite disturbance; suicidal thoughts; or recurrent thoughts of death. Women affected frequently show obsessive worry about the baby's health and well-being or conversely show a lack of attachment or express negative feelings about the infant. The woman with postpartum depression may worry or fantasize about harming or abandoning her baby. She may have trouble coping with her daily tasks. Typically, postpartum depression develops gradually over the first 3 postpartum months, although symptoms can occur with unexpected suddenness and severity anytime during the first year. Counseling and medication often successfully treat this condition.

Postpartum Psychosis

Childbirth can trigger psychotic episodes in approximately 1–2 women per 1,000 after childbirth. Postpartum psychosis usually presents abruptly as early as 48–72 hours after delivery and usually within the first 2 postpartum weeks. The woman with postpartum psychosis presents with confusion, agitation, hyperactivity, irrationality, delusions, and hallucinations. The mother may have delusional beliefs about her baby or may hear voices telling her to harm herself or her baby. Women with postpartum psychosis are at high risk for suicide and infanticide. This condition can be successfully treated with hospitalization, medication, psychotherapy, electroconvulsant therapy, and removal of the infant from danger.

PEARLS As you would any other psychiatric patient, carefully assess whether the woman with postpartum depression has plans to hurt herself or others and whether her depression has caused her to abuse her children.

As with any psychiatric patient, carefully assess whether the woman with postpartum depression has plans to hurt herself or others and whether her depression has caused her to abuse her children. Be comforting and nonjudgmental. Use restraints as indicated if she is a threat to herself or others. Report your findings to the hospital personnel so that they might appropriately follow up with psychiatric and social services.

Initiating Breastfeeding

There are many important reasons to breastfeed the infant. Breastfeeding protects the baby from many illnesses, including ear infections, respiratory infections, gastrointestinal infections, childhood cancers, and sudden infant death syndrome. Breastfeeding protects against hereditary allergic disease, obesity, diabetes, and hypertension and promotes development of the baby's jaw and teeth. Breastfeeding has even been shown to increase the infant's intelligence.

Breastfeeding benefits prehospital care by triggering uterine contractions that may reduce postpartum bleeding, especially during a long transport of a woman with a persistently boggy uterus. Putting the baby to breast can help stabilize both mother and infant. Not only will the mother's bleeding decrease, but the infant will also stay warmer and be less likely to become hypoglycemic. Skin-to-skin contact with the mother helps to regulate the infant's vital signs. Of course, breastfeeding should be attempted only if mother and infant are clinically stable.

Most mammals unerringly begin to nurse without assistance, but human breastfeeding is a learned skill for mother and baby alike. The newborn in her arms has practiced sucking *in utero* on his hands, fingers, and even his tongue and may display ingrained sucking habits from birth that can interfere with his ability to nurse. First-time mothers are often insecure and awkward about putting the baby to breast, however, and experienced mothers may find that this particular baby does not nurse the way previous children have done.

Breastfeeding is best accomplished with respect for a woman's privacy. Help the woman into a comfortable position, as upright as possible. The mother should support her breast with her hand, her fingers curved above and below the nipple in a "C" hold, her fingers well back from the **areola**. To encourage the baby to latch onto the breast, position the baby

areola
The pigmented ring around the nipple.

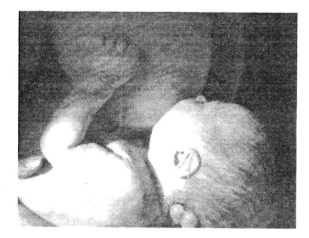

FIGURE 8-2
Latched to the Breast.
The breastfeeding baby should hold the nipple at the back of the tongue and take as much areola in his mouth as possible.
Photographed by Bonnie U. Gruenberg

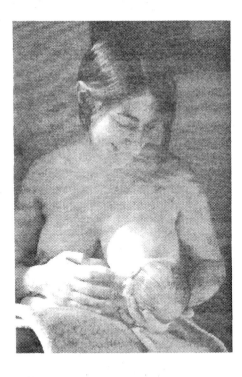

FIGURE 8-3
Breastfeeding Is Beneficial.
Breastfeeding is not only beneficial to the infant and rewarding to the woman; it also encourages the uterus to contract, making hemorrhage less likely.
Photographed by Bonnie U. Gruenberg

sideways across the mother's chest, belly in full contact with the mother. See Figure 8-2. The infant's ear, shoulder, and hip should be in alignment. If the baby will not face the breast, have the mother tickle his cheek with her nipple; he will usually turn toward the breast.

Ask the mother to tickle the baby's lips with her nipple. The baby will eventually open his mouth wide and search for the nipple. At this time, bring the baby in close until his nose and chin touch the breast. See Figure 8-3. The object is to direct the nipple to the back of the tongue and allow the baby's gums to encircle the areola. He should have as much areola in his mouth as possible. His lips should be widely flanged. If the first nursing is extremely painful to the mother, the baby is not on the breast correctly.

If the breast occludes his nose completely, lifting up the breast will usually clear the airway. A healthy baby will not passively allow himself to be smothered—if he cannot breathe, he will pull his head away from the breast.

PEARLS Do not grasp a breast in one hand and the baby in the other to establish a latch. Have the mother support her own breast and use the baby's reflexes to initiate nursing.

Although the baby may eagerly take to the breast, he is more likely to make faces, lick the nipple, try to suck his hands instead, or spit out the nipple before latching. Even this mild stimulation gets maternal hormones flowing and may reduce bleeding substantially. Many babies will latch and nurse successfully within 15–20 minutes of birth. You may allow the baby to feed on one side for as long as he is interested and then try the other side. To detach the baby, insert a gloved finger between the gums to break the suction. Monitor to make sure that the baby is breathing well, has a good pulse, and has good color while feeding. Breastfeeding should not delay transport. It can be accomplished en route after mother and infant are stabilized.

Summary

The postpartum period is usually a time for healing, familial bonding, showing off the new baby, and returning to the comfort of routine activity. The puerperium can also become physically and emotionally stressful, and a variety of conditions and complaints may arise during the postpartum period. The astute EMS provider interferes as little as possible in natural processes, while remaining on the alert for conditions that require rapid intervention.

REVIEW QUESTIONS

1. You are called to the home of a woman who is 6 hours postpartum. She has been bleeding steadily. You feel for her fundus and find it just beneath the lower margin of her right ribs. What is your clinical impression?

2. You are called for a woman 10 days postpartum who has been running a low-grade fever for days. Today she has spiked a temperature of 102.4° F. She has shaking chills, malaise, and red vaginal bleeding soaking a pad every three hours. Her fundus is 3 fingerwidths below her umbilicus and tender to the touch. What is your clinical impression, and how would you treat this patient?

3. What is lochia? Describe lochia rubra, lochia serosa, and lochia alba and the usual duration of each.

4. Describe the signs and symptoms of thrombophlebitis.

5. What are the signs and symptoms of postpartum depression?

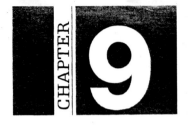

CHAPTER 9

The Neonate

Objectives

By the end of this chapter you should be able to

- Care for the newborn at delivery

- Perform a basic physical assessment of the newborn infant

- Perform a gestational age assessment of the neonate

- Manage common illnesses of the neonate in the field

- Prevent hypothermia from developing in the neonate and treat hypothermia that has already occurred

CASE Study

Susan was panting and moaning when Alison and Elijah loaded her into the ambulance for transport. She was 38 weeks pregnant and clearly in active labor. Susan was a 35-year-old gravida 3 para 2 who had developed insulin-dependent diabetes with every pregnancy, but had normal blood glucose readings when she was not pregnant. Her other two babies were over 9 lb, but had birthed easily.

Susan had presented to prenatal care at the beginning of her third trimester. Because of irregular cycles and poor record keeping, she did not know at that time how far along she was in her pregnancy. She had avoided seeking care because she dreaded the insulin injections that she knew she would require. As expected, her fasting blood sugar was 200 at her first visit, and she was started on insulin and blood glucose monitoring. An ultrasound performed at that time had dated her fetus at 28 weeks' gestation.

When it appeared that Susan was progressing quickly, Alison opened the obstetrical kit and prepared suction and oxygen. En route to the hospital, Susan delivered a baby girl who began to cry immediately, with Apgar scores of 8 and 9. At 5 minutes of life her heart rate was 160—up to 180 with crying—and her respirations were 56 per minute. The placenta showed no calcifications.

As Alison examined the infant, she took note of her physical characteristics. She guessed that the baby was about 5 lb. The infant had thin, smooth skin, and was somewhat hairy and covered thickly with vernix. Her ear cartilage was soft, but had some recoil. Her feet were mostly smooth, especially the heel. Her inner labia and clitoris protruded conspicuously from between her labia majora. She had good mobility of her limbs, but her resting tone was somewhat loose. The baby's limbs were yielding and pliant—when Alison gently drew the baby's arm across her chest until resistance was met, the elbow was slightly beyond the midline.

Questions

1. Is this baby small for gestational age or premature?

2. What are immediate concerns Alison will have in caring for this baby?

3. Diabetes can cause heart defects and other structural anomalies in the fetus. Should Alison expect this baby to have a birth defect?

4. Are this infant's vital signs in the normal range?

Introduction

neonate
An infant less than 4 weeks old.

At the time of birth, the fetus becomes a **neonate**, undergoing dramatic physical changes necessary to sustain life outside the uterus. In the first hours after delivery, the newborn stabilizes respiratory and circulatory functions, establishes feeding and elimination patterns, and finds a new homeostatic equilibrium. Most full-term neonates need little more than supportive care, but deviations from normal processes can quickly become life threatening. Every newborn therefore requires close observation.

The EMS professional must become familiar with the physical, physiological, and behavioral characteristics of the normal newborn to promote and facilitate a normal transition to extrauterine life. It is also essential to recognize pathological processes so that appropriate intervention can be initiated. By evaluating the infant's history, gestational age, physical features, behavior, and physiology, the prehospital provider can assess how well the infant is making the transition to extrauterine life and anticipate problems that may arise.

KEY TERMS

biophysical profile, p. 238

caput succedaneum, p. 232

fontanelles, p. 232

hyperbilirubinemia, p. 230

kernicterus, p. 230

lanugo, p. 236

milia, p. 231

neonate, p. 226

nonstress test (NST), p. 238

periodic breathing, p. 228

postmaturity syndrome, p. 237

uteroplacental insufficiency, p. 237

Care of the Newborn at Delivery

ON TARGET *Attending to the infant's basic needs immediately after delivery circumvents most life-threatening problems.*

Most babies are healthy and vigorous at birth and make the transition from fetus to neonate uneventfully. Attending to the infant's basic needs immediately after delivery circumvents most life-threatening problems. Whenever possible, the infant should be delivered into a warm environment and protected from heat loss. After the infant emerges, place him on a blanket or towel that you have draped over the maternal abdomen. If the cord is intact and pulsing, he is still receiving oxygen from his mother. Suction the fluids from his mouth and nose. Vigorously dry the baby with warm towels or blankets, then place a cap on his head to retain warmth. He may start breathing and crying immediately or may appear momentarily stunned. Firmly but gently rub his back and the soles of his feet. Most babies will be breathing and perfusing well, pink, and responsive by 1 minute of age.

Apgar Scoring

The Apgar scoring system provides a framework for assessing how well the infant is adapting to extrauterine life. Five characteristics and behaviors are scored at the ages of 1 and 5 minutes. Apgar scores say little about the child's overall health, however. Many mentally handicapped infants have excellent Apgar scores; and many healthy, normal children have started life with poor Apgars.

Resuscitation should not be delayed or interrupted to obtain Apgar scores. Rather, as the responder stimulates and suctions the infant, he or she should note whether the infant has a good pulse and whether he is breathing or crying, pink or cyanotic, limp or kicking and flailing. The Apgar score can be tabulated later, after the infant is stable.

Table 9-1 Neonatal Vital Signs	
Heart rate	120–160 beats per minute
Respiration	30–60 respirations per minute
Axillary temperature	97.5–99.0°F (36.4–37.2°C)
Rectal temperature	97.8–99.0°F (36.6–37.2°C)
Blood pressure at birth	80–60/45–40 mmHg

Healthy babies usually have initial Apgars of 7–10. Apgars of 4–6 indicate mild depression, and Apgars of 0–3 denote severe depression with a need for full resuscitation.

In the minutes following birth, the EMS provider should scan the infant for obvious anomalies. Is he alert and responding to stimuli? Is he moving his arms and legs equally? Document any deviations from normal.

Vital Signs

The neonate's heart and respiratory rates are greater than those of an older child, and his blood pressure is lower. See Table 9-1. The newborn's heart rate should always remain above 100 beats per minute, and it usually remains in the fetal range of 120–160. A neonate breathes about 30–60 times a minute, and crackles (rales) are not uncommon in the first minutes of life. **Periodic breathing** is a respiratory pattern considered normal for many babies, consisting of short pauses in respiration lasting up to 12 seconds (without bradycardia or oxygen desaturation) followed by a burst of faster breaths. Cyanosis of the face and trunk, gasping, and grunting indicate respiratory compromise. It is normal for a newborn's hands and feet to be pale or even blue; only central cyanosis indicates a problem. Facial bruising can resemble cyanosis—if you are unsure, look closely at the color of the mucous membranes of the mouth and watch the infant for other signs of respiratory distress. The average blood pressure in the first day of life is 72/47 for a full-term infant and 64/39 for a preterm infant. Blood pressure can increase 20 mmHg with crying. Typically, the neonate's blood pressure is not measured in the field.

periodic breathing
Intervals of rapid respiration interspersed with very slow breathing and pauses.

Physical Assessment of the Newborn

Normal healthy newborns do not much resemble the chubby, smiling babies depicted in formula or diaper commercials. It is important to recognize which features are considered normal in a newborn infant in order

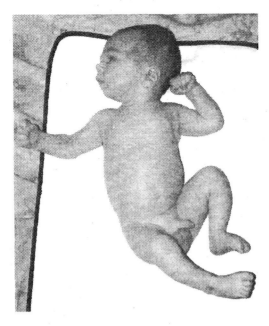

FIGURE 9-1
Tonic Neck Reflex.
The asymmetric tonic neck reflex is a normal newborn reflex that causes the infant to extend the arm and the leg on the side of the body to which his head is turned and flex the limbs on the opposite side. This reflex prevents him from rolling over until about 3–4 months of age, when he is neurologically ready for rolling.
Photographed by Bonnie U. Gruenberg

to better recognize pathology. The full-term newborn infant is generally between 5.0 and 10.5 lb. Many newborns lose up to 10% of birth weight during the first 3 to 5 days of life, then regain their birth weight by the seventh day. Subsequent weight gain is usually about 25–30 g per day for the first 3 months. Approximately one-fourth of the total body length is head. The limbs usually maintain an attitude of flexion. Babies born in a face or frank breech position may maintain these positions for days after birth. See Figures 9-1 and 9-2.

The Skin

A newborn's skin should be smooth, creamy, and opaque. If it is thin and red, the infant may be premature. A baby with pale skin and mucous membranes may be hypovolemic, perhaps from a tight cord or placental abruption.

Jaundice is common in newborns. Physiologic jaundice peaks at day 4 of life and affects about half of all newborns to some extent. The fetus has extra red blood cells in utero to pick up as much oxygen as possible from his mother. After birth, these extra red cells are no longer needed and are destroyed by the body. A by-product is the yellow pigment bilirubin, which must be metabolized by the liver and excreted in the urine and feces.

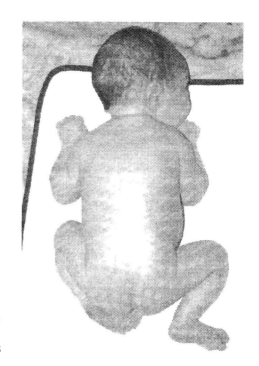

FIGURE 9-2
Crawling Reflex.
The neonate will draw up his
legs and attempt to crawl when
placed prone.
Photographed by Bonnie U. Gruenberg

hyperbilirubinemia
Elevated levels of
bilirubin (a by-
product of the
breakdown of red
blood cells) in the
newborn's blood,
often evidenced by
jaundice.

A baby with an immature liver, excessive bruising from birth, or poor feeding is more likely to develop **hyperbilirubinemia**—elevated blood levels of bilirubin that increase over the first days of life until the liver is able to process it. Jaundice can also be caused by maternal–fetal blood incompatibilities, neonatal hepatitis, biliary atresia, bacterial infection, metabolic disease, or other causes.

If bilirubin levels are high enough, brain damage can result, but in most cases the infant is able to handle his bilirubin load without assistance. Babies with high bilirubin levels are kept under blue "bili-lights" to help them break down and excrete bilirubin. To check for jaundice, press the baby's forehead or sternum with your finger for 5 seconds, then lift. Before the capillaries refill, the blanched skin will appear yellowish in a jaundiced baby. Yellowness can also be noted in the whites of the eyes. Use good light when checking for jaundice. Meconium can also stain the skin yellow or green.

kernicterus
Irreversible brain
damage caused by
hyperbilirubinemia.

A baby with significant jaundice who is hard to wake and feeding poorly needs to be evaluated immediately at a hospital before brain damage or other morbidity occurs. Severe jaundice can result in **kernicterus** (irreversible damage of brain tissue by bilirubin), which is one cause of cerebral palsy. Any jaundice in an infant less than 24 hours old is potentially serious. A baby born with jaundice needs rapid evaluation for blood disorders and other serious problems.

- **Cyanosis.** The fetus is usually somewhat purple *in utero;* but after a few seconds of crying at birth, he should rapidly turn pink. It is normal for the hands and feet to remain blue or pale for hours after delivery. The face and mucous membranes should be pink. A bluish face and trunk—central cyanosis—denotes inadequate oxygenation.

  Sometimes the infant will have bruising on its face, especially after a rapid delivery. This should not be confused with cyanosis. When in doubt, check the color of the mucous membranes inside the mouth.

- **Vernix caseosa.** A coating of vernix caseosa thickly coats the skin at 35 weeks' gestation, usually decreasing with gestational age until it remains only in creases by the due date. Some babies are so thickly frosted in vernix at birth that it is necessary to wipe it away to let them open their eyes. If stained with meconium, the vernix may be green or yellow. Vernix is best left in place so that it might absorb into the skin, moisturizing and protecting it.

milia
Pinhead-sized lesions across the nose, forehead, and cheeks of an infant caused by sebaceous glands blocked with vernix.

- **Skin lesions.** It is common for babies to have skin pores blocked by vernix, called milia. **Milia** are visible as pinhead-sized lesions across the nose, forehead, and cheeks. Babies can also have enlarged sebaceous glands that resemble acne.

- **Erythema toxicum.** This newborn rash appears between 2 and 10 days after birth. It has the appearance of flea bites and can been seen anywhere on the infant. Its cause it unknown, but it seems to be a skin reaction to clothing.

- **Mongolian spots.** These blue or purple spots are usually found over the lumbar or sacral area. They are more common in dark-skinned infants, but occur in 5–10% of Caucasian infants. They can be easily confused with bruising, but are benign and usually fade gradually.

- **Nevus flammeus or "stork bite."** This collection of distended capillaries is commonly seen on the nape of the neck, eyelids, forehead, and upper lip. It is a flat pink lesion with irregular borders that fades with finger pressure and darkens with crying. Most fade by 18 months, but some persist.

- **Petechiae.** Petechiae, or pinpoint hemorrhages, are sometimes seen on the face of a newborn who was born with a tight nuchal cord.

The Head

The infant's head compresses during birth in order to better fit the pelvis. This process is called molding. The suture lines (connections between the bones of the head) in an infant's skull are not fused as they are in an adult's, but instead consist of strong, flexible fibrous tissue. This structure allows bones of the head to slide over and under one another to facilitate birth, and overriding sutures may be noted in the first days of life. The newborn may have an elongated head the first day or so of life, especially if born to a primigravida.

At the intersection of the sutures are spaces called **fontanelles,** or "soft spots," which are normally slightly concave and may pulsate. The largest is the anterior fontanelle, or bregma, the diamond-shaped "soft spot" located at the junction of the coronal and sagittal sutures. The posterior fontanelle is triangle shaped and is palpated at the top and to the back of the head at the junction of the occipital bone and the two parietal bones. A bulging fontanelle can indicate abnormally high intracranial pressure, whereas a depressed fontanelle can indicate dehydration. Fontanelles are often difficult to palpate immediately after birth because of the molding of the head.

Caput succedaneum is a soft swelling at the part of the head that dilated the cervix. On most babies this will be the vertex. It feels soft and spongy; it may appear purple, and it crosses the suture lines of the skull. Cephalohematoma is a subperiosteal hemorrhage, or bleeding between the skull bone and the membrane that surrounds it. It is similar to caput succedaneum, but does not cross suture lines.

The posterior fontanelle is also easily palpated, although it is the size of a fingertip. It is triangular and found between the lambdoid and sagittal sutures.

fontanelles
Gaps between fetal and infant skull bones covered with thick connective tissue that allow the bones to overlap during birth; "soft spots."

caput succedaneum
A soft, spongy temporary swelling on the part of the baby's head that pushed open the cervix.

Eyes

Eyelids may be swollen after delivery, but most babies will open their eyes if the lights are dimmed or if you support their heads and sit them upright. Scleras are normally white, but may appear yellow in the jaundiced infant or have dramatic, but harmless, red hemorrhages (subconjunctival hemorrhage) from the pressures of birth. Iris color at birth does not reliably predict eye color later in life. Pupils should be black and not gray. Newborns do not usually produce tears in the first weeks of life.

The newborn can focus about 8–12 in., about the distance from the mother's breast to her face. Objects beyond that range are a blur. The eyes of normal newborn can follow a bright moving object.

Ears and Nose

Low-set ears can be associated with genetic problems and other abnormalities. Diabetic mothers sometimes have babies with hairy ears. Premature babies have soft, flexible ears.

Aggressive suctioning can cause overproduction of mucus and swelling of the nasal passages. The newborn infant is an obligatory nose breather.

Neck, Trunk, and Genitals

The infant's neck is short and unable to support the head for more than a few seconds. The abdomen is protuberant. Some babies have umbilical hernias.

It is normal for a newborn girl to have bloody mucous discharge from her vagina the first few days. Newborn boys often have disproportionately large genitals. Both conditions are reactions to maternal hormones in the infant's system. Lingering maternal hormones can cause babies of either sex to have swollen breasts and even milky nipple discharge. A nonretractable foreskin covers the glans of a boy's penis. If he is circumcised, the glans of the penis will be red and sore for 4–5 days after the procedure.

PEDIATRIC NOTES

A hydrocele is a pathological accumulation of serous fluid in the scrotum. Boys born with a hydrocele will have a very large, edematous scrotum that is painless and transilluminates if a penlight it held to it. Hydroceles generally decrease in size and resolve over the first year of life. Other causes of neonatal testicular swelling are testicular torsion (transillumination will be negative), scrotal abscess, testicular tumor, hematoma or infarction, or incarcerated hernia.

Extremities

The fetus spends much of his waking time *in utero* mouthing and sucking its hands, and this behavior continues after birth, especially when he is hungry. Some babies are born with sucking blisters on hands, fingers, or arms. The limbs of the newborn are usually flexed and adducted. The baby with Down syndrome may have decreased muscle tone.

Clavicular fracture is not uncommon during delivery, especially following shoulder dystocia. You may suspect a fractured clavicle if you hear a click or pop with the delivery of a shoulder (although the maternal pubic bone sometimes makes a similar popping noise as the shoulder passes beneath it). Babies with clavicle fractures are usually reluctant to move the affected arm.

Reflexes

The infant is born equipped with many reflexes, most of which help him to feed and position himself. The presence of these reflexes is a good indicator of an intact nervous system. If the infant's cheek is stroked, he will turn toward the touch and open his mouth. A newborn will open his mouth if his lips are brushed and suck anything that comes into the mouth. The infant will grasp with fingers and toes if the palm or sole is pressed with a finger. If held upright over a firm surface, he will make stepping motions.

The Moro or "startle" reflex is stimulated if the baby is jostled or feels himself falling. Sometimes a loud noise will trigger the Moro reflex. The arms spread and hands open, then the arms adduct and hands close. Often the infant cries.

Behavior

The newborn is usually alert for the first hour of two after delivery, then falls into a deep sleep for about the next 6 hours. Behavior varies with personality. Some babies cry incessantly; others are interested and alert, seldom crying at all.

Gestational Age Assessment

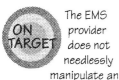

The EMS provider does not needlessly manipulate an unstable infant to determine gestational age, but instead observes characteristics while performing necessary tasks.

If gestational age is unknown, the EMS provider can roughly estimate maturity by the infant's physical appearance. Maturity develops in a linear fashion, from viability at about 24 weeks to postterm at 42 weeks. See Figure 9-3. Size is not always a reliable indicator of gestational age—a severely growth-restricted infant at term may be extremely small, and the preterm infant of an uncontrolled diabetic may be both large and physically immature.

It is possible to estimate the degree of prematurity in a small infant by observing and assessing several features. See Figure 9-4. Many of these assessments are done more appropriately in the hospital than in the field, but it is helpful for the EMS provider to understand the physical characteristics associated with prematurity.

• **Posture.**   Muscle tone improves week by week *in utero*. A very premature infant has poor tone and will passively allow any positioning of its limbs. The term infant holds arms and legs flexed tight against the body. If a limb is straightened, the term infant will actively resist or

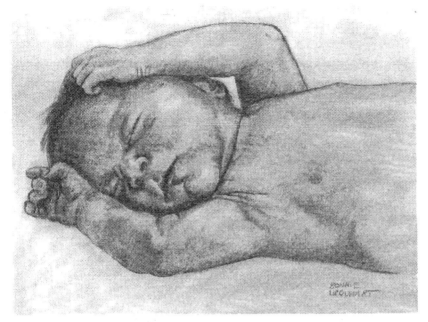

FIGURE 9-3
The Full-Term Newborn.
The full-term infant usually has plenty of subcutaneous fat, and there is little lanugo or vernix on his skin.
Illustration by Bonnie U. Gruenberg

even fight the procedure, immediately bringing the limb back into a flexed position against the body.

 PEARLS The extremely preterm infant has poor muscle tone and lies with arms and legs straight. The term infant holds arms and legs flexed tight against the body.

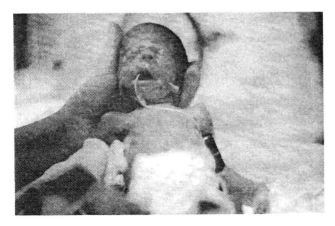

FIGURE 9-4
The Premature Newborn.
The preterm infant is small and thin-skinned and has floppy muscle tone. There is little subcutaneous fat, ear cartilage is soft, and the feet and scrotum are smooth.

The Neonate 235

• **Flexibility.** An extremely preterm infant has soft joints with weak muscles and poor tone. If his hand is grasped, his arm can be gently pulled until the elbow passes the midline of his chest. In very immature babies, it can even be draped around his neck like a scarf. A full-term baby's elbow will not cross the midline of the chest if this same maneuver is attempted. Likewise, the leg of a very early baby can be extended until the foot reaches the ear. A full-term baby cannot do this unless it was born frank breech. (In that case, intrauterine posture persists for some time after birth.) An EMS provider does not generally perform these manipulations in the field for the purpose of determining gestational age, but makes note of the infant's tone and flexibility while performing necessary tasks.

• **Skin.** The skin of a premature baby is red, transparent, prominently veined, and gelatinous at the cusp of viability. As he matures, subcutaneous tissue thickens and he adds a layer of fat beneath the skin, causing the skin to become opaque and veins to become less visible as he approaches term. The premature baby is often coated in white, pasty vernix, which diminishes in amount as he matures. The postterm baby tends to have leathery, wrinkled skin with no visible blood vessels and sometimes even deep cracks.

Premature babies are often thickly covered in downy fetal hair called **lanugo**, which serves to hold the protective vernix close to the delicate skin. Lanugo is most abundant at 28–30 weeks of gestation, then becomes sparser close to term, lost first from the face, then the trunk and limbs. Some term babies retain significant lanugo on their cheeks and upper backs.

lanugo
Fine, downy hair that covers the fetus until shortly before or after birth; especially abundant on a premature infant.

• **Feet.** The soles of an immature baby's feet are smooth and uncreased, and with advancing gestational age creases appear over distal sole, then the heel. His full-term counterpart has obvious creases over his entire sole.

• **Breast.** The extremely preterm infant has a barely perceptible nipple. The term baby has not only a pronounced nipple and areola but also palpable breast tissue beneath the surface.

• **Ear.** The very immature baby has soft ears; if folded over, they remain folded. The ears of a term baby are thicker and recoil instantly if folded.

• **Genitals.** The scrotum of a very immature boy is smooth, and the testicles have not yet descended from the body into the scrotal sac. The testes of a term boy are large and palpable within the creased, rough-skinned scrotum. A very preterm girl has a very prominent clitoris and labia minora. By term, unless she is very small for gestational age, increased body fat plumps her labia majora until they completely cover her clitoris and labia minora. If she is low birth weight, however, her labia minora and clitoris may remain exposed even if she is term.

- **Grasp.** The preterm infant has a weak grasp reflex, whereas the term baby usually grips so strongly it is possible to lift the child's shoulders from the mattress without breaking the grip.

Postmaturity

postmaturity syndrome
A condition occurring in infants of prolonged gestation (usually beyond 42 weeks) who exhibit signs of perinatal compromise related to diminished intrauterine oxygenation and nutrition resulting from placental insufficiency.

uteroplacental insufficiency
Insufficient oxygen and nutrient exchange between the uterus and the placenta.

Postmaturity syndrome is a condition of pregnancy that extends beyond 42 weeks of gestation involving an aging placenta that can no longer meet the nutritional and metabolic demands of the fetus. Without intervention, about 10% of pregnancies continue 14 or more days beyond the due date. Twenty to 40% of babies born after 42 weeks' gestation are considered postmature.

The placenta begins to age at about 36 weeks of gestation, and by 42 weeks placental function has often begun to decline. Amniotic fluid volume declines because decreased blood flow to the fetus results in less fetal urine production.

The postmature baby is at higher risk for **uteroplacental insufficiency** and cord compression, both of which can cause hypoxia. Impaired nutrition may result in fetal weight loss, causing his skin to become loose and wrinkled. The skull becomes harder and less malleable, sometimes making birth more difficult. As his bowels mature, he is increasingly likely to pass meconium into the amniotic fluid, increasing the risk for meconium aspiration syndrome. The aging placenta may be unable to sustain the fetus during the rigors of labor, increasing the risk for intrapartum asphyxia.

Often to circumvent the dangers of postterm pregnancy, many obstetrical providers induce labor whenever a woman exceeds her due date by a certain number of days or weeks. Others use fetal surveillance methods such as **biophysical profiles** and **nonstress tests** (**NST**) to monitor the growth and well-being of the unborn child. Accurate dating of the pregnancy is crucial when determining risk to the fetus and determining how best to proceed.

Common Illnesses of the Neonate

Hypoglycemia

In the full-term neonate, hypoglycemia is defined as a blood glucose level below 40 mg/dl in the first 24 hours of life and 40–50 after this. The full-term infant deposits glycogen stores in the liver, heart, and

biophysical profile
An ultrasound
exam to assess fe-
tal well-being,
which is inter-
preted alongside
the nonstress test.
During the bio-
physical profile,
the sonographer
evaluates fetal
movement, fetal
tone, breathing
movements, and
the amniotic fluid
volume.

nonstress test
(NST)
A test that assesses
fetal well-being by
graphing the fetal
heart rate while
monitoring for
uterine contrac-
tions. Reassuring
features of a fetal
heart rate include
accelerations when
the baby moves,
variability or fluc-
tuations above and
below the normal
baseline rate, and
lack of pathologi-
cal decelerations.

skeletal muscles during the last trimester of pregnancy. These stores are usually sufficient to last until regular feedings are established.

Babies who suffer respiratory distress, cold stress, infection, or other stressors may increase glucose utilization and deplete glycogen stores. If his need for glucose is greater than his ability to take feedings, his blood sugar may plummet. Premature infants and babies small for gestational age may be especially vulnerable to hypoglycemia due to increase in metabolic rate in response to heat loss and low glycogen stores. Infants large for gestational age or who were born to diabetic mothers are also vulnerable to hypoglycemia. These babies may have increased insulin levels at birth, and in the absence of frequent feedings, blood sugar may decrease precipitously.

Signs and symptoms of hypoglycemia are vague. The infant may be jittery, lethargic, hypotonic, or excessively sleepy and may show a weak or high-pitched cry, poor feeding, respiratory distress, apnea, or seizures.

Ensure an open airway and adequate oxygenation, and resuscitate as indicated by the infant's cardiopulmonary status. Determine blood glucose levels, contact medical control, and administer dextrose ($D_{10}W$ or $D_{25}W$). Keep the infant warm and transport rapidly.

Hypovolemia

Hypovolemic shock is not uncommon in the neonate, most frequently resulting from dehydration or hemorrhage. Babies may be hypovolemic following placental abruption; intracranial or intra-abdominal hemorrhage; fluid shifts as seen in sepsis, diarrhea, vomiting; or following prolonged cord compression, such as with a tight nuchal cord or after shoulder dystocia. Hypovolemic babies will show cool, pale skin, tachycardia, weak peripheral pulses, decreased urine output, lethargy, or irritability.

Early recognition and volume expansion with the intravenous fluid is the key to successful resuscitation. If hypovolemia is suspected, the EMS provider should bolus 10 mL/kg of an isotonic crystalloid solution such as Ringer's lactate or normal saline (never a solution containing dextrose) over 5–10 minutes. Reassess and consider additional boluses. The hypovolemic infant may need 40–60 mL/kg of fluid during the first hour of resuscitation, but guard against causing hypervolemia by excessive volume replacement.

Sepsis

Sepsis, or septicemia, is a bacterial infection of the bloodstream. Neonates are highly susceptible to infection, but do not react to pathogens in obvious ways as do older children and adults. Neonates often do not develop fever in response to infection, and temperature elevation above 100.4°F (38°C) can indicate a potentially life-threatening condition.

Symptoms of infection may be vague and nonspecific in the neonate, and it may be difficult to pinpoint the source. Whereas a toddler may have inflammation at the site of an infection, an infant may not. Boys are more vulnerable to infection than girls and suffer greater mortality. Premature infants are more susceptible than full-term babies, and chronically ill babies are at greater risk than their healthy counterparts. Microorganisms, many of which are resistant to antibiotics, are abundant in hospitals, so babies who have spent their early weeks in an NICU setting are at increased risk for acquiring infections that may be difficult to treat.

The microorganisms that cause diseases such as cytomegalovirus and toxoplasmosis can cross the placenta and infect the fetus. Neonatal sepsis can arise *in utero* from the ascent of bacteria after rupture of membranes, especially if prolonged. Babies may become septic following direct contact with microorganisms during birth, especially if the mother harbors group B streptococci or *E. coli* in her genital tract. The infant can contract infection though the umbilical stump, skin, mucus membranes, circumcision site, or internal systems such as the respiratory, gastrointestinal, and urinary tracts.

Early signs and symptoms of systemic neonatal infections are usually vague. The septic infant may present with lethargy and unwillingness to feed, but many babies are excessively sleepy for the first day or so after birth. Conversely, the infant may be inconsolably irritable. Tone may be poor. There may be respiratory distress or apnea, tachycardia or bradycardia, hypoglycemia, or unexplained hypothermia. The infant may appear pale or mottled. An experienced mother may report the baby "just isn't acting right." Fever is seldom present. Babies with meningitis will not show the classic nuchal rigidity (stiff neck) demonstrated by other individuals with the disease, so the provider should suspect this disease in neonates with signs of sepsis.

EMS treatment involves supportive care and maintaining stable vital signs through resuscitation and fluid therapy as appropriate. If body temperature is assessed, tympanic, rectal, or axillary sites may be appropriate—follow local protocols. Never allow a febrile infant to chill rapidly, but be careful not to increase the body temperature by overdressing the infant.

Neonatal Seizures

Seizures in the newborn often indicate significant underlying disease that may produce permanent brain damage. The most common cause of neonatal seizures is hypoxic ischemic brain injury, but seizures may also be caused by electrolyte imbalance; hypoglycemia; extremely high bilirubin levels; drug withdrawal; infections such as toxoplasmosis, herpes simplex, hepatitis, meningitis, or septicemia; brain hemorrhage; or congenital malformations, especially of the central nervous system. Any seizure in a newborn is clinically significant.

Seizures in the neonate can be subtle and seldom present as tonic-clonic activity. Owing to the immaturity of the nervous system at birth, neonatal seizures can include behaviors that are normal for a sleeping infant, such as sucking or grimacing, or they may occur with few or no observable signs. Seizures commonly involve abnormal rhythmic movements; alterations in tone such as rigidity, swimming, or bicycling movements; abnormal facial, tongue, or eye movements; and alterations in breathing pattern.

As with any seizure, ensure an open airway and adequate oxygenation. Suction if necessary, and monitor oxygen saturation with a pulse oximeter. Check glucose levels and administer dextrose ($D_{10}W$ or $D_{25}W$) for hypoglycemia. Consider consulting medical control about the use of anticonvulsants. Maintain warmth and transport rapidly. Document the physical manifestations of the seizure activity and the time they occurred.

Jitteriness

Jittery babies show tremulousness of extremities, especially with crying or stimulation. Almost half of all babies show some jitteriness in the first 4 days of life, and a provider unfamiliar with babies may wonder whether the child is seizing. Jitteriness can be distinguished from seizures by several assessments. With jittery tremors, there is no associated ocular movement; seizures usually involve the eyes. The tremors of the jittery baby can usually be stopped by flexion of the affected extremities and may be triggered by stimulation; seizures are rhythmic and not influenced by manipulation of the limbs. Jitteriness may indicate an abnormality if it persists longer than 4 days or if it is prolonged or very easily elicited. Jitteriness can also indicate hypoglycemia.

Apnea

Breathing is intermittent in the fetus, but after delivery rhythmic continuous breathing is necessary to sustain life. All premature newborns and many full-term babies display periodic breathing, or intervals of rapid respirations interspersed with very slow breathing and pauses in respirations lasting up to 10 or 12 seconds. About one-third of neonates less than 32 weeks' gestation and virtually all infants less than 30 weeks' gestation have apnea spells. They appear to related to neurological immaturity and are often associated with the rapid eye movement stage of sleep.

Pathologic apnea is defined as apnea lasting 20 seconds or longer or a pause in breathing of shorter duration accompanied by bradycardia, cyanosis or pallor, or oxygen desaturation. Bradycardia in a premature baby is considered significant if it is at least 30 beats per minute less than the baseline rate. An oxygen saturation level less than 85% lasting for 5 seconds is considered pathologic in this age group.

Reasons for Apnea in Premature Infants

- Central apnea is caused by an immature nervous system that fails to supply sufficient neural impulses from the respiratory centers in the medulla to the respiratory muscles—the baby "forgets" to breathe.

- Obstructive apnea is caused by an airway occlusion, often from mucus or a head or neck position that kinks the airway.

- Problems in other organs can also affect the breathing control center in the brain. Other causes of apnea include hypoglycemia, hemorrhage or tissue damage in the brain, respiratory disease, infections, gastrointestinal problems such as reflux, electrolyte imbalances, heart problems, hypothermia, and overstimulation.

An infant may be discharged from the hospital with a home apnea monitor, especially if he or she has had occasional episodes of apnea in the hospital or has had a sibling die from sudden infant death syndrome. An apnea monitor should sound an alarm if there are no respirations for more than a predetermined limit (usually 20 seconds) or if the heart rate falls below a certain baseline rate. Documentation of the apnea events can be obtained by downloading information from the monitor.

Some medications are helpful in stimulating the infant's central nervous system to reduce apnea episodes, most commonly aminophylline, theophylline, and caffeine. Babies are discharged on these medications and continue to take them daily until the nervous system matures and the apnea is outgrown. Side effects of apnea medications include tachycardia, vomiting, and irritability.

If an apnea episode occurs, gently stimulate the baby by changing its position slightly or rubbing the back or feet. Remember, overstimulation can also trigger apnea in the premature infant. If the infant does not respond, open the airway, suction the mouth and nose, and start blowby 100% oxygen. If the infant still does not breathe, initiate ventilation by bag and mask with the pop-off valve disabled. Watch the baby's response and discontinue if the baby begins breathing on his own again. If the baby does not resume breathing or the heart rate remains below 60 despite adequate oxygenation, intubate and continue to ventilate, initiate intravenous access, monitor the heart rate, and perform compressions as indicated. Consider administration of naloxone if the child was recently exposed to narcotic drugs. Naloxone is contraindicated in neonates born to mothers who are narcotic addicted or who used large quantities of narcotic analgesics late in pregnancy.

 Naloxone is contraindicated in neonates born to mothers who are narcotic addicted or who used large quantities of narcotic analgesics late in pregnancy.

Hypothermia

The neonate is at high risk for hypothermia because of the large ratio of surface area to body weight, inadequate insulating fat, and inability to shiver. Heat loss can be caused by evaporation of amniotic fluid from the wet newborn. Convective loss can occur through drafts, and conductive loss occurs when the infant is placed on cool surfaces and handled with cold hands. Cold stress begins a downward spiral of compensatory processes that can be life threatening for the infant. If the infant's body temperature drops below 95°F, serious problems can develop. Even a typical room temperature of 70°F can cause profound hypothermia in the newborn, especially if he is wet.

Although some heat is produced by the metabolic processes of the liver, heart, brain, and skeletal muscles, neonates cannot shiver; so, if chilled, they will burn brown fat stores to generate heat. The infant releases norepinephrine when stressed by cold, and this hormone stimulates the metabolism of brown fat, increasing metabolic rate and oxygen consumption. A small baby with immature lungs may become hypoxic if he is unable to meet the demand for additional oxygen.

Norepinephrine also causes pulmonary vasoconstriction, which leads to hypoxemia and pulmonary hypertension. Hypoxemia means that less oxygen is available for glucose metabolism, so glucose is broken down by an alternative hypoxic pathway (anaerobic glycolysis), which forms lactic acid. The baby develops metabolic acidosis. Anaerobic metabolism metabolizes glycogen at an accelerated rate, causing hypoglycemia. The very immature infant born in the field should not be allowed to breastfeed, so there is no caloric intake to offset this energy depletion in the preterm infant.

Maintaining warmth is a crucial component of the care of any neonate, but thermoregulation is especially important for the premature infant. Preterm babies have smaller muscle mass, less brown fat, less insulating fat, and poor reflex control of skin capillaries, all of which contribute to less heat production and greater heat loss.

The hypothermic neonate may be lethargic or irritable and appear pale and cool to the touch. Acrocyanosis is a normal finding in the first few hours of life, but thereafter it can indicate cold stress. Respiratory distress, apnea, bradycardia, and cyanosis may be seen as the infant's condition worsens.

The prehospital provider should seek to prevent hypothermia by maintaining a neutral thermal environment for the infant, which allows the infant to maintain the optimal temperature without increasing caloric or oxygen requirements. The skin of the mother's abdomen is a convenient warming table that can keep the baby's temperature at the optimal level if mother and infant are topped with additional blankets.

If the baby must be placed elsewhere, as for resuscitation, it is crucial to be mindful of the risks of heat loss and devise some other method of maintaining warmth. Chemical hot packs can be used to prewarm blankets before they are used on the infant. Hot water bottles (no hotter than 104°F) may be helpful if the provider is certain that they will not overheat the infant or make contact with his skin. It may be practical to run the ambulance heater to create a very warm environment. Drafts and moving air, including blowby oxygen, can cause convective heat loss. All blankets, towels, and the like that come in contact with the infant should be prewarmed if possible, perhaps by holding them in front of the heat vents or wrapping them around hot packs.

The hypothermic infant needs rapid transport in a warm ambulance. Maintain adequate ventilation and oxygenation during transport, and resuscitate as necessary. Medical control may advise the administration of warmed IV fluids through an IV heater. Check glucose levels and administer dextrose ($D_{10}W$ or $D_{25}W$) if the infant is hypoglycemic.

Vomiting

Vomiting may be associated with many different conditions of the newborn. New parents may confuse vomiting with "spitting up" or regurgitation, a sudden reflux of stomach contents mixed with mucus that can appear copious and often occurs after burping. Spitting up often occurs after overfeeding or placing the infant flat after a large meal.

Vomiting in the neonate can indicate obstruction in the gastrointestinal tract, increased intracranial pressure (as may occur with intraventricular hemorrhage; see Chapter 10), or infection. While bloody vomitus may indicate life-threatening illness, it is not unusual for babies to swallow maternal blood during delivery (particularly if the mother had heavy bloody show) and then regurgitate red or brown mucus for hours or days following birth.

When transporting the vomiting neonate, the EMS provider should ensure a clear airway with suction if necessary, remembering that suctioning can trigger bradycardia. Oxygenate as indicated. Intravenous fluids may be necessary if the infant is dehydrated. Transport in a side-lying position.

Diarrhea

Diarrhea can result from infection, food intolerance, or other causes, but is usually viral. A newborn with diarrhea can very quickly become dehydrated and decompensate, develop electrolyte imbalances, and lapse into hypovolemic shock.

Assessment of diarrhea can be difficult. Diarrhea is rare in a baby who is totally breastfed. A breastfed baby will normally have as many as 6–10 moist, semiliquid, yellow, often large stools every day. Inexperienced parents may confuse this normal product with diarrhea. These stools have a mild odor similar to that of yogurt. Formula-fed babies may have only 1 or 2 (but as many as 5) semisolid stools per day that have a stronger odor.

An infant with diarrhea will have very frequent stools that are usually green and full of mucus (or specks of blood), and are usually foul-smelling. Bowel movements may be so liquid that they leave a water ring in the diaper. Diarrhea may be accompanied by fever and irritability. Signs of dehydration include decreased urination, dry mouth, lethargy, and sunken eyes and fontanelles. Field management involves stabilizing vital signs, including intravenous fluid replacement if indicated. Transport to a facility capable of treating high-risk infants.

 Newborns do not usually produce tears in the first weeks of life, so tearless crying is not a reliable indicator of dehydration in the neonate.

Sudden Infant Death Syndrome

Sudden infant death syndrome (SIDS) is the sudden death of a child during the first year of life for which postmortem examination fails to determine a cause. SIDS is responsible for 30% of all deaths for babies between the ages of 1 week and 1 year, making it the leading cause of death for this age group. Risk increases in lower socioeconomic groups, with prematurity, in infants with underlying respiratory pattern abnormalities, in siblings of SIDS victims, and in smokers' households. Because soft bedding can enfold the head and trap CO_2, some SIDS deaths appear similar to suffocation.

In most cases, the infant is put down for a nap and never awakens. The bedcovers are often in disarray, and the child often has worked himself into a corner or has wrapped blankets around his head and is clutching the sheets. Frothy pink fluid often fills the baby's mouth and nose.

Research has been unable to pinpoint the etiology of SIDS, but it appears to be related to a neurological failure of the regulation of breathing, though multiple mechanisms are probably responsible. Babies who sleep on their stomachs are more likely to experience SIDS, so mothers are cautioned to put infants to sleep on their backs and avoid soft bedding that may pose a suffocation risk. SIDS is largely a diagnosis of exclusion, made after autopsy rules out other causes of death. Babies at high risk for SIDS often spend their early months on home apnea monitoring and taking medications that stimulate the respiratory system, such as caffeine.

Losing a child to SIDS is devastating to the parents. The death is utterly unexpected and the inability to determine a cause exacerbates feelings of guilt and helplessness. Investigations to exclude the possibility of abuse as a cause of death only increase this guilt and frustration.

The reactions of prehospital providers can either begin healing or worsen pain and anxiety in the grieving parents. If called to the scene of a child with SIDS, is important to avoid any statements or questions that suggest responsibility or blame. If the death was caused by abuse or neglect, that will be addressed later; accusatory statements serve no purpose in the field. Avoid disturbing the scene before law enforcement officials have investigated. If the parents have attempted to resuscitate the baby, the child may have bruises and rib fractures that mimic abuse injuries. Use tact and sensitivity in your determination whether to start resuscitation. Ask only objective questions, such as when they found the baby and in what position. If appropriate, you may explain that it appears to you that the baby died of a condition called sudden infant death syndrome, which cannot be foreseen or prevented.

ON TARGET When an infant has died of SIDS, allegations of abuse, neglect, or wrongdoing will add to the parents' long-term burden of grief and guilt.

Summary

For the neonate, the physiological changes of birth are abrupt and dramatic, and successful negotiation of this transition is necessary to his survival. Within minutes of leaving the uterus, he is an independent individual, meeting his own oxygen and nutritional requirements, maintaining his own temperature, and keeping his body in homeostasis.

In most cases, the neonate will transition to extrauterine life with little more than supportive care, but the EMS professional should realize that any newborn can develop life-threatening problems and decompensate rapidly. Basic assessment of the neonate will often allow the provider to identify the infants at greatest risk. Early recognition of existing or potential complications allows the prehospital provider to stabilize and transport the infant with speed and efficiency.

REVIEW QUESTIONS

1. Describe the signs and symptoms of hypoglycemia in the neonate.

2. What are the normal ranges for vital signs in the newborn infant?

3. Describe how hypothermia in the neonate can lead to hypoglycemia, hypoxia, and metabolic acidosis.

4. Describe common presentations of seizure activity in neonates and how this can be distinguished from jitteriness.

5. You are called to the home of a 6-day-old infant with diarrhea. Describe how you will assess this baby and what signs and symptoms would indicate true diarrhea instead of a normal stooling pattern.

The High-Risk Neonate

Objectives

By the end of this chapter you should be able to

- Resuscitate the newborn with primary apnea

- Manage the infant who has aspirated meconium

- Recognize the conditions that cause respiratory distress in the neonate

- Recognize birth trauma in the neonate

- Manage the care of a premature infant

CASE Study

After a tense 90 seconds of attempting to resolve a shoulder dystocia, Andrew finally freed the large baby and placed him on the bed between his mother's legs. The infant was limp, showed no respiratory effort, and made no response to stimulation, but had a pulse of 80. His purple head contrasted sharply with his pale body.

Andrew left the cord intact and pulsing while he dried the boy briskly with a soft blanket. His partner, Ginny, suctioned the baby's airway with a bulb syringe and massaged his back and feet. The baby did not cry, but lay inert, appearing lifeless. They removed the wet linens and replaced them with dry bath blankets. Andrew hooked a resuscitation bag to 100% oxygen and began to breathe for the baby while keeping him warm. His chest rose with the ventilations, but he did not attempt to breathe on his own.

"It's been 1 minute," Ginny said, fingers gently palpating the cord stub for a pulse. "He still has a pulse of about 80, but no respiratory effort, poor color, no tone. Grimaced a little at the bulb, but that's it."

Ginny cut the cord, repositioned the infant, and stimulated him again. After a full minute of ventilation, the baby made an odd noise, then inhaled, flinging his hands up and grimacing. He began to cry weakly, then more vigorously. His heart rate was 120, and his tone was improved. By the time he was 5 minutes old, he was crying strongly and moving actively. He still showed central cyanosis, so Andrew supplied blowby oxygen. A few minutes later, the baby's face and trunk were pink and remained so even without the benefit of supplemental oxygen.

Questions

1. What Apgars would you give this baby at 1 and 5 minutes?
2. If the amniotic fluid had been meconium stained, how would resuscitation have differed?
3. This baby had suffered a shoulder dystocia. What physical findings do Ginny and Andrew need to assess and chart?

Introduction

Every infant must make profound physiological changes while transitioning from fetus to neonate. The minutes following birth may well be the most critical and vulnerable moments of his entire life. If the neonate is unable to adapt satisfactorily to extrauterine life, he will die. At highest risk are infants already compromised by problems such as prematurity, birth defects, birth trauma, perinatal hypoxia, or infection. Serious complications, however, can arise even after the uncomplicated birth of an apparently healthy baby.

The signs and symptoms of a compromised newborn are often nonspecific, and it can be difficult to pinpoint etiology. Management of the distressed newborn requires sharp assessment skills and a good working knowledge of physiology. Prudent management by proficient prehospital providers can be lifesaving for the compromised neonate.

KEY TERMS

atelectasis, p. 263

brachial plexus, p. 267

ductus arteriosus, p. 250

foramen ovale, p. 250

gastroschisis, p. 284

intrauterine growth restriction (or retardation; IUGR), p. 268

meconium aspiration syndrome (MAS), p. 263

neural tube defect, p. 276

pulmonary hypoplasia, p. 280

surfactant, p. 253

virilization, p. 282

Care of the High-Risk Newborn

In most cases, the newborn will spontaneously begin to breathe and will need minimal assistance in his transition to the extrauterine environment. However, about 10% of newborns require resuscitation following delivery, and 1% require extensive resuscitative measures to survive.

The high-risk neonate is a newborn who has a higher risk of morbidity or mortality due to the conditions before, during, or following birth or has some congenital anomaly that will require medical or surgical treatment to resolve or stabilize. Certain conditions are more likely to result in a depressed newborn, including prematurity or postmaturity, prolonged rupture of membranes, lack of prenatal care, fetal distress during labor, malpresentations, multiple gestation, substance abuse, fetal heart-rate abnormalities, meconium in the amniotic fluid, and maternal problems such as diabetes and preeclampsia. Sometimes a tight nuchal cord at delivery or shoulder dystocia will result in a depressed baby. Babies with some congenital anomalies may also be at greater risk. Some are born without incident, but require resuscitation or transition poorly to extrauterine life.

About 40% of babies that require resuscitation come as a surprise to the birth attendant, having shown no risk factors during the antepartum or intrapartum period. At every delivery the EMS professional should be prepared to launch full-scale resuscitation if the infant requires assistance. A crew with ALS capacity is best suited to respond to a delivery, and there should be ideally at least three crew members involved in patient care—one to attend to the mother postpartum and two to resuscitate the baby if necessary. All items of equipment required for infant resuscitation should be kept together in a readily accessible location, and ideally there should be enough equipment to work on two or more babies simultaneously.

 PEARLS All items of equipment required for infant resuscitation should be kept together in a readily accessible location, and ideally there should be enough equipment to work on two or more babies simultaneously.

The American Heart Association and the American Academy of Pediatrics have created the Neonatal Resuscitation Program (NRP) to train health care professionals to resuscitate newborns, and EMS professionals (and their patients) stand to benefit from maintaining NRP certification. The Pediatric Education for Prehospital Professionals (PEPP) Course is a training program specifically designed to enhance proficiency in managing prehospital neonatal and pediatric emergencies. Pediatric Advanced Life Support (PALS) is also valuable for learning and practicing neonatal resuscitation skills.

Some infants will require prolonged care at a hospital in a neonatal intensive care unit (NICU) if they are to survive or have a good prognosis. Many serious conditions are diagnosed ultrasonographically during the antepartum period, and the parents may plan to deliver at a facility that specializes in the treatment of high-risk children. A fast-moving labor may force the woman to deliver her high-risk infant in the field or at a hospital unequipped to handle the needs of a critically ill infant.

The EMS provider should learn which local and regional hospitals offer neonatal intensive care and the local protocols regarding transport to these facilities. A hospital with level I neonatal intensive care facilities can manage normal newborn and maternal care, identify high-risk pregnancies, and provide basic emergency services. A level II facility can handle most maternal and neonatal complications. A level III facility offers the full range of maternal and neonatal services and can provide care for critically ill infants. At least one full-time neonatologist is on staff. In addition, certain regional facilities provide special services for the sickest of babies, manage rare conditions and diseases with high mortality rates, and often perform fetal surgery and other procedures to begin treatment for certain anomalies while the fetus is still in utero. When in doubt about which facility is most appropriate, seek the advice of your medical control.

foramen ovale
An opening between the atria of the fetal heart that ordinarily closes on its own shortly after birth.

ductus arteriosus
A fetal blood vessel that connects the pulmonary artery to the ascending aorta, allowing the circulating blood largely to bypass the pulmonary circulation. It normally closes at birth.

The Transition from Fetus to Neonate

The first breath of air taken at delivery marks not only a transition to independent existence outside the mother's body but also a major anatomical and physiological transformation. Before birth, the fetus obtains all required oxygen from the mother's blood, which diffuses across the placenta into the fetal bloodstream. The unborn child does not need his lungs to survive, and they receive just enough blood supply to allow them to grow and develop. A hole between the atria of the heart (**foramen ovale**) and a shunt between the pulmonary artery and the aorta (**ductus arteriosus**) divert blood from the fetal lungs. To ready them for the task of breathing and to encourage lung expansion, the fetus breathes amniotic fluid in the absence of air. See Figure 10-1.

At birth, the infant suddenly must obtain his own oxygen, and his lungs become vital to life support. The changes in pressure and temperature stimulate him to draw his first breath, which distends the alveoli with air. The pressures of birth squeeze much of the fluid and mucus from his respiratory tract, and then as the baby draws a breath the lungs

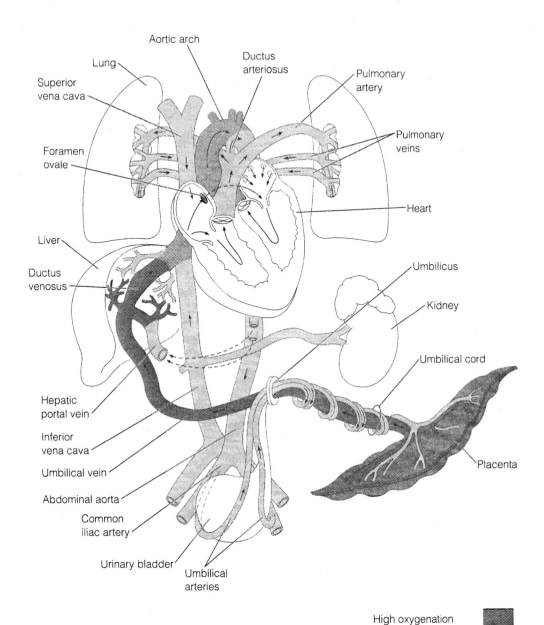

Aortic arch
Lung
Superior vena cava
Foramen ovale
Liver
Ductus venosus
Hepatic portal vein
Inferior vena cava
Umbilical vein
Abdominal aorta
Common iliac artery
Urinary bladder
Umbilical arteries
Ductus arteriosus
Pulmonary artery
Pulmonary veins
Heart
Umbilicus
Kidney
Umbilical cord
Placenta

High oxygenation
Moderate oxygenation
Low oxygenation
Very low oxygenation

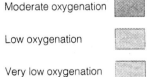

FIGURE 10-1
Fetal Circulation.
Blood returns to the fetus from the placenta through the umbilical vein and returns to the placenta through the umbilical arteries. The ductus arteriosus, foramen ovale, and ductus venosus allow the blood to largely bypass the fetal lungs and reduce flow through the liver.

absorb any retained amniotic fluid. Oxygen from the air begins to diffuse into the newborn's bloodstream in much greater quantities than he was able to absorb from his mother *in utero*. See Figure 10-2.

The distention of the alveoli and the abundant oxygen cause the network of tiny blood vessels in the lungs to relax, creating a dramatic

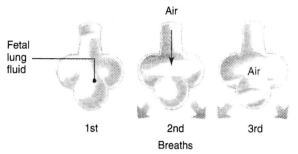

Air

Fetal lung fluid

1st   2nd   3rd
Breaths

Following birth, the lungs expand as they are filled with air. The fetal lung fluid gradually leaves the alveoli.

Arterioles dilate and blood flow increases

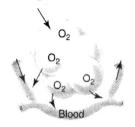

O_2

O_2

O_2 O_2

O_2

Blood

At the same time as the lungs are expanding and the fetal lung fluid is clearing, the arterioles in the lung begin to open, allowing a considerable increase in the amount of blood flowing through the lungs.

Pulmonary blood flow increases

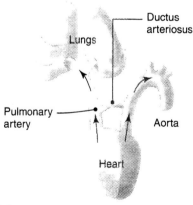

Ductus arteriosus

Lungs

Pulmonary artery

Aorta

Heart

Blood previously diverted through the ductus arteriosus flows through the lungs where it picks up oxygen to transport to tissues throughout the body. Soon there is no need for the ductus and it eventually closes.

FIGURE 10-2
Hemodynamic Changes in the Newborn at Birth.
(a) With the first breath, the lungs fill with air and any remaining fluid within them begins to absorb.
(b) The influx of oxygen dilates arterioles, increasing blood flow to the alveoli. (c) The ductus arteriosus constricts, sending increased blood flow through the lungs. Blood oxygen levels increase dramatically.

increase in blood flow through the lungs. The baby breathes deeply or cries to bring air into the lungs and expand more and more alveoli. The climbing levels of blood oxygen have a relaxing effect on pulmonary vessels and cause the ductus arteriosus to constrict, sending blood flow from the heart to the lungs as in adult circulation. These pressure changes also close the foramen ovale. Abundant oxygen causes the infant's skin to turn pink quickly.

The first breath requires more effort than the breaths that follow. In the term infant, a **surfactant** within the alveoli reduces surface tension and prevents these small air sacs from collapsing with each exhalation, thus decreasing the work of breathing.

Blood pressure also increases in the minutes following birth. Recall that the blood in the placenta and umbilical cord is fetal in origin and is circulated by the fetal heart. The placenta is typically one-sixth the size of the infant and holds a substantial amount of blood. When the umbilical vessels spasm and the cord is cut, the newborn is freed from the vast network of placental vessels and needs only to perfuse his own body. Consequently, the blood pressure rises.

If the baby is compromised at birth, this normal transitional process is disrupted. If the baby does not breathe deeply at birth, the lung vessels remain constricted and the blood continues to course through the ductus arterious, largely bypassing the lungs. Small arteries in the intestines, kidneys, muscles, and skin then constrict to maintain adequate blood flow to the heart and brain. But if the newborn does not begin breathing, soon, compensatory mechanisms begin to fail, leading to organ damage and death.

surfactant
A substance secreted by the alveolar cells of the lung that reduces surface tension of fluids that coat the lung, allowing the lung to remain expanded.

Neonatal Resuscitation

Apnea in a newborn is classed as primary or secondary, and it can begin before, during, or after delivery. When a baby suffers a hypoxic episode, either in *utero* or after birth, heart rate and tone decrease, and the baby either gasps ineffectively or shows no respiratory effort. This is primary apnea. In the neonate, primary apnea can be corrected with oxygen and stimulation. Resumption of oxygen delivery to the fetus will correct primary apnea in *utero*. Often the prehospital provider will be unaware that there is a problem with the unborn baby. But if a bradycardic fetal rhythm is identified, maternal position change, oxygen administration, and an intravenous fluid bolus will often correct the problem.

Secondary apnea can occur if hypoxia is persistent, or if the baby is not resuscitated. The heart rate and blood pressure decrease further, and the baby shows no respiratory effort. Aggressive resuscitation is necessary to reverse this condition.

There is no way for the emergency responder to determine whether the depressed neonate is in primary or secondary apnea. A fetus can

FIGURE 10-3
Inverted Pyramid of Neonatal Resuscitation.
When resuscitating a neonate, the provider should begin with the interventions described at the top of the pyramid and move down to the lower levels as needed. Most babies will respond to basic life support measures.

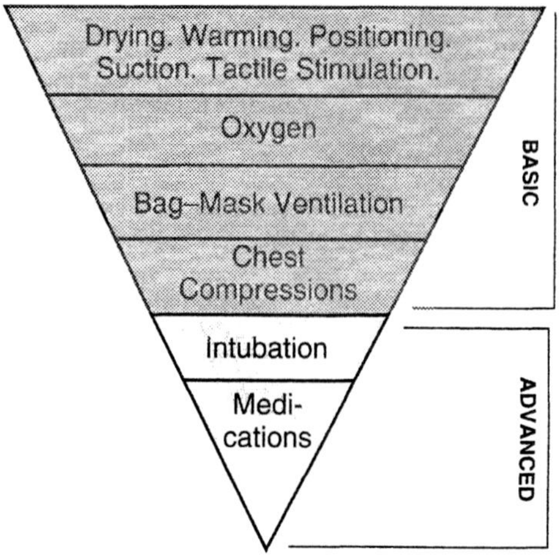

pass through primary apnea *in utero* and be in secondary apnea at delivery. No amount of stimulation and oxygen will initiate spontaneous breathing in the baby with secondary apnea. Therefore, if an infant does not respond immediately to back rubs and brisk toweling, the responder should immediately initiate more aggressive resuscitation efforts. See Figure 10-3.

Neonatal resuscitation can be anxiety provoking for even the most seasoned professional. The provider who memorizes the steps of resuscitation and mentally rehearses them on the way to a delivery is likely to find that the events flow smoothly and is more likely to have a successful outcome.

Immediately after birth, assess the infant:

- Is the baby clear of meconium? (If meconium is present, skip to the section Meconium.)
- Breathing or crying?
- Good tone?
- Color pink or cyanosis confined to hands and feet?
- Is baby full term?

The ABCs
As with adult patients, neonatal resuscitation follows the ABCs.

- Airway, warm, and stimulate.   Open and clear the airway. Dry and stimulate the baby and provide warmth; reposition the head to open the airway. See Figure 10-4. Give oxygen if indicated by cyanosis. Flick or rub his feet and rub his back. These steps should be accomplished in the first 30 seconds following birth.

  After 30 seconds, assess.

CORRECT

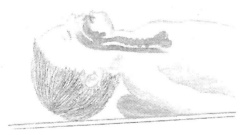

Neck slightly extended

Care should be taken to prevent hyperextension or underextension of the neck since either may decrease air entry.

INCORRECT

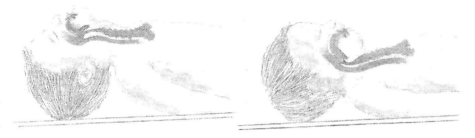

Neck hyperextended   Neck underextended

FIGURE 10-4
Positioning the Newborn to Open the Airway.
If the infant's neck is hyperextended or flexed, air entry may be blocked.

- **Breathing.** If breathing is ineffective and gasping or not spontaneous, or if the heart rate is under 100, assist respirations with a bag and mask connected to 100% oxygen for the next 30 seconds. Oxygen ideally should be warmed and humidified.

  After 30 seconds of ventilation have passed (1 minute after delivery), reassess.

- **Circulation.** If pulse is less than 60 after 30 seconds of positive pressure ventilation, begin chest compressions while continuing positive pressure ventilation.

  Reassess. If heart rate remains below 60 after 30 seconds of compressions, continue compressions and positive pressure ventilation, and administer epinephrine.

If heart rate increases above 60 after 30 seconds of chest compressions, stop compressions, but continue positive pressure ventilation until the heart rate remains above 100 and the baby is breathing on his own.

- Any obvious anomalies?

Steps of Resuscitation

- **Warm, dry, suction, and stimulate the infant for the first 30 seconds after birth while he rests on his mother's abdomen.** Position the baby so that the airway remains open and bulb suction the mouth, then nose—or use a DeLee suction trap or mechanical suction set at 80–100 mmHg. Use an 8 or 10 French catheter. See Figure 10-5. Do not suction for more than 5 seconds. Suctioning may cause vagal stimulation resulting in bradycardia. Replace the wet linen beneath the baby with dry to reduce heat loss. Reposition to open the airway, placing him on his back with his head slightly lower than his body and his neck slightly extended. If the baby is not on the mother's abdomen, place a 1-in. thickness of folded blanket beneath his shoulders, especially if the baby is large and has a molded or edematous occiput. While accomplishing these steps, determine the baby's heart rate by palpating the cord, and note color, tone, and respiratory efforts. All this should be accomplished within the first 30 seconds after delivery.

- **If the baby is gasping or not breathing, or if the pulse is below 100 bpm, immediately start positive pressure ventilation with 100% oxygen (5–10 L/min) and a bag and mask for 30 seconds.** Select a mask that fits the baby's face properly without air leakage, and then extend the neck slightly to the "sniffing" position. This is best accomplished with the baby placed on a firm surface (while taking care to avoid chilling). With light downward hand pressure, the mask should seal evenly on the infant's face without air leakage. A correctly sized mask covers the tips of the chin, mouth, and nose without putting pressure on the eyes. See Figure 10-6.

 Oxygen toxicity is a concern in the long-term care of infants, but resuscitation with 100% oxygen is lifesaving and essential in the prehospital setting.

The self-inflating bags carried in most ambulances are easy to use and frequently disposable. Bags used for newborns should have a volume of 200–750 cc (optimal is 450 cc). Remember that infants' tidal volume is only 20–30 cc. Larger bags increase the risk of lung

When head is delivered

As soon as the baby's head is delivered (prior to delivery of the shoulders) *the mouth, oropharynx, and hypopharynx should be thoroughly suctioned*, using a 10 Fr. DeLee suction catheter or other flexible suction catheter. Any catheter used should be no smaller than a 10 Fr.

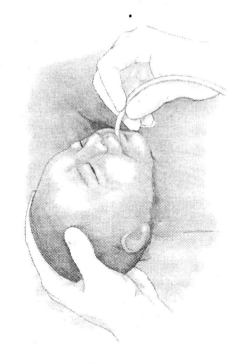

(a)

Following delivery

After delivery of the infant, if a great deal of meconium is present, the trachea should be intubated and any residual meconium removed from the lower airway.

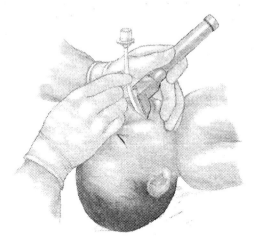

(b)

FIGURE 10-5
The Infant with Meconium Stained Fluid Needs Thorough Suctioning at Birth.
(a) Suctioning of the mouth using a flexible suction catheter. (b) Intubation for the removal of residual meconium.

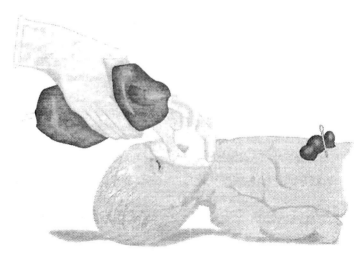

FIGURE 10-6
Use of a Bag Valve Mask.
A properly fitting mask and a good mask seal are essential to successful ventilation.

overinflation. The bag should also have a pop-off valve set to 30–45 cm H2O to release pressure if the bag is squeezed too vigorously. The pressure required for the initial breath may be as high as 60 cm H2, so for the first few breaths it may be necessary to deactivate the pop off.

The addition of an oxygen reservoir allows the rescuer to deliver nearly 100% oxygen to the baby. Self-inflating bags cannot be used to deliver free-flow oxygen; so if the patient is breathing, use a mask or blowby to ensure oxygen delivery.

Compress the bag until the chest rises, taking care not to overinflate the lungs. The first breath requires more pressure than the breaths that follow, and premature infants may have more lung resistance. If the chest does not rise, check mask size and positioning for air leaks and equipment for proper functioning. Ventilate 40–60 times per minute. You are likely to maintain the correct rate if you repeat to yourself, "BREATHE . . . two . . . three . . . BREATHE . . . two . . . three. . .," as you ventilate, compressing the bag every time you say, "BREATHE," then allowing the baby to exhale while you finish the count.

Reassess after 30 seconds of positive pressure ventilation. If the heart rate increases to more than 100 BPM and the baby begins breathing effectively on his own, you may discontinue ventilation. Continue to provide supplemental oxygen until the baby's trunk and face are pink. If the heart rate exceeds 100 BPM, but the baby is still not breathing effectively, continue ventilation. If you must provide positive pressure ventilation for more than a few minutes or the stomach appears distended, insert an orogastric or nasogastric tube. Consider intubation if positive pressure ventilation with bag and mask is ineffective, if ventilation is likely to continue for a prolonged period, or if diaphragmatic hernia is suspected. Intubation maintains an open airway but eliminates PEEP—the physiologic positive end-expiratory pressure created when the baby cries or coughs, necessitating the addition of a PEEP valve (set at 2–4 cm H_2O) to the bag valve outlet. Always use an uncuffed endotracheal tube on a neonate.

 PEARLS Always use an uncuffed endotracheal tube on a neonate.

- **After 30 seconds of positive pressure ventilation, check the pulse by grasping the umbilical stump.** If the infant remains apneic with a heart rate below 60 bpm, start chest compressions. This intervention will compress the heart against the spine, increasing intrathoracic pressure and helping to perfuse vital organs. One crew member should compress the chest while another ventilates.

Two hand positions are acceptable, either encircling the baby's chest with the thumbs over the sternum below the nipple line and above the xyphoid, or with two fingers of one hand positioned over the same location. The baby should be on a firm surface and protected against heat loss. The downstroke of each compression should be quicker than the release. Keep your fingers or thumbs on the sternum at all times while performing compressions. Compressions should be approximately one-third the depth of the chest. See Figure 10-7.

Babies must be ventilated when chest compression is deemed necessary, and ventilations must be timed to avoid simultaneous delivery of compressions and ventilations. The ventilation should be administered after every third compression, yielding a total of 30 breaths and 90 compressions every minute. It helps if the person giving compression repeats the words "One-and-Two-and-Three-and-BREATHE-and-One-and . . ." with the bag squeezed for a breath on the cue "BREATHE-and," with compressions suspended to allow for the breath.

After 30 seconds of good compressions, reassess heart rate and breathing efforts. If the heart rate is above 80, you may discontinue compressions, but continue to breathe for the baby at 40–60 breaths per minute. Once the heart rate surpasses 100 bpm, gradually stop ventilation and provide oxygen until the baby remains centrally pink.

- **If the baby does not improve, reassess the effectiveness of CPR techniques.** If the baby is not breathing effectively, consider intubation (always performed with an uncuffed tube in a newborn). Check to

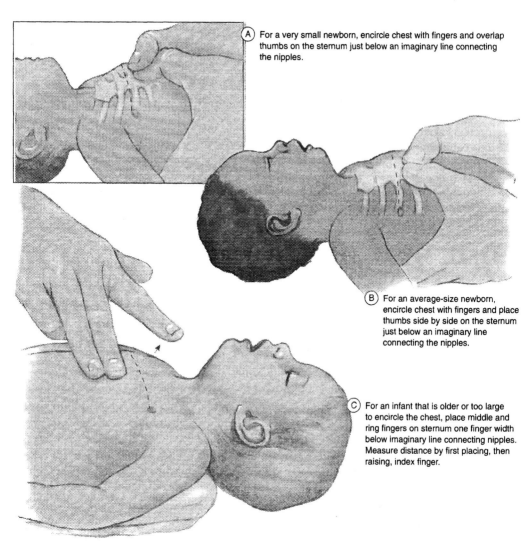

A) For a very small newborn, encircle chest with fingers and overlap thumbs on the sternum just below an imaginary line connecting the nipples.

B) For an average-size newborn, encircle chest with fingers and place thumbs side by side on the sternum just below an imaginary line connecting the nipples.

C) For an infant that is older or too large to encircle the chest, place middle and ring fingers on sternum one finger width below imaginary line connecting nipples. Measure distance by first placing, then raising, index finger.

FIGURE 10-7
Position of the Fingers for Chest Compressions on the Neonate.
Correct finger position is essential for effective chest compressions and minimizes harm to the infant.

be sure that 100% oxygen is being delivered to the infant—did the tubing disconnect from the oxygen source or has the tank run out?

If CPR is effective and the infant is not responding, administer epinephrine via the endotracheal tube with a 1 ml saline flush, and ventilate. Epinephrine increases the rate and strength of cardiac contractions and raises the blood pressure through vasoconstriction. Newborns should receive 0.1–0.3 mg of a 1:10,000 concentration of epinephrine hydrochloride per kilogram of weight. Follow with several deep ventilations to move the drug into the lungs.

- **Continue CPR and reassess in 30 seconds.** The infant should improve markedly. If the heart rate is still below 60, reevaluate the effectiveness of CPR and make sure the endotracheal tube is still in the trachea. Epinephrine may be repeated every 3–5 minutes.

At this point, if the baby shows little improvement, establish venous access through a peripheral vein, intraosseus cannulation, or umbilical vein cannulation. If local protocols permit access through the umbilical vein, trim the cord to 1 in. above the abdomen and identify the three vessels. Normally the opening of the umbilical vein will be large and obvious, while the two umbilical arteries are smaller. Some babies have only one umbilical artery. Do not attempt cannulation if you cannot clearly identify the vein. Do not allow this procedure to delay transport.

Prepare a sterile field and a 5 French umbilical catheter or (20 gauge intravenous catheter) with the needle removed. Flush a three-way stopcock and connect to a normal saline extension set. Insert the catheter into the vein until the tip is just below the abdominal skin and you can observe free flow of blood. Attach a 10 cc syringe partially filled with normal saline and aspirate gently to confirm lack of resistance. If blood does not reflux into syringe, withdraw the catheter slightly and aspirate again. Inject a small amount of saline and check for resistance. Secure with umbilical tape.

- **If the baby still has not responded to resuscitation efforts, consider other causes for depression.** In the case of placental abruption, placenta previa, or cord accident, the baby may be in hypovolemic shock. In this case a fluid bolus of 10 mL per kilogram of lactated Ringer's or normal saline given by slow IV push can be lifesaving. Overhydration may cause a brain hemorrhage, so use caution.

Sometimes after resuscitation the baby regains adequate heart rate, but remains floppy and cyanotic and breathes poorly or remains apneic. Consider that the mother might have taken a narcotic before the birth, which may have been recreational or therapeutic. If the mother of a depressed infant has taken a narcotic within 4 hours of delivery and is not addicted to narcotics, naloxone administration may be indicated.

Naloxone administration is contraindicated when resuscitating the newborn of a mother who used narcotics in the weeks prior to delivery. The fetus becomes physically dependent on the narcotic, and naloxone administration will cause instant withdrawal and seizures in the infant. When in doubt, support respirations and transport. If Narcan is ordered by medical control, the dose for neonates is 0.1 mg/kg IV, IM, ET, or SC. It may be repeated every 2 or 3 minutes as needed.

Once a baby has been successfully resuscitated, expedite transport. Monitor the infant en route and frequently reassess vital signs, color, and tone. Ensure that the baby remains warm and that his airway remains clear. Newborn babies are often very mucusy for several days after birth and may gag or even develop an obstructed airway while attempting to expel tenacious globs.

Respiratory distress in a newborn can develop rapidly and unexpectedly, even if the baby had good Apgars and was initially doing well. It is especially common in deliveries involving meconium-stained fluid. Listen to the respirations. If you identify a grunting "uh . . . uh . . . uh . . ." with each breath, he is having trouble breathing. If you watch his chest move, you may see retractions, or a sinking in of the flesh between the ribs and above and below the sternum as he inhales, and a seesawing motion between the chest and the belly with breathing. Nasal flaring also indicates difficulty breathing. The child with respiratory distress needs rapid transport to the hospital. Supply blowby oxygen as needed and stand ready to use positive pressure ventilation if needed.

Meconium

The normal fetus continuously drinks amniotic fluid and urinates into the amniotic sac. Amniotic fluid is mostly fetal urine. Floating in this fluid are fetal hair, bits of vernix, and dead skin cells. When ingested, this debris passes into the fetal digestive tract where it forms the first stool, a sticky, tar-like substance called meconium.

The fetus ordinarily does not move its bowels until after it is born. Sometimes, however, a hypoxic event can cause the anal sphincter to relax and expel meconium into the amniotic fluid. A healthy postterm baby may pass meconium in *utero* as his intestines mature and start to function. Breech babies often pass meconium as the fetal abdomen is squeezed through the maternal pelvis. Meconium, like the fetus and everything else within the amniotic sac, is sterile, so it does not pose the threat of infection.

Meconium is such a dark green color that it appears black and tar-like on a diaper, but diluted in fluid it can range from a light brown or yellow-green to particulate pea soup. Consistency varies with the amount of meconium passed and the amount of fluid present. It is important to determine the color of the fluid when a woman reports rupture of the membranes.

When meconium enters the amniotic fluid, the fetus may inhale it and develop lower airway obstructions. A distressed fetus may gasp in utero, drawing meconium deeper into the lungs. If meconium is inhaled into the lower airway, meconium aspiration syndrome (MAS) may result. Not

atelectasis
Alveolar collapse
resulting from in-
sufficient ventila-
tion. It can also
represent incom-
plete expansion of
the lungs in the
neonate.

all babies with meconium-stained fluid will develop MAS, but the ones who do may suffer severe respiratory distress. Complete bronchial obstruction may lead to **atelectasis** whereas partial blockage leads to air trapping that can progress to tension pneumothorax.

If meconium-stained fluid is noted, prepare to suction the infant aggressively at delivery. When the head is born, ask the mother to stop pushing. Suction the infant's mouth, oropharynx, hypopharynx, and nares with a 10 French catheter attached to wall suction or with a bulb syringe.

Deliver the infant to the maternal abdomen or the bed and briefly observe his activity. If the baby is vigorous, defined as having a heart rate over 100, spontaneous crying or breathing, and flexed or flailing extremities, then care proceeds routinely unless the baby subsequently declines. The Apgar score for a vigorous baby will be 8 or greater. If the infant is not vigorous, cut the cord and move the baby *with minimal stimulation* to a surface where resuscitation can be readily performed. Take care not to chill the infant.

**ON
TARGET**

*Caution!
Endotra-
cheal suc-
tioning can
trigger a vagal
response that can
drop the infant's heart
rate to dangerously
low levels.*

Quickly intubate the infant and perform suctioning through the endotracheal tube itself, using a meconium suction adapter. Occlude the suction control port on the aspirator and gradually withdraw the tube. Do not apply suction for more than 3–5 seconds. If no meconium is removed, do not resuction, but ventilate the infant. If suctioning yields meconium and the heart rate is not significantly bradycardic, reintubate and repeat until little or no meconium is extracted or the heart rate begins to drop. Ventilate and stimulate the infant as usual.

Caution! Endotracheal suctioning can trigger a vagal response that can drop the infant's heart rate to dangerously low levels. If the infant becomes significantly bradycardic, the responder may need to stop suctioning and provide positive pressure ventilation, even though ventilation could drive the meconium deeper into the respiratory tract.

Respiratory Distress in the Neonate

*meconium aspira-
tion syndrome
(MAS)*
Hypoxia and other
problems that oc-
cur when meco-
nium is inhaled
into the tracheo-
bronchial airways.

Meconium Aspiration Syndrome (MAS)

Meconium aspiration syndrome (MAS) can develop when meconium is aspirated into the lower airways. Approximately 20% of all infants with moderate to thick meconium-stained amniotic fluid will develop MAS. Meconium can create a partial obstruction that allows air to flow into the lungs on inspiration but blocks exhalation, causing hyperinflation of the lungs distal to the blockage. The baby develops air hunger and gasps, potentially bringing more meconium into the lungs as he struggles to breathe. Hyperinflation, hypoxemia, and acidemia cause increased pulmonary vascular resistance, which shunts blood through the ductus arteriosus and away from the lungs. Hypoxemia worsens as blood moves through the fetal circulation circuit rather than the neonatal system. Hyperinflation of the lungs predisposes the baby to pneumothorax. Babies with MAS, especially if postterm, frequently develop persistent pulmonary hypertension of the newborn (see later).

Babies with MAS are often hypoxic and depressed at birth, showing floppy "rag doll" tone, retractions, grunting, tachypnea or apnea, cyanosis or pallor, and nasal flaring similar to infants with respiratory distress syndrome (see RDS later in this chapter). A barrel chest may develop from hyperinflation of the lungs. Increased work of breathing leads to hypoglycemia, hypothermia, respiratory and metabolic acidosis, and electrolyte imbalance. These conditions may progress rapidly to respiratory failure.

Babies with MAS are admitted to the NICU for ventilatory support, intravenous fluids, chest percussion, and postural drainage. Some babies must receive specialized treatments such as extracorporeal membrane oxygenation (ECMO) (see Pediatric Notes), available only in certain regional hospitals, if they are to survive.

Transient Tachypnea of the Newborn

Transient tachypnea of the newborn usually affects infants that are full term and of average weight. The infant is born vigorous, then develops progressive respiratory distress. Auscultation of the lungs reveals crackles from excessive fluid, which may result from a failure to empty the lungs of fluid during birth or from aspiration of amniotic fluid. Dyspnea gradually worsens, until by 6 hours of life the infant may have respirations of 100 to 140 breaths per minute. Prehospital treatment is the same as with any condition that compromises respiration.

Persistent Pulmonary Hypertension of the Newborn (Persistent Fetal Circulation)

Persistent pulmonary hypertension of the newborn (PPHN) is when the baby fails to make the changes necessary to convert from fetal to neonatal circulation. Instead, his pulmonary arterioles remain constricted, and he diverts blood flow away from the lungs before it can pick up oxygen. The foramen ovale and ductus arteriosus remain open, causing severe hypoxemia even when the infant is breathing 100 percent oxygen.

PPHN occurs most often in term or postterm infants who have suffered cold stress or perinatal asphyxia, babies with congenital cardiac anomalies, and infants with diaphragmatic hernia. Hypoxia constricts blood vessels in the lungs, creating pulmonary hypertension that shunts blood away from the lungs. Babies with PPHN will show dyspnea and poor oxygen saturation, and they should be treated as appropriate for any infant in respiratory distress. Diagnosis is made at the hospital through history, physical findings, X-ray results, and laboratory data. Hospital treatment includes vasodilating medications and mechanical ventilation with 100% O_2, because oxygen effectively dilates pulmonary arteries. Some cases may require extracorporeal membrane oxygenation.

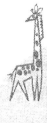

PEDIATRIC
NOTES

Extracorporeal membrane oxygenation (ECMO), an adaptation of conventional cardiopulmonary bypass technique, is a treatment method used to support infants with severe respiratory compromise. ECMO therapy acts as an artificial heart and lung to maintain oxygenation until the infant improves and can resume independent respiratory function. Typically ECMO is offered only at large regional facilities, where it is used to treat conditions such as respiratory distress syndrome, sepsis, meconium aspiration syndrome, persistent pulmonary hypertension of the newborn, and other disorders.

Hypoxic-Ischemic Encephalopathy

Hypoxic-ischemic encephalopathy is a fairly common cause of neurologic impairment. Asphyxia can occur before, during, or after delivery, and can cause brain damage. After an episode of asphyxia, blood flow may remain decreased, causing cerebral ischemia. The amount of damage is variable, with some infants profoundly affected and others surviving with no apparent deficit.

Neurologic symptoms commonly begin within the first few hours of the hypoxic episode and may include lethargy or stupor, poor tone, difficulty with sucking and swallowing, muscular weakness, and seizures. Treatment includes adequate ventilation and measures to maximize cerebral perfusion, but damage is often irreversible.

Birth Trauma

It can be disheartening to realize that an otherwise healthy infant was injured during the birth process. The EMS provider may arrive at a scene to find that bystanders have pulled and twisted the baby in an attempt to "help" with the delivery, causing serious harm to the infant. Or the birth attendant may rectify a severe shoulder dystocia only to find the baby is not moving his arm after birth. Some birth injuries are caused when the baby encounters bony pelvic obstructions during a normal birth. Birth trauma is sometimes unavoidable even when the delivery is accomplished by prudent, experienced providers.

Certain antepartum or intrapartum factors can predispose the infant to birth injury. Macrosomia, malpresentations, prolonged labor, and prematurity carry a higher incidence of injury to the newborn.

Skin

Petechiae may be present and localized to the site of injury, such as head, neck, or lower back. A baby's face may have petechiae after a rapid second-stage labor or a tight nuchal cord. Bruising may be present, especially if the infant is premature.

Head

Cephalohematoma is a large swelling without associated bruising caused by bleeding beneath the periosteum overlying a single cranial bone. It might not appear for days after birth. Skull fracture is sometimes associated with this injury. This injury usually resolves on its own between 2 weeks and 3 months.

Subgaleal hemorrhage is bleeding into the soft tissue above the periosteum. Swelling may begin as a small hematoma and then extend slowly or rapidly to involve the neck and ears and even the eye sockets. Babies with subgaleal hemorrhage may show poor tone, seizures, pallor, and, a few days later, jaundice. The infant may become hypovolemic. Intracranial hemorrhage may or may not be symptomatic.

Face

The most common facial injury is nasal fracture or dislocation of the nasal cartilage, which may result from the pressure of the maternal sacrum or pubis during second-stage labor. This injury can present with respiratory distress. Edema and bruising of the eyelids can occur. Subconjunctival hemorrhage is common and usually benign, resolving spontaneously in 1–2 weeks. Facial nerve paralysis may occur from the pressure of the mother's sacrum against the fetal face.

Neck, Shoulder, and Extremities

The clavicle is the bone most commonly broken in delivery. These injuries are most common in macrosomic infants with shoulder dystocia and in breech presentations in which the arms are extended. The infant with a clavicular fracture may be unable or unwilling to move the affected arm and will often have an asymmetrical Moro reflex. Crepitus and deformity may be present at the site of injury. Sometimes the doctor or midwife will deliberately fracture the clavicle of an infant with severe shoulder dystocia if the infant will not deliver by any other means.

The humerus is the second most common bone broken in delivery, most often after a shoulder dystocia or breech presentation. Infants with humerus fracture usually cannot or will not move the affected arm, and tenderness and crepitus may be present at the site. The femur might fracture in a breech delivery.

brachial plexus
A network of nerves located in the neck and axilla supplying the chest, shoulder, and arm.

Trauma to the **brachial plexus** can cause motor disabilities to the arm. These injuries can occur with excessive traction applied to the head, neck, and arm to free a shoulder dystocia or breech presentation. With Erb's palsy the arm is adducted and internally rotated, with an intact grasp reflex and an absent or unilateral Moro. Klumpke's palsy involves hand and wrist paralysis. Some babies will evidence a complete paralysis of the arm. Infants with brachial plexus injuries may also injure the phrenic nerve where it crosses the brachial plexus. Babies with phrenic nerve damage may show respiratory distress. Most babies with brachial plexus injury recover by 3 months of age, but some may have long-term injury.

Spinal cord injuries are unusual, but are more likely to result from a breech delivery, face presentation, or shoulder dystocia.

Abdomen and Genitals

Grasping a breech baby around the abdomen to facilitate delivery can cause damage to abdominal organs such as rupture of liver and spleen, adrenal hemorrhage, and kidney damage. Babies with injuries to abdominal organs often present with shock, abdominal distention, and irritability. Often symptoms do not occur until hours after birth.

Boys born breech may suffer swelling of the scrotum and penis. Bleeding into the scrotum can cause it to distend markedly.

Carefully document any evidence of birth injury in great objective detail. It may help to draw a map of the extent of bruising or swelling with certain injuries. Document the infant's vital signs and motor function, and behavior (quietly alert, sleeping, crying loudly).

The Infant with Low Birth Weight

Intrauterine Growth Restriction (IUGR)

Growth failure can develop early in pregnancy, resulting in underdeveloped body organs, or later in pregnancy, resulting in normal organs that are smaller than usual. There is a higher risk of morbidity and mortality for both the fetus and the neonate when the weight falls below the 10th percentile. Common causes of **intrauterine growth restriction (IUGR)** include multiple gestation, maternal smoking, chronic maternal disease, high altitude, excessive exercise, abnormal placenta structure or placement, certain antepartal infections such as rubella or syphilis, and fetal chromosomal abnormalities.

intrauterine growth restriction (or retardation; IUGR) **Fetal weight below the 10th percentile with poor growth due to insufficient nutrition and oxygenation** *in utero.*

Symmetric IUGR results in chronic, prolonged restriction of the growth of organs, weight, length, and sometimes head circumference. Symmetric IUGR can be caused by any chronic maternal condition that diminishes blood flow or nutrients to the fetus, including long-standing hypertension, malnutrition, anemia, or tobacco use. Symmetric IUGR can also be associated with fetal genetic abnormalities. This condition can be diagnosed on ultrasound as early as the early second trimester.

Asymmetric IUGR reflects an acute compromise in the blood flow to the placenta, such as with placental infarctions and pregnancy-induced hypertension. The fetus with asymmetrical IUGR shows a normal head circumference and length, but decreased weight and abdominal circumference.

It is thought that the stressed fetus produces elevated levels of norepinephrine and epinephrine, which cause loss of fat stores, muscle mass, and glycogen stores and increase blood flow to the brain, heart, and adrenal glands. The fetus retains a normal head circumference as it attempts to protect brain development, but suffers weight loss and poor growth elsewhere.

After delivery, the fetus with IUGR becomes an infant with limited reserves. He is at increased risk for hypoxia during labor and delivery and is more likely to need resuscitation at birth. He shows poor thermoregulation and is more likely to suffer hypoglycemia.

Managing the Premature Infant

The premature infant born in the field requires careful management. Babies born before the 37th week of gestation are considered premature, regardless of weight. See Table 10-1. Infants are considered viable after the 24th week of gestation, but some children have been saved when born as early as 21 or 22 weeks. In 2002, 1 out of every 8 babies (12.1% of live births) was born preterm in the United States. Between 1992 and 2002, the rate of infants born preterm in the United States increased 13%. The majority of premature babies under 35–36 weeks will need resuscitation or specialized supportive care following birth.

Preterm infants born out of the hospital are often delivered with unexpected swiftness. Women in preterm labor often feel minimal pain until labor is advanced. The baby is often delivered shortly after the water breaks

Table 10-1 Terms Commonly Used with the Chronology of Pregnancy and Birth

Preterm or premature	Born before 37 completed weeks of gestation
Low birth weight	Less than 2,500 g at birth regardless of gestational age
Very low birth weight	Less than 1,500 g at birth
Extremely low birth weight	Less than 1,000 g at birth
Perinatal death	Death that occurs after 22 weeks of gestation (or 500 g if gestational age is not known), but before 28 days following delivery
Neonatal death	Death that occurs within 27 days following birth
Infant mortality	Death between birth and 1 year of age
Fetal death	Death after 20 weeks of gestation, either *in utero* or upon delivery

and is more likely to assume a nonvertex position for birth. Premature babies are extremely delicate, and even grasping the body at delivery can damage the delicate skin and organs. Allow the baby to deliver with as little assistance as possible, and if possible position the mother on her side to reduce pressure on the fetal head.

The earlier the gestational age, the more the preterm baby will differ from the term infant. Energy is best spent staying warm and growing, so the preterm infant is weak and not very active. Reflexes may be only partially developed, and sucking may be uncoordinated and ineffective. The preemie is easily overstimulated and may respond to noise or rough handling with apnea or bradycardia.

The 36-week infant will be very much like a small-term baby, but may have initial breathing and feeding problems and more jaundice by day 4. The 32–34-week baby will be thin-skinned and gaunt because of minimal subcutaneous fat. Infants of this gestational age will often cry vigorously at birth, though they frequently need assistance to sustain adequate respirations.

The extremely premature baby will need aggressive intervention if he is to have any chance of survival. Babies born on the cusp of viability usually have severe, lifelong health problems, including cerebral palsy and blindness, if they survive. If a child is extremely premature, his organ systems may be insufficiently developed to sustain life. The mother may report a reliable gestational age if she has had an early ultrasound scan or is sure of the conception or last menstrual date. Gestational dating is not always accurate, however, even if the woman has had prenatal care, the infant may prove more or less mature than expected.

Premature infants require resuscitation more often than full-term infants. Other important considerations include

* **Warmth.** Small babies become chilled easily, and hypothermia can start a spiral of complications ending in cardiovascular collapse. Temperature management is crucial.

* **Immature lungs.** The lungs of the very immature baby may be stiff and require more pressure when using a bag and mask. A lack of surfactant in the lungs may cause them to collapse after each breath.

* **Brain hemorrhage.** Delicate blood vessels in the brain may break during delivery and cause intracranial hemorrhage. Hypoxia, rapid changes in intravascular volume, and rough handling can also cause bleeding in the brain.

* **Blood sugar.** Preterm babies are more likely to develop hypoglycemia soon after delivery.

Neonatal intensive care units are best suited for stabilizing and supporting any preterm infant. Ideally the baby should be directly transported to a hospital with a neonatal intensive care unit if it does not greatly prolong transport to do so.

Conditions Associated with Prematurity

Respiratory Distress Syndrome (RDS or Hyaline Membrane Disease)

Respiratory distress syndrome (RDS) is a syndrome caused by insufficient surfactant, which causes respiratory distress in the preterm infant and in some full-term infants as well. RDS kills more babies than any other disease and causes the most long-term complications.

RDS is most likely to develop in the infant born before 37 completed weeks of gestation, the risk increasing with earlier gestational age or in the presence of maternal diabetes. Fetuses exposed to chronic intrauterine stress, such as those born to women with chronic hypertension or prolonged rupture of the membranes, are less likely to develop RDS than are other babies of the same gestational age. This difference is probably due to stress triggering the release of endogenous steroids, which accelerates lung development.

PEDIATRIC
NOTES

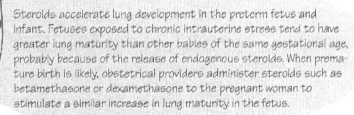

Steroids accelerate lung development in the preterm fetus and infant. Fetuses exposed to chronic intrauterine stress tend to have greater lung maturity than other babies of the same gestational age, probably because of the release of endogenous steroids. When premature birth is likely, obstetrical providers administer steroids such as betamethasone or dexamethasone to the pregnant woman to stimulate a similar increase in lung maturity in the fetus.

Respiratory distress syndrome is a condition primarily involving babies who are born before the lungs are mature. Structurally, the lungs of a preterm baby contain many undeveloped and uninflatable alveoli that would have matured late in gestation had the pregnancy continued. Pulmonary blood flow is reduced due to immature vascular development and incompletely formed capillary beds surrounding the alveoli.

Pulmonary surfactant is secreted by the lungs near term to decrease surface tension and keep the lungs partially inflated between breaths after delivery, reducing the work of breathing. The preterm newborn lacks sufficient surfactant and has a more flexible chest wall that restricts air entry. Alveoli inflate unevenly and collapse on exhalation. Atelectasis develops, and the infant displays rapid, labored, grunting respirations either immediately or within a few hours after delivery.

Fibrin-rich fluid in the alveoli and necrotic alveolar cells form a membranous layer termed a hyaline membrane, which blocks gas exchange and reduces lung expansion. This stiffening of the lungs necessitates increased ventilation pressure to achieve acceptable blood gases. The increased pressure exacerbates damage to the lungs and progression of the disease.

Progressive atelectasis increases pulmonary vascular resistance, sending blood away from the lungs through the persistent ductus arteriosus. Hypoxemia and hypercapnia cause vasospasm in the pulmonary arterioles, further increasing pulmonary vascular resistance. Atelectasis and severity of respiratory failure progressively worsen with time, and the increasing struggle to breathe leads to hypoxia, CO_2 retention, and respiratory and metabolic acidosis. Preterm infants with RDS are also at risk for pneumothorax, retinopathy of prematurity, necrotizing enterocolitis, and stroke.

Preterm infants also have a high proportion of fetal hemoglobin. Fetal hemoglobin has a much higher affinity with oxygen to function well in the low-oxygen environment in the uterus. Fetal hemoglobin binds and holds oxygen effectively, but releases less to the tissues at normal oxygen tension than would adult hemoglobin. Fetal hemoglobin binds oxygen until the infant's arterial oxygen concentration drops, so the infant with a large proportion of fetal hemoglobin will show excellent saturation on a pulse oximeter, but remain hypoxic at the cellular level.

Babies with RDS can develop symptoms immediately or over a period of hours. Often the babies will become pink and show good respiratory effort at birth, then with time show tachypnea, retractions, and color changes. Infants in respiratory distress increase the rate of breathing rather than the depth, so with time the respiratory rate escalates to 80–120 breaths per minute. Retractions increase, nostrils flare, crackles may be heard in the lung fields, and there is an audible grunt as the baby attempts to increase end-expiratory pressure in the lungs to maintain alveolar expansion. Central cyanosis is a late and ominous sign.

A very immature baby may not show dyspnea but simply fail to breathe at all at birth, due to an inability to overcome the resistance of lung and chest wall to take that first breath. In either case, respiratory support can be lifesaving.

With treatment in a modern NICU, the infant will usually begin to produce surfactant, and respiratory function will improve within days or weeks. Pulmonary surfactant can also be administered intratracheally to improve respiratory status, and is often given prophylactically at birth to preterm babies at high risk for developing RDS. Surfactant administration improves survival by reducing the risk of tension pneumothorax and decreasing the incidence and severity of bronchopulmonary dysplasia.

Bronchopulmonary Dysplasia (BPD)

Bronchopulmonary dysplasia (BPD) involves chronic lung damage that may develop in babies who have been treated for respiratory distress with oxygen and mechanical ventilation for a prolonged period, or who have developed pneumonia soon after birth. The lifesaving treatments that sustain babies who cannot breathe effectively without assistance can also cause pulmonary inflammation, which progresses to the breakdown of alveolar walls and scarring. BPD occurs most frequently in premature babies, often following RDS, but may develop in full-term neonates who require mechanical ventilation and oxygen under pressure for problems such as neonatal pulmonary hypertension or meconium aspiration syndrome.

BPD is one of the most common chronic infant lung diseases in the United States. Babies with a history of BPD are at increased risk for lower respiratory tract infections in early childhood and may rapidly grow severely ill when infection occurs. They also may suffer severe bronchospasm and decreased respiratory reserve. The first 2 years of life may be marked by delayed growth and generalized susceptibility to illness. Some babies may require a ventilator and/or oxygen therapy throughout early childhood and suffer functional lung impairment even as adults.

Bradycardia

Bradycardia is more common in premature infants than in full-term infants, but it can occur in neonates of any gestational age. Often a slow pulse is secondary to hypoxia and can be improved by adequate oxygenation. Metabolic or neurological abnormalities can also cause bradycardia. Field treatment involves emphasis on airway management, suctioning, ventilation, and intubation as necessary, with cardiac monitoring and thermoregulation. If adequate oxygenation fails to correct the problem, epinephrine may be indicated.

Intraventricular Hemorrhage (IVH)

Intraventricular hemorrhage (IVH) is bleeding into the ventricles of the brain, a condition that is common in premature infants and potentially a threat to life and long-term health. Young fetuses have a network of fragile, well-perfused blood vessels in the region of the ventricles of the brain. Hypoxemia, changes in venous pressure, and metabolic imbalances can cause these vessels to rupture, precipitating IVH. Babies under 3.5 lb are more vulnerable, especially in the first days of life. Some cases of IVH proceed to hydrocephalus and can permanently damage brain tissue.

Symptoms of IVH include apnea, bradycardia, respiratory distress, poor tone, bulging anterior fontanelle, stupor, and seizures. Diagnosis is by computer tomography or magnetic-resonance imaging.

Necrotizing Enterocolitis (NEC)

Necrotizing enterocolitis (NEC) is an acute inflammatory disease of the intestines. The cause appears multifactorial; NEC is most likely to develop in babies who have experienced ischemia of the bowel, have been formula fed, and have been colonized by certain pathogenic bacteria. This condition primarily affects preterm or other high-risk infants.

The disease process begins when some insult reduces blood supply to the intestines, causing the cells of the bowel to die in great numbers. The thin bowel wall is attacked by enzymes, causing further breakdown and inflammation. Bacteria colonize the damaged intestines and release gas, which bloats the abdomen. The feeding of formula and hypertonic medicines seems to contribute to or exacerbate this process by stressing the bowel.

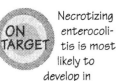

Necrotizing enterocolitis is most likely to develop in preterm babies and is treated in a neonatal intensive care unit (NICU) setting.

Retinopathy of Prematurity (ROP)

Retinopathy of prematurity (ROP) is a condition involving abnormal growth of blood vessels in the eye, causing blindness or vision impairment.

It affects primarily premature babies of young gestational age. It was once thought to be an iatrogenic disease related to abnormally high oxygen levels in the blood. Current research indicates that although oxygen therapy is contributory, ROP is a complex disease with multiple influences including hypocarbia and hypercarbia, intraventricular hemorrhage, infection, vitamin E deficiency, lactic acidosis, maternal diabetes, prenatal complications, and genetic factors.

In ROP, constriction of the immature vasculature of the infant's retina causes hypoxia of the retinal tissues. This process apparently triggers the proliferation of new capillaries into the hypoxic areas. The capillaries begin to leak and cause the retina to separate. Scar tissue forms within the eye and causes irreversible blindness.

Congenital Anomalies

Abnormalities of structure, function, or metabolism affect many babies, although the likelihood of encountering any specific anomalie is low. See Table 10-2. A comprehensive discussion on congenital anomalies is beyond the scope of this book. At delivery, the EMS provider should scan each newborn for obvious anomalies.

If there is a problem, gently tell the parents what you have found, at your level of understanding. "It seems your baby has problems with her legs and feet. I don't know how serious her problem is or what to expect. Her doctor can tell you more. Otherwise, she's breathing and alert, and

Table 10-2	Estimated Incidence of Common Birth Defects
Heart and circulation	1 in 115 births
Muscles and skeleton	1 in 130 births
Club foot	1 in 735 births
Cleft lip/palate	1 in 930 births
Genital and urinary tract	1 in 135 births
Nervous system and eye	1 in 235 births
Anencephaly	1 in 8,000 births
Spina bifida	1 in 2,000 births
Chromosomal syndromes	1 in 600 births
Down syndrome (trisomy 21)	1 in 900 births
Respiratory tract	1 in 900 births
Metabolic disorders	1 in 3,500 births

Source: Adapted from www.marchofdimes.com.

seems to be doing well." Do not offer false hopes or empty promises. Do not offer information unless you are sure it is accurate.

Airway, breathing, and circulation remain the primary concerns when caring for any baby. Some babies are born with body wall defects that expose internal organs—intestines, spinal cord, and so forth. These should be covered with saline gauze and protected from injury and infection, while ensuring that the infant does not become hypothermic. Do not use tape on an infant's tender skin. If possible, transport to a hospital with a neonatal intensive care unit.

Some of the more common congenital abnormalities follow.

Nervous System

Hydrocephalus

Hydrocephalus, or enlargement of the head due to excessive accumulation of cerebral spinal fluid, may be congenital or acquired. It usually arises from an obstruction in the ventricles of the brain and can cause compression and stretching of brain tissue, cerebral ischemia, anoxia, edema, and dysfunction of the blood–brain barrier. It is often associated with other congenital defects.

Often hydrocephalus is not apparent in the newborn but develops later. The affected child will often show enlarged head circumference, bulging anterior fontanelle dilated scalp veins (especially with crying) and widely separated sutures between skull bones. Setting sun sign is a downward rotation of the eyes.

Treatment includes placement of a shunt that drains the cerebral spinal fluid and relieves pressure.

Cerebral Palsy

Cerebral palsy involves mild to severe damage to parts of the brain that control movement and posture, and is a group of nonprogressive disorders that affects control of movement and posture. The disorder is not progressive and may be accompanied by other abnormalities of brain function, such as mental retardation, learning disabilities, seizures, and sensory impairment.

- Spastic cerebral palsy is characterized by muscular rigidity, which makes movement difficult.
- Athetoid or dyskinetic cerebral palsy is characterized by fluctuations in muscle tone from flaccid to rigid, sometimes with uncontrolled movements or difficulties with swallowing and speech.
- Ataxic cerebral palsy is characterized by poor balance and coordination.

Most cases of cerebral palsy represent brain damage from antepartal insults such as infections (most notably rubella, toxoplasmosis, or cytomegalovirus). Premature babies weighing less than 3⅓ pounds are up to 30 times more likely to develop cerebral palsy than full-term infants. Severe hyperbilirubinemia can cause permanent brain damage resulting in cerebral palsy, as can Rh disease or blood-clotting disorders and certain genetic diseases. Occasionally, brain injuries in early childhood (such as from meningitis or head injury) can result in cerebral palsy. A 2003 report issued by the American College of Obstetricians and Gynecologists (ACOG) and the American Academy of Pediatrics (AAP) asserts that less than 10% of the kinds of brain injury that can result in cerebral palsy are caused by intrapartum hypoxia or anoxia. Often the cause remains unknown.

Neural Tube Defects

The neural tube is the part of the embryo that develops into the brain and spinal cord by the 28th day of gestation. Malformation of the neural tube results in disorders such as spina bifida or anencephaly. The woman carrying a fetus with a **neural tube defect** is likely to develop polyhydramnios due to the continual leaking of fetal cerebrospinal fluid into the amniotic sac.

neural tube defect Any of various congenital anomalies resulting from incomplete closing of the neural tube in an embryo, such as spina bifida or anencephaly.

Spina Bifida   Spina bifida occurs when closure of the neural tube is incomplete, creating a vertebral malformation through which the spinal cord and spinal nerve roots may protrude. This defect can cause paralysis, impairment in bladder and bowel function, and hydrocephalus. Spina bifida may have a genetic component, and risk increases with lack of folic acid in the maternal diet, certain anticonvulsant medications (such as phenytoin or phenobarbitol), uncontrolled maternal diabetes, or with chromosomal anomalies. The defect is usually in the lumbar or sacral region, and may involve severe disability or may be so minor as to escape detection.

Spina bifida occulta involves a minor vertebral anomaly, usually without damage to the spinal cord or nerves. Children with this malformation might show a tuft of hair, freckle, dimple, skin tag, or other lesion over the site of the defect, but often show no signs or symptoms. The condition may be discovered as an incidental finding when the patient is X-rayed later in life for some other reason.

A meningocele involves herniation of the spinal meninges through the vertebral defect. The child who undergoes surgical correction of the problem may develop normally. Myelomeningocele occurs when the meninges as well as the spinal cord and its nerve roots herniate into the vertebral defect, or the spinal cord and nerves are completely exposed. Myelomeningoceles are surgically repaired within the first day or two of life to minimize infection and further nerve damage from trauma, but permanent nerve damage is typical, and most children with this condition suffer lower extremity paralysis.

If a child with spina bifida is delivered in the field, protect the infant from hypothermia and infection and do not touch any open lesions. Protect the lesion with a sterile dressing—check with your medical control to confirm the treatment required by your institution. Some protocols favor sterile plastic covering and prefer to avoid contact with gauze or any other material that might stick to the exposed tissue. In other cases gauze may be acceptable. The lesion should be kept moist and sterile. Do not use tape on the infant's tender skin. Position prone or on the side to reduce pressure on the lesion. If resuscitation is necessary, resuscitate infant while maintaining a side-lying position if possible. Monitor vital signs as with any infant.

Anencephaly   Anencephaly is a defect that occurs when the upper end of the neural tube does not close normally during the 3rd or 4th week after conception, resulting in severe malformation of the skull and brain. The anencephalic infant has a very small, oddly shaped head with a minimally developed or absent cerebrum and cranial vault with an intact lower brain stem.

The same genetic and environmental factors that cause spina bifida can also cause anencephaly. About 75 percent of babies with anencephaly are stillborn, and most of the rest do not survive beyond 2 weeks of age. Infants with anencephaly are given supportive care until they succumb.

Cardiovascular

Congenital Heart Defects
In the United States, about 1 of every 125 to 150 babies are born with cardiac defects each year, and most are diagnosed in the first week of life. The heart is formed during the first 7 weeks of gestation, and any disruption of normal development can result in a cardiac anomaly. Cardiac defects can be caused by chromosomal abnormalities, hereditary conditions, environmental influences, exposure to certain medications *in utero* (such as Accutane or lithium), or maternal conditions (such as hyperglycemia, infection, or hyperthermia), but most cases are multifactorial. Between 1987 and 1997, the death rates from congenital heart problems decreased 23% due to advances in diagnosis and surgical treatment.

Some common cardiac defects include

- **Patent ductus arteriosus (PDA).**   This affects 5–10% of full-term infants and the majority of preemies weighing less than 1,500 g. This condition involves a reversal in blood flow that allows blood to reenter the pulmonary vessels and flood the lungs. The increased blood flow can cause increased pulmonary vascular resistance, pulmonary hypertension, and right ventricular hypertrophy. The developing lungs of the fetus do not require much blood supply, so most of the circulating volume is diverted from the pulmonary artery through the ductus arteriosus to the aorta. This routing allows oxygenated blood from the placenta to largely bypass the lungs. At birth, the ductus arteriosus should constrict, sending blood to the lungs to acquire oxygen and release carbon dioxide as with adult circulation. If the ductus fails to close within 96 hours of birth, the condition is termed a patent ductus arteriosus (PDA). The neonate is more likely to develop PDA following respiratory distress syndrome, intravenous fluid overload, asphyxia, or if premature or born at high altitudes.

PDA presents with a murmur that persists beyond 3 or 4 days of life, bounding peripheral pulses, dyspnea arising over the course of hours or days, tachypnea, episodes of apnea, or audible crackles. The infant with PDA is managed in the hospital by restricting fluids, supporting ventilation, increasing hematocrit, and administration of medication such as indomethacin or ibuprofen, and surgical ligation.

- **Ventricular septal defect (VSD).**   This is a flaw or opening in the ventricular septum caused by imperfect ventricular division during early embryonic development. VSD is the most common congenital heart anomaly, accounting for 20–25% of babies born with cardiac defects. The child with a symptomatic VSD shunts oxygenated blood back to the right heart rather than to the aorta, increasing pressure in the right ventricle and pulmonary artery. A small defect may be asymptomatic, whereas an infant with a large VSD may display decreased exertional tolerance (such as difficulty feeding), poor weight gain, pulmonary infections, and congestive heart failure.

- **Atrial septal defect (ASD).**   This is a flaw or opening in the atrial septum that results from an error in atrial formation in embryonic development. Blood flow shifts from the left ventricle to the right during systole, gradually increasing pulmonary artery pressure and sometimes leading to congestive heart failure if the ASD is large. Spontaneous closure occurs in almost half of all cases by age 5, but surgical closure is sometimes indicated.

- **Coarctation of the aorta.**   This is a narrowing of the aortic arch, most commonly below the origin of the left subclavian artery. It usually occurs alongside other defects such as VSD, PDA, or aortic valve anomalies. The blood pressure in the segment of aorta proximal to the constriction is elevated, causing an increase in left ventricular pressure and workload, which may lead to congestive heart failure. Bounding pulses may be present in the upper extremities. Blood pressure beyond the constriction is decreased, and pulses may be weak or absent in the lower limbs. The infant's legs may be cool and pale. Affected babies can deteriorate rapidly. Surgical correction is often required.

- **Tetralogy of Fallot (TOF).** This is a congenital heart defect accounting for 10% of all congenital heart anomalies. The condition includes four abnormalities: pulmonary stenosis, ventricular septal defect, aorta positioned directly over the VSD, and right ventricular hypertrophy. In TOF, deoxygenated blood flows through the VSD and out the aorta rather than to the lungs for oxygenation. The affected baby will usually show respiratory distress and persistent cyanosis from birth, and a loud, long murmur may be audible.

Surgical repair under cardiopulmonary bypass may be attempted in infancy. Affected children may show exercise intolerance and poor feeding. The EMS provider may encounter the decompensating child with TOF at delivery or when parents call the ambulance for a hypoxic event. Increased activity, feeding, crying, or defecation can trigger an episode of severe oxygen desaturation, which can lead to coma, seizures, and death. Children with TOF are also at increased risk for cerebrovascular accident.

The EMS professional called to the home of a decompensating child diagnosed with TOF should fold the child's legs to the chest while transporting to trap blood in the extremities and reduce systemic venous return, decreasing cardiac workload and increasing pulmonary blood flow. (Children with TOF will instinctively squat if they suffer mild hypoxia while at play.) Treat as appropriate for the child with cardiorespiratory compromise.

- **Transposition of the great arteries (or transposition of the great vessels).** This is a reversal of the normal attachment of arteries that directly receive cardiac output. With this defect, the pulmonary artery is connected to the left ventricle and the aorta is connected to the right ventricle. Deoxygenated blood comes into the right heart through the vena cava and is pumped out through the aorta, while oxygenated blood is circulated from the lungs, to the left heart, and back to the lungs.

Transposition of the great vessels could be quickly fatal, but most affected children have associated defects such as septal defects or PDA that allow some of the oxygenated blood to enter the systemic circulation and sustain life. However, these defects may also increase pulmonary blood flow and cause congestive heart failure and pulmonary hypertension.

Babies with transposition of the great vessels may be cyanotic and depressed at birth or show signs of congestive heart failure. The amount of decompensation depends on how much oxygenated blood is able to reach the systemic circulation and the degree of increased pressure in the lungs and heart. Definitive treatment is surgery to switch the arteries to their proper positions, or to divert blood flow to promote oxygenation. Patients who have undergone surgical treatment for transposition of the great vessels may be at greater risk throughout life for arrhythmias and ventricular dysfunction.

Alimentary Tract

Cleft Lip or Palate

Cleft lip or palate is a division of the lip, hard palate, or soft palate resulting from failure of these structures to close in early fetal development. Cleft lip or lip and palate affects approximately 1 in 1,000 babies, males more often than females. More than 70% of babies with cleft lip also have cleft palate. Babies with clefts often have other abnormalities as well.

Every embryo has a divided lip and palate early in gestation. Normally the two halves of the lip fuse by 5–6 weeks after conception, and the palate about 4 or 5 weeks later. A cleft lip may be unilateral or bilateral, manifesting as a small notch in the upper lip, or a division of the lip that extends into the nostril or upper gum.

The EMS provider may have difficulty sealing a mask around the defect if the child requires resuscitation, and intubation should be considered as appropriate. The cleft lip defect is often surgically repaired by 3 months of age, and the cleft palate usually between 9 and 18 months. Babies with clefts may initially have difficulty feeding.

Genitourinary

Renal Agenesis

Renal agenesis is the congenital absence of one or both kidneys. In most cases babies born with a single kidney have a good prognosis, although they may be at increased risk for pyelonephritis, renal calculi, hypertension, and renal failure throughout life. Unilateral renal agenesis can also be associated with syndromes that include other malformations of the urogenital tract or other organs.

About 1 in 4,000 babies is born with bilateral renal agenesis. This condition is universally fatal, with all affected babies dying before birth or within the first days of life. Because the fetus with bilateral renal agenesis cannot produce urine, severe oligohydramnios develops. When fluid is decreased around the fetus, he cannot inhale enough to fully expand his growing lungs and suffers abnormal lung development. **Pulmonary hypoplasia** develops, and at birth these infants are unable to obtain sufficient oxygen to sustain life. Oligohydramnios also causes fetal compression, resulting in flattened facial features and limb deformities. The affected child may also have low-set ears, skeletal anomalies such as lack of a sacrum, eye malformations, or cardiac anomalies.

pulmonary hypoplasia
Underdeveloped lungs.

Newborns with bilateral renal agenesis develop severe respiratory distress (due to pulmonary hypoplasia) shortly after birth and may also develop spontaneous pneumothorax.

Renal agenesis is often identified antepartally through routine sonogram. Because bilateral renal agenesis is fatal, some parents opt to terminate the pregnancy when the condition is discovered. In other cases, the babies are carried to term. The hospital will usually withhold life support from these newborns, and the EMS provider should consult medical control for instructions if a baby with known bilateral renal agenesis is delivered in the field.

Hypospadias and Epispadias

Hypospadias in males occurs when the urethral opening is located along the underside of the penis, not at the tip. This condition affects nearly 1 in 300 male infants and can involve a meatus placed slightly below the usual location, or a severe malformation wherein the urethral meatus is located between folds of the scrotum or on the perineum. Often the foreskin wraps only partly around the penis, forming a dorsal hood. Without surgical correction, the patient may be unable to urinate while standing and may experience pain with intercourse. Neonates with hypospadias are not usually circumcised, because the tissue of the foreskin can be used to repair the defect. Surgical correction is usually performed between 9 and 15 months of age. Hypospadias in females occurs when the urethra opens into the vaginal introitus.

Epispadias in males is a condition wherein the urethral opening is located on the dorsal aspect of the penis, rather than at the tip. The penis is often short and flat, and may be associated with other conditions such as a bladder exstrophy (the bladder opens directly to the outside of the body) and separation of the pubic bone. In females, the defect involves an abnormally placed urethral opening, often with a divided clitoris.

Ambiguous Genitalia

Ambiguous genitalia are external genital organs that do not appear obviously male or female, or have features of both. For the first 6 weeks of gestation, the embryo has a chromosomal gender, but there are no observable physical differences between male and female embryos. All embryos have two genital ducts—one with the capability of developing into a male reproductive system, the other able to become a female reproductive system.

During the 7th and 8th weeks of development, the primitive genitalia of the embryo differentiate. Homologous male and female structures are derived from the same undifferentiated embryonic tissues; the labia and scrotum arise from the same structures, as do the clitoris and the penis. If the embryo is male, genes on the Y chromosome differentiate the primitive gonads into testes that produce testosterone. Testosterone causes the gender-neutral embryonic genitalia to develop into a penis and scrotum and the male genital duct system (Wolffian) to form a male reproductive tract, while the genital duct system that would produce a female (Müllerian) regresses. If no testosterone is produced, the Müllerian tract will develop and the embryo will grow ovaries and female genitals.

Ambiguous genitalia are seen in about 1 or 2 babies per 1,000 births. This condition can be caused by chromosomal anomalies, hormonal imbalances, enzyme deficiencies, and unexplained disruptions in fetal development. Ambiguous genitalia are most commonly caused by adrenal hyperplasia, a hereditary enzyme deficiency involving an overproduction of androgens by the fetal adrenal glands. If the fetus is female, the excess androgens cause **virilization** such as hypertrophy of the clitoris until the organ resembles a penis. Girls with adrenal hyperplasia may undergo surgery to give their genitals a more feminine appearance.

Androgen insensitivity syndrome occurs when an embryo is genetically male (XY) and has testes that produce androgens, but the cells of the embryonic genitals resist testosterone and do not develop into normal male genitalia. In most cases, the infant with complete androgen insensitivity will have testes that remain within the abdominal cavity and normal female labia, clitoris, and vaginal introitus. Uterus and fallopian tubes are rudimentary or absent, and the vagina is usually a blind pouch. Most children with complete androgen insensitivity are raised as girls, and they are medically, legally, and socially considered female, but will never menstruate or bear children. Breast development and other female secondary sex characteristics occur at puberty when testosterone is converted to estrogen by the body. Infants with partial androgen sensitivity have some response to androgens, but not enough to masculinize the fetus; the result is often ambiguous external genitals.

Androgen insensitivity is often identified in the newborn by the presence of inguinal masses that are identified as testes during surgery. Sometimes this condition is not discovered until the girl fails to experience menarche. In most cases the testes are removed to prevent malignancy, but often not until after puberty. Thereafter, hormonal replacement therapy is required.

If following a field delivery there is any doubt to the child's gender, do not guess. Assignment or verification of gender can involve physical examination, chromosomal analysis, measurement of hormonal levels, and ultrasound scanning. Sometimes surgery or hormone therapy is initiated after gender assignment to help the child to live a more normal life. In the past, a boy with a very undeveloped penis was usually raised as a girl and treated with feminizing hormones and surgery. More recently, physicians have begun to recognize the role of gender in the physiology of the brain and watch the child's development to ascertain whether he feels more like a boy or a girl before permanently assigning gender.

virilization
Development of male secondary sex characteristics.

PEARLS Even normal infant genitals can look anomalous to the inexperienced provider. A preterm girl can have a very prominent clitoris and labia minora and thin, retracted labia majora. Girls often have hypertrophied hymenal tags. An uncircumcised boy can look unusual to a provider who has seen only circumcised penises.

Musculoskeletal/Limbs/Body Structure

Dwarfism

There are many different syndromes and disorders that cause dwarfism, including

- **Achondroplasia.** This is a genetic disorder of bone growth affecting 1 in every 25,000 births. In the majority of cases, the disorder is not inherited but arises as a new mutation in the chromosomes of the egg or sperm. It is the most common form of dwarfism. In affected individuals, cartilage cells in the growth plates of the long bones are slow to transform into bone. People with achondroplasia have normal-sized torsos with shortened limbs, have a separation between the middle and ring fingers, and often have large heads, prominent foreheads, and flat noses. In infancy, hydrocephalus can develop.

  Respiratory and airway problems are more likely in babies with achondroplasia because the head is proportionally larger and can cause airway obstruction if flexed or hyperextended. The neck is also more flexible than that of a normal newborn, while the spinal cord is more vulnerable to damage if the neck is hyperextended or hyperflexed; handle a baby with achondroplasia carefully and with secure neck support.

- **Ellis–van Creveld (EvC) Syndrome.** This is another type of dwarfism that is rare in the general population, but occurs as frequently as 1 in 200 births among the Old Order Amish in Pennsylvania. It bears mention because babies born with this type of dwarfism suffer a 50% mortality rate from heart defects (usually atrial septal defects or lack of an atrial septum) and pulmonary hypoplasia. Many of the Old Order Amish babies are born at home, so EMS may be called if a baby with EvC develops respiratory distress at birth. Children with EvC who have a normal heart, lungs, and chest have a normal life expectancy. The disorder is readily recognizable because there are always six fingers on each hand and sometimes six toes on each foot. Adult height is about 42–60 in.

Talipes Equinovarus (Clubfoot)

Clubfoot is a common birth defect, with an incidence of 1–4 cases per 1,000 infants. Children with this disorder show a foot or feet that are exaggeratedly plantar flexed, with the forefoot swung medially and the sole facing inward. The deformity involves many related problems including muscle shortening and abnormal formation and placement of foot and ankle bones. Treatment includes manipulation, casts, and sometimes surgery. Treatment is frequently begun in the first week of life, and the child usually remains in casts for 3–6 months.

Abdominal Wall

Omphalocele

Omphalocele involves the herniation of the intestines and sometimes other abdominal organs into the umbilical cord. Omphalocele is often detected on ultrasound antepartally. The condition is usually obvious at birth, although sometimes a small omphalocele may be difficult to distinguish from a large, thick gelatinous umbilical cord.

In the normal embryo, by the 6th week of gestation, the growth of the intestines and liver outpaces the growth of the body, resulting in a scarcity of space in which the abdominal contents can develop. At about 7 weeks' gestation, intestinal segments begin to herniate into the umbilical cord. By about 10 weeks' gestation, the abdominal cavity has grown large enough to accommodate the liver and the intestines in their entirety, and the loops of intestine are retracted into the abdomen. With omphalocele, this process fails to occur. At birth abdominal organs, enclosed in a membrane, protrude through a defect at the opening at which the umbilical cord enters the abdomen.

Omphalocele frequently is associated with other malformations and lethal chromosomal anomalies. Babies with omphalocele are often premature.

EMS management of the newborn with omphalocele includes thermoregulation because babies with exposed organs lose heat at an accelerated rate. Do not allow the baby to feed. The defect should also be protected from trauma, infection, and fluid loss with a moist dressing. Protocols may vary, but most guidelines specify that the EMS provider, wearing sterile gloves, should wrap sterile warm, moist saline-soaked gauze loosely around the defect—two fingers should fit easily between the infant and the dressing. A dry outer layer of gauze may then be applied, and the dressing then topped with sterile plastic wrap. If transport time is long, medical control may request that EMS providers start intravenous fluids to counteract fluid loss. The infant should be comforted to reduce crying to prevent the swallowing of air.

gastroschisis
A condition in which the abdominal wall is incompletely formed and the intestines protrude through the gap without a protective membrane.

Gastroschisis

Gastroschisis is a condition in which the abdominal wall is incompletely formed and the intestines protrude through the defect without a protective membrane surrounding them. While this defect is often more dramatic in appearance than omphalocele, the incidence of associated malformations of systems other than the GI tract is low, and prognosis is generally good. Babies with gastroschisis are often premature.

The defect is usually about 2 to 5 cm in size and is typically located to the right of the umbilicus. The umbilical cord shows a normal insertion. By the time of birth, the unprotected intestines have been damaged by amniotic fluid and appear as a swollen, matted mass rather than pink loops.

Most deaths that occur in newborns with gastroschisis can be attributed to shock, infection, or hypothermia. Prehospital care is the same as with omphalocele (covered previously).

Chromosomal Abnormality

Down Syndrome (Trisomy 21)

Individuals with Down syndrome have three copies of chromosome 21. Distinctive facial features and physical characteristics often makes this condition identifiable in the field, but some individuals are more profoundly affected than others. A patient with Down syndrome may show epicanthal folds, upward slanted palpebral fissures, flattened nasal bridge, protuberant tongue, lowset ears, short fingers and toes, Simian crease (transverse line across the palms), and other characteristic features. Babies with this condition tend to have floppy muscle tone and a poor Moro reflex. About 40% of infants with Down syndrome also have congenital cardiac defects, and many have gastrointestinal anomalies, increased susceptibility to infection, visual or hearing impairment, and other health concerns. Mental retardation can range from mild to severe, and degree of mental impairment cannot be determined by physical appearance. An individual who has many obvious features of Down syndrome may be much higher functioning than another individual with more subtle physical manifestations.

Trisomy 18

Individuals with trisomy 18 have three copies of chromosome number 18. Affected children have distinctive features including rocker-bottom feet, overlapping fingers, hypoplastic nails, small jaw, low-set ears, and intrauterine growth restriction and profound mental retardation. This syndrome is fatal. Most babies die before birth, and only 5% survive beyond the first year.

Respiratory

Choanal Atresia

Choanal atresia is obstruction of the nasal passages from the back of the nose to the throat by bone or tissue, rendering the baby unable to breathe through the nose. Choanal atresia may be unilateral or bilateral and may be associated with other abnormalities. The normal neonate is an obligate nose breather, because the oral airway is not developed enough to allow for mouth breathing, except when crying.

The baby with choanal atresia may show signs of respiratory distress such as cyanosis, retractions, or apnea due to an inability to maintain airflow through the mouth. The infant may be unable to feed and breathe simultaneously, and is at high risk for aspiration. If a shiny metal object like the back of a stethoscope is held under the baby's nose, the baby with choanal atresia will not create the double semicircles of mist that a nose-breathing infant would produce. The provider will be unable to pass a catheter from the nares into the oropharynx.

Newborns with bilateral choanal atresia may require resuscitation at birth. Respiratory arrest can occur even if the baby seems to be stable. Babies with respiratory problems can decline rapidly. Some babies with choanal atresia require intubation to maintain an airway. Surgical correction can resolve the problem, but restenosis can recur, necessitating dilation or repeat surgeries.

Diaphragmatic Hernia

Diaphragmatic hernia involves a defect in the diaphragm that allows intestine and often other abdominal organs to enter the chest cavity, compressing the lung and pulmonary and visceral vasculature. Babies are born with marked pulmonary hypoplasia and pulmonary hypertension on the affected side and to a lesser degree on the contralateral side.

At birth, affected infants usually show marked respiratory distress, cyanosis, and shock. If the infant gulps air at birth, the viscera expand with air and further compromise respiration. The abdomen appears flat and hollowed, and breath sounds are absent on the side of the defect (usually the left). Bowel sounds may be heard in the chest, and the heart sounds may be heard on the right because of mediastinal shift away from the hernia.

Oftentimes diaphragmatic hernia is diagnosed ultrasonographically before birth. Polyhydramnios is common, resulting from fetus swallowing little fluid.

If a child with a known diaphragmatic hernia is born in the field, or the condition is strongly suspected, the provider should elevate the infant's head and thorax. Do not initiate bag and mask ventilation because it can fill the digestive tract with air and worsen the condition. If a diaphragmatic hernia is suspected, the infant should be intubated and ventilated at birth, and a nasogastric or orogastric tube attached to low intermittent suctioning should be placed to vent air from the digestive tract. Monitor oxygen saturation with a pulse oximeter. Ventilation should proceed at a rapid rate and low volume to reduce lung trauma.

Transport the infant with the head and chest elevated above the abdomen to encourage downward displacement of the abdominal organs. Surgical correction of the defect is necessary, but the prognosis is poor for infants who show severe respiratory compromise at birth.

Summary

A distressed baby requires quick, decisive action, including rapid transport to an appropriate facility. Almost half of neonatal deaths occur within 24 hours of delivery, and many of these occur within the first hour. Effective management of respiratory compromise in the first few minutes of life may profoundly influence long-term outcome.

Any provider who may be responsible for the delivery of a newborn—that is, virtually all prehospital providers—must possess the knowledge and skills to perform successful resuscitation during the first few precarious minutes after delivery. An effective resuscitative effort requires the provider to understand transitional physiology and adaptation, recognize deviations from normal, confidently initiate appropriate treatment, and understand the infant's possible responses to resuscitation.

REVIEW QUESTIONS

1. What are some risk factors that might predict a baby who will require resuscitation at birth?

2. Describe meconium aspiration syndrome. What signs might an infant with MAS show?

3. You have just delivered a baby with an abdominal-wall defect. Compare and contrast gastroschisis and omphalocele and describe the field management of these defects.

4. What is cerebral palsy, and what are its most common causes?

5. You are transporting a woman who is in her 30th week of pregnancy, and you realize she will probably give birth en route. Describe some of the challenges of managing a preterm infant in the field.

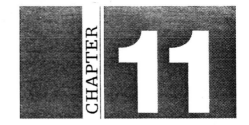
Gynecology

Objectives

By the end of this chapter you should be able to

- Implement emergency treatment for vaginal bleeding

- Distinguish between cyclic and noncyclic pelvic pain

- Manage the patient with toxic shock syndrome

- Provide treatment for the woman with genital trauma

- Recognize the signs of domestic violence

- Manage the victim of sexual assault

CASE Study

After being turned out for an "assault victim," Louis and Debbie arrived on scene to find numerous police cars parked at the address. Upon entering the well-kept suburban home, they heard loud wailing issue from the kitchen.

A policewoman crouched helplessly in front of a deep cupboard that contained a sobbing young woman. The patient had not responded to the best efforts to calm her. As Louis questioned the other policemen on the scene, Debbie joined the female officer in trying to calm the patient. The victim's name was Kaitlyn. Her friend had arrived after work to drive her to an evening class and found her hysterical and inconsolable in the cabinet. Her friend's 911 call had brought the police, and the police had summoned the ambulance. So far, the officers had been unable to determine the exact nature of the crime, but the evidence indicated a struggle and injury that had caused bleeding.

It seemed that Kaitlyn was still reliving the trauma and did not yet realize that she was safe. Debbie cautiously placed her hand on Kaitlyn's arm, knowing that touch could either ground and comfort Kaitlyn, or intensify her panic. "Open your eyes," Debbie crooned in a soft voice. "It's safe now. Nobody can hurt you now. Open your eyes." Kaitlyn did not withdraw her arm from Debbie's touch, and in time her sobs began to quiet and she appeared to be listening to Debbie's reassurance. She opened her eyes and looked blankly at the paramedic.

Debbie was patient. Kaitlyn slowly reconnected with her environment and began to answer questions. Finger bruises were already noticeable on her neck; her arms and cheek were reddened, and there was a hematoma on her inner thigh. There was a lot of blood on her legs and on the living room rug, where the assault had apparently taken place, but Kaitlyn reported that she was having a menstrual period, and she wasn't sure how much of the blood was attributable to injury.

Questions

1. What kinds of question should Debbie ask Kaitlyn? What kinds of question should she avoid?
2. How should Debbie perform a physical assessment of this patient?
3. How should Louis and Debbie manage transport of this patient?
4. How should Debbie document this transport?

Introduction

Women and girls make up slightly more than half the population, but they account for a larger majority of people who seek health care. From infancy to postmenopause, however, a woman's health care needs change greatly. Women seek treatment for common gynecological and urinary problems, including abnormal bleeding, pelvic pain, trauma, and infection. To form a correct clinical impression and provide proper care, the prehospital provider must be well versed in a wide range of topics in female anatomy and physiology; understand what problems and processes a patient's symptoms may represent; and implement appropriate treatment modalities.

KEY TERMS

adhesion, p. 296

atrophic vaginitis, p. 292

diverticulitis, p. 299

dysmenorrhea, p. 298

menorrhagia (hypermenorrhea), p. 291

necrotizing fasciitis, p. 300

primary amenorrhea, p. 301

salpingitis, p. 294

secondary amenorrhea, p. 301

somatization disorder, p. 296

Abnormal Vaginal Bleeding

Abnormal vaginal bleeding is one of the most common gynecological complaints encountered in emergency medicine. The term *abnormal* applies to bleeding that occurs at intervals of less than 21 days or greater than 36 days or that produces more than 80–130 cc of blood lost with each menstrual cycle. A woman who soaks a thick pad in an hour or less for several hours is considered to be bleeding heavily. Excessive or prolonged menstrual bleeding that occurs at normal intervals is **menorrhagia, or hypermenorrhea.**

menorrhagia (hypermenorrhea) Excessive or prolonged menstrual bleeding that occurs at normal intervals.

Ten to 20% of women experience abnormal bleeding at some point during their reproductive lives. It is most likely to occur at either end of the childbearing years, during adolescence, and in the years preceding menopause. About 95% of the time, dysfunctional uterine bleeding (DUB) occurs when the woman fails to ovulate or ovulates very early in her cycle.

 PEARLS Always consider pregnancy a possible cause of vaginal bleeding, even if the patient has had a tubal ligation, denies having had intercourse, or has not reached menarche.

Always consider pregnancy a possible cause of vaginal bleeding, even if the patient has had a tubal ligation, denies having had intercourse, or has not reached menarche. Her medical history alone may be undependable when the woman is unaware she is pregnant, has irregular cycles, or is ashamed to admit the possibility of pregnancy. A history of breast tenderness, frequent urination, nausea, and vomiting may indicate pregnancy, and bleeding may be related to spontaneous abortion or bleeding behind the placenta. It is also possible to miscarry one twin and continue to gestate the other. Hydatidiform molar pregnancy can cause persistent bleeding. Bleeding with abdominal pain or fainting spells may indicate ectopic pregnancy. A woman may hemorrhage weeks after an abortion or miscarriage if all the products of conception have not been passed.

Hormonal contraceptives can cause irregular bleeding, especially progesterone-only methods such as Depo-Provera (an injectable medication given every 3 months), the "minipill" Micronor (a daily oral medication), or the progesterone IUD (an intrauterine device that releases progesterone and may remain in place for as long as 5 years). Oral contraceptives are more likely to cause abnormal bleeding if the woman misses one or more pills, but certain medications such as antibiotics may decrease the efficacy of the pill. Hormone-replacement therapy can also cause changes in bleeding.

Other causes of vaginal bleeding include

- Injury or disease of the vagina (caused by intercourse, trauma, infection, warts, ruptured polyps, or varicosity)
- Vaginal injury from insertion of foreign objects
- Malignancy
- Trauma related to **atrophic vaginitis** (damage to thin, dry vaginal walls caused by a lack of estrogen after menopause)
- Hormonal imbalance
- Thyroid disorder
- Recent procedures on cervix, such as cone biopsy
- Ovarian cysts or polycystic ovarian syndrome
- Blood-clotting disorder
- Medication or herbal use
- Chronic liver disease
- Intrauterine devices
- Sexually transmitted infections
- Weight gain
- Stress
- Irregular menses
- Uterine fibroids

atrophic vaginitis
Irritation of thin, dry vaginal walls caused by a lack of estrogen after menopause.

PEARLS Whenever a woman presents with bleeding after intercourse, consider abuse as a possible cause.

Postmenopausal Bleeding

Because uterine cancer is most common between the ages of 50 and 75, vaginal bleeding in a postmenopausal woman can indicate uterine or cervical cancer, but it may also result from cervical polyps. Some older women with poor pelvic muscle tone experience prolapse of the cervix or bladder, conditions that may present with minor spotting.

The vagina of an elderly woman may atrophy from lack of estrogen, especially if she is not sexually active. Resuming intercourse can cause the vagina to tear and bleed. A younger woman who has had her ovaries removed and is not on hormone therapy or a woman who has been lactating for many months may also experience atrophic vaginitis.

Prehospital Management of Vaginal Bleeding

Profuse vaginal bleeding can be very frightening to both the woman and her provider. A woman may lose a significant amount of blood through vaginal bleeding, and the EMS responder must remain vigilant for signs of decompensation.

Begin by taking a history of the complaint, including onset, duration, amount (including clots and gushing), menstrual history and date of last period, contraception and likelihood of pregnancy, medical history, medications (especially warfarin, aspirin, or other anticoagulating medicines), and allergies. The OLDCART method works well for this purpose. Assess for associated symptoms, such as pain, dizziness or fainting, bruising or petechiae, nausea, or vomiting. Assess for the presence of a coagulation disorder (abnormal bruising, wounds that do not stop bleeding), which often remains undiagnosed until a young girl reaches menarche and heavy periods begin. Observe for pallor, clamminess, diaphoresis, or altered consciousness. Monitor vital signs. Assess her abdomen for tenderness or distension. *Never perform a vaginal exam.*

A woman's perception of blood loss is highly subjective, and it can be difficult to quantify. Ask whether she is passing clots and if so, how many and how large: The size of a dime? The size of a lemon? A patient may be able to describe blood loss in terms of household measurements—a cup, a tablespoon—but research has demonstrated that even medical professionals tend to miscalculate blood loss using this method.

Ask how many hours it took her to soak a pad, whether her pad is thick or thin, and whether the pad contains a spot of blood or is thoroughly saturated when she changes it. Generally pads hold more fluid than tampons. An average superabsorbency sanitary pad holds about 20–30 ml when fully saturated. A woman used to light cycles may panic over a period that would be normal for another woman. Conversely, a woman who ordinarily has very heavy cyclic bleeding may assume that such bleeding is normal. One study showed that almost half of women with excessive bleeding considered their periods normal or even light.

If vital signs, pad count, and level of consciousness indicate that the patient is at risk for hypovolemia, transport in the position that maximizes her blood pressure with oxygen and cardiac monitoring. Establish an intravenous line of normal saline or lactated Ringer's and infuse as vital signs indicate. If local protocols specify, draw blood for a CBC and coagulation panel. Monitor for shock and treat accordingly.

Upon arrival at the hospital, some women with severe vaginal bleeding will require a dilation and curettage (D&C) procedure to stop the hemorrhage. In other cases, a Foley catheter may be inserted into the uterus and the balloon distended with saline to tamponade the bleeding. Many cases of vaginal bleeding can be treated with hormonal therapy.

Pelvic Pain

Pelvic pain is a common complaint that is frequently encountered in the field. It may be acute, chronic, or recurrent and may originate in the reproductive tract or other organs or structures. Acute pelvic pain may be a surgical emergency. Chronic pain can be severe and debilitating and may also require surgical intervention.

Acute Pelvic Pain

Sudden onset of pelvic pain may indicate a potentially serious or even life-threatening problem. The EMS professional can often form an accurate clinical impression of the problem by taking a careful history.

GERIATRIC NOTES

Endometrial cancer is the most common gynecologic malignancy in the United States. It occurs mostly in older women with a peak incidence between the ages of 55 and 65. Risk factors include age, obesity, nulliparity, and prolonged use of exogenous estrogen without progesterone supplementation. The most common symptom is post-menopausal vaginal bleeding.

Ectopic Pregnancy

Always consider ectopic pregnancy as a cause of pelvic pain until it is proven otherwise. Ectopic pregnancy can be difficult to diagnose and quickly fatal if missed. Most commonly, the woman will report that her period is a week or two late and often that she has been spotting, but presentation varies widely. Pain is usually unilateral and may radiate to the shoulder. A ruptured ectopic pregnancy will rarely present with periumbilical ecchymosis, known as Cullen's sign. Five percent of cases result in severe hemorrhage with hypovolemic shock. Ectopic pregnancy is more likely among women with a history of pelvic inflammatory disease, prior ectopic pregnancies, or tubal surgery and those who use intrauterine devices. If pregnancy occurs after tubal ligation, it is likely to be ectopic. Consider ectopic pregnancy as a possible source of pelvic pain in any woman of childbearing age.

Pelvic Inflammatory Disease

salpingitis
Inflammation of the fallopian tube.

Pelvic inflammatory disease (PID) is the generic term for a variety of infections of the female reproductive tract, including endometritis, **salpingitis,**

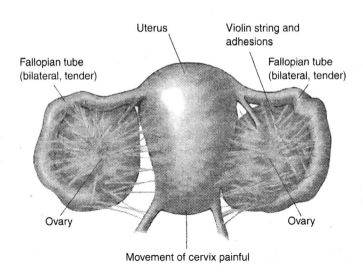

Uterus

Violin string and adhesions

Fallopian tube (bilateral, tender)

Fallopian tube (bilateral, tender)

Ovary

Ovary

Movement of cervix painful

FIGURE 11-1
Pelvic Inflammatory Disease.
In pelvic inflammatory disease, adhesions can increase pain and cause infertility.

tubo-ovarian abscess, and peritonitis. PID accounts for about 20% of acute pelvic complaints in women and can occur at any age, but is especially prevalent in women younger than age 25. It is caused by microorganisms that ascend from the vagina and cervix into the usually sterile upper reproductive tract. The most common culprits are the sexually transmitted disease organisms *Chlamydia trachomatis* and *Neisseria gonorrhoeae*, but other microorganisms can cause PID, including those normally present in a woman's vaginal flora. The presence of an intrauterine contraceptive device facilitates the ascent of harmful bacteria into the upper reproductive tract, and vaginal douching can push bacteria through the cervix into the uterus. After infection with PID, tubal scarring may cause infertility, predispose to ectopic pregnancy, or cause chronic pelvic pain. See Figure 11-1.

Initially the causative infection may be asymptomatic for weeks or months after exposure to an infected partner, becoming severely painful when the infection has spread into the fallopian tubes and lymphatic system. PID is uncommon in pregnancy, but can occur during the first trimester. Pain is usually bilateral, although one side may be more painful than the other, and is often accompanied by fever, chills, back pain, tachycardia, nausea and vomiting, spotting, vaginal discharge, and pain during intercourse. Enlarged pelvic lymph nodes may be palpable as a row of tender, firm, marble-sized lumps running transversely across the groin.

The patient with PID will require intravenous antibiotic therapy. If the responsible microorganism was sexually transmitted, treatment of her sexual partner is indicated. Prehospital treatment includes transport in the position of comfort. If vital signs indicate sepsis, oxygen via nasal cannula and an infusion of normal saline (at a rate indicated by vital signs) are appropriate.

Other Causes of Noncyclic Pelvic Pain

Endometritis is an infection of the endometrial layer of the uterus. This condition presents similarly to PID and may follow a D&C, miscarriage, childbirth, or insertion of an IUD. Vaginal bleeding, foul-smelling discharge, and suprapubic tenderness are common.

Adhesions from previous surgery or pelvic infection can cause pelvic pain. Pain from adhesions can be aggravated by defecation, urination, menstruation, or intercourse.

Pelvic pain can be musculoskeletal. Inquire about straining, lifting, or trauma. Ovarian and uterine pain often radiate to the anterior thigh, but any other pattern of radiation down the legs suggests a musculoskeletal origin. Musculoskeletal pain generally worsens with palpation or movement. Backache can be caused by trauma, poor posture, lack of exercise, osteoporosis, disk problems, or malignancy.

Somatization disorder is a common psychogenic cause of pelvic pain. Because health professionals often cannot find a physical cause for the pain, patients are often dismissed as attention seekers or malingerers. A holistic perspective of health, however, recognizes that the nervous system, the endocrine system, the immune system, and all other body functions are inextricably entwined. This is why simply harboring specific thoughts can raise blood pressure or cause sexual arousal independently of the immediate physical situation.

Often, if a woman has experienced emotional trauma or suffers other psychological imbalance, blocked or diverted emotions apparently emerge as physical complaints that have no identifiable physical origin. Most frequently, the complaints involve chronic pain and problems involving many seemingly unrelated body systems. These symptoms are very real to the patient and may even be disabling. The EMS provider should not consider this a voluntary or "faked" condition. Treatment often involves psychological counseling, but medications such as serotonin selective reuptake inhibitors and alternative therapy such as acupuncture, myofascial release, chiropractic, and reiki may be of benefit.

Ovarian Cysts

Ovarian cysts can develop in females of any age, from fetuses to postmenopausal women, and may be present at any point in the menstrual cycle and during pregnancy. Thirty percent of women with regular menses and 50% of those with irregular menses develop ovarian cysts, as do 6% of postmenopausal women. Most cysts develop during the reproductive years and are benign and self-limiting. Others can result from malignancy or create a surgical emergency such as ovarian torsion.

adhesion
Union of normally separate parts, as during healing of a wound or infection. Surgery, inflammation, or trauma may create adhesions—scar tissue that binds tissues together abnormally, causing pain and organ dysfunction.

somatization disorder
A condition characterized by physical symptoms that have no apparent physiological cause and are attributable to psychological factors.

With every normal monthly cycle during the childbearing years, hormonal stimulation causes many follicles to develop. One follicle quickly becomes larger and more mature than the rest and continues to flourish while the others wither. After the egg is released, the empty follicle transforms into the corpus luteum, which manufactures progesterone until the beginning of the next cycle.

Two types of functional cysts can develop during the normal progression of monthly cycles. A follicular cyst develops when fluid surrounds the maturing ovum in the first 2 weeks of the cycle, sometimes expanding the follicle to 8–10 cm in size. Corpus luteum cysts develop when the opening where the ovum escaped from the follicle seals and allows blood and fluid to collect inside, usually in the last 2 weeks of the cycle. A luteal cyst may measure as much as 4 in. in diameter and may cause considerable pain, but tends to resolve spontaneously.

A hemorrhagic ovarian cyst occurs when a small blood vessel in the cyst wall bursts and blood distends the cavity. Infrequently, a hemorrhagic cyst may rupture and spill blood into the abdominal cavity, usually causing great pain. Most hemorrhagic cysts are self-limiting, but some require surgical intervention.

A cyst may also form when ovulation fails to occur and the mature follicle collapses on itself. Polycystic ovarian syndrome can cause the ovaries to enlarge with multiple cysts from follicles that fail to ovulate.

Ovarian cysts are usually asymptomatic. They may cause aching heaviness or pressure or pain that can be sudden, intermittent, sharp, and severe. Sudden, severe unilateral pain can indicate hemorrhage into a cyst or rupture and leakage into the pelvic cavity. Pain may be localized to one side of the abdomen, or it may be more diffuse across the lower abdomen. Activity such as walking, exercise, or intercourse will often increase the pain. Light vaginal spotting many occur, and uncommonly peritonitis or septic shock may develop after the rupture of a cyst. Anticoagulant use may increase the amount of associated external or internal bleeding. Sometimes the woman will have a low-grade fever and tachycardia.

The weight of a cyst can twist the ovary and fallopian tube, cutting off blood supply and causing extreme ischemic pain to the sensitive ovary. Sometimes the woman with tubal or ovarian torsion will report vigorous exercise, abrupt change in position, or sexual activity occurred before the onset of pain. Differential diagnoses include appendicitis and ectopic pregnancy.

Ovarian cysts are usually diagnosed by pelvic ultrasound. A ruptured or twisted cyst may require surgery. If torsion compromises blood flow to the ovary, the organ may be saved if surgery is performed within 6 hours of onset.

Cyclic Pain

Mittelschmerz

Some women suffer sharp pain when the follicle ruptures upon ovulation. This discomfort is termed *mittelschmerz*, or "middle pain." This pain may be stabbing or crampy in nature, and is felt low in the abdomen on either side, often radiating into the back and down the front of the thigh. It is similar to the pain of an ovarian cyst, but generally lasts only a few hours. Some women experience light spotting with ovulation.

Dysmenorrhea

dysmenorrhea
Pain just before or during a menstrual period.

Fifty to 90% of women experience **dysmenorrhea**, or menstrual pain, at some point. For some it is a monthly bane.

Primary dysmenorrhea involves no physical abnormality. It most commonly occurs just before menses begin, lasts through the first few days, and is felt as a suprapubic cramping that may radiate to the back and anterior thighs. Nausea, vomiting, diarrhea, and migraines are sometimes associated. The most common cause is overproduction of prostaglandins, which stimulate uterine contractions.

Secondary dysmenorrhea results from abnormal conditions that increase the severity of menstrual cramps, sometimes causing intense pain. Some of these disorders include

- **Cervical stenosis.** Severe cramps can occur when the uterus ejects menses through a narrowed cervical opening.

- **Endometriosis.** In this condition endometrial tissue implants and grows outside the uterus, usually within the pelvic cavity, including the fallopian tubes; ovaries and outer walls of the uterus; and even the intestines, bladder, and peritoneum. These tissues bleed minuscule amounts of blood during monthly menses, but the blood cannot escape the body, causing irritation and scarring within the pelvis. Endometriosis often causes severe pain, usually with menses, and can cause infertility. Pain may be worse with intercourse or defecation. It is most common in women aged 30–40 and is treated with hormonal therapy, anti-inflammatory medications, and laparoscopic surgery.

- **Adenomyosis.** This abnormal condition occurs when endometrial glands and supporting tissues are present in the uterine muscle. This tissue swells and sloughs during menses, trapping blood in the uterine muscle and causing severe cramps and sometimes abnormal bleeding.

- **Endometrial polyps.** These are localized outgrowths of the endometrium that project into the uterine cavity or through the cervix, sometimes causing pain and bleeding.

- **Fibroids (leiomyomas).** These benign tumors of the uterus can increase monthly bleeding and pain. The woman may report painful or heavy periods, back pain, and constipation. About half of all women develop fibroids in their lifetimes; 20–25% percent of these develop before age 40. Because estrogen causes fibroids to grow, pregnant women, those with naturally high estrogen levels, and those using high-estrogen contraceptive methods are especially susceptible to fibroid enlargement.

GERIATRIC

NOTES

Fibroids usually shrink with the low estrogen levels after menopause and are unlikely to be the cause of pain or bleeding in an elderly woman.

Nongynecological Pelvic Pain

diverticulitis
Inflammation of small outpouch-ings of the colon.

Pelvic pain can frequently be attributed to nongynecological causes.

Gallbladder or ureteral stones can radiate pain to the pelvis. Chronic constipation can cause pelvic pain and pressure. **Diverticulitis** (inflammation of small outpouchings of the colon) presents as left lower quadrant pain with fever, usually in the woman over the age of 40. A history of alternating diarrhea and constipation with relief of pain after moving the bowels, urge to defecate following eating, or increased pain during stress indicates irritable bowel syndrome or spastic colon.

Urinary tract infections are common in women and usually present with pain and burning on urination; cramping; frequency; urgency; and sometimes fever, chills, hematuria, or foul-smelling urine. Flank pain can indicate pyelonephritis (kidney infection) and can be elicited by lightly tapping down the back with the flat of a fist, first down one side, then the other. The patient with tenderness at the costovertebral angle (where the bottom ribs join the spine) may have kidney inflammation.

Appendicitis classically begins with epigastric to midabdominal pain that eventually localizes to the right lower quadrant, suprapubic area, or flank. Some patients may present with left lower quadrant pain or bilateral pain. In the pregnant patient, pain may be localized to the right upper quadrant or elsewhere. Rebound tenderness, guarding, malaise, nausea, vomiting, and fever are common.

Prehospital Management of the Woman with Pelvic Pain

When called to the home of a patient with pelvic pain, take a complete history of the complaint using the OLDCART method or similar approach. Is there any chance that she might be pregnant? Is the pain related to menses, movement, urination, defecation, or sexual activity? Has she had any surgical procedures; PID; recent trauma; or history of fibroids, ovarian cysts, or urinary tract infections? Has she ever experienced this pain before, and if so, what was the diagnosis? If cyclic, how does it relate to menses, and how long has she experienced this pain? Gently palpate the abdomen, assessing for tenderness, distention, and discoloration.

The patient with gynecological pelvic pain usually requires little more than supportive care, a position of comfort, and a compassionate attitude. If the pain is severe or the vital signs are altered, establish intravenous access, oxygen, and cardiac monitoring as appropriate. It is inappropriate to administer analgesic medications to the patient with abdominal or pelvic pain, because eliminating discomfort may make diagnosis difficult in the emergency department and mask a worsening of the condition, such as a rupturing appendix or ectopic pregnancy.

Toxic Shock Syndrome

Toxic shock syndrome (TSS) is a multisystem disease caused by toxins produced by *Staphylococcus aureus* or *Streptococcus pyogenes* (group A strep). TSS is commonly associated with tampon use in women of childbearing age, but it does not always originate in the vagina. It can result from infections such as pneumonia, from sinusitis, and from surgical wounds and skin lesions (such as those from chicken pox); it can involve the cardiovascular, renal, integumentary, gastrointestinal, musculoskeletal, hepatic, hematologic, and central nervous systems; and it can afflict men, children, and nonmenstruating women.

Toxic shock syndrome from *Staphylococcus* begins with acute onset of vomiting, fever above 102°F (38.8°C), syncope, diarrhea, headache, sore throat, and muscle aches. Most patients show signs of soft-tissue infection, such as swelling and erythema that can progress to **necrotizing fasciitis.** As the disease progress, the patient may develop a sunburn-like rash, bloodshot eyes, desquamation, or petechiae. As shock sets in, the patient may display hypotension; pale, cool, moist skin; confusion; thirst; weak, rapid pulse; and tachypnea. The liver and kidneys may fail, and DIC, adult respiratory distress syndrome, dysrhythmia, or persistent, prolonged hypovolemic and septic shock may develop.

necrotizing fasciitis Severe infection with toxin-producing bacteria that leads to necrosis of subcutaneous tissue and adjacent fascia.

Suspect TSS in any patient with a sudden onset of fever, rash, hypotension, and apparent systemic toxicity. If the patient is in shock, transport rapidly, following shock protocols. In toxic shock syndrome capillaries leak copiously, and aggressive fluid infusion of 0.9% normal saline may be necessary to maintain an acceptable blood pressure. High-flow oxygen and cardiac monitoring are indicated.

Hospital treatment usually involves admission to intensive care and aggressive intravenous antibiotic therapy. Mortality rates for streptococcal TSS are 30–70%, and patients who survive often undergo fasciotomy, surgical debridement, laparotomy, amputation, or hysterectomy.

Amenorrhea

Amenorrhea is the absence or cessation of menses. It is unlikely that an ambulance would be called for this symptom, but understanding common causes of amenorrhea may shed insight on related emergencies.

During the childbearing years, the most common and obvious reason for lack of menses is pregnancy, and this diagnosis must always be considered, even if the patient denies the possibility. Pregnancy is even possible after tubal ligation sterilization, though it is more likely to be ectopic than intrauterine. A woman may also conceive after her partner has had a vasectomy.

Amenorrhea may also be normal for the woman using certain birth-control methods. Depo-Provera, injectable progesterone that is given every 3 months to prevent pregnancy, is expected to produce erratic bleeding for the first two or three injections; thereafter a total lack of menses is likely. The Marina intrauterine device (IUD) similarly releases progesterone, which may cause scanty or missed menses.

primary amenorrhea
Failure of menstruation to begin by age 16.

Primary amenorrhea occurs when a girl fails to menstruate despite showing physical signs of readiness or reaching the age of maturity. Sometimes this lack of bleeding may indicate a hormonal imbalance or endocrine failure; or there may be a problem with the reproductive system, such as an obstruction to menstrual outflow or lack of a uterus. Pregnancy is not out of the question, because a girl may also conceive before her first period.

secondary amenorrhea
Cessation of menstruation after menses established.

Secondary amenorrhea is when a previously menstruating woman fails to have periods. Many conditions can cause this symptom. Women with eating disorders or athletes with very low body fat often experience cessation of menses. Stress can cause irregular or missed periods. Thyroid dysfunction, polycystic ovarian disease, ovarian failure, and pituitary tumor are all possible reasons for lack of menstruation. Breastfeeding also often suppresses menses.

Menopause occurs for most women between ages 45 and 55, and for years before menses stop, irregular and skipped periods may be commonplace.

Vulvar Itching

Candida albicans (yeast) infection is one of the most common causes of vulvar itching. The vagina, like most body surfaces and cavities, is home to many species of microorganism, which generally live together in harmony. Populations of "good" bacteria such as lactobacilli ordinarily keep the harmful microorganisms in check. Any condition that upsets the balance can allow one species to overgrow, causing symptoms of infection. A woman with a yeast infection will usually complain of itching, burning, or an odorless, white, often lumpy discharge. It occurs in many healthy women, but more commonly in pregnant or immunocompromised patients and in women with diabetes. Vaginal itching can be extreme, and a woman may scratch herself raw in a desperate attempt to get relief.

Other causes of itching include sexually transmitted diseases such as trichomonas, human papilloma virus, and herpes. Infestation with lice or scabies mites can cause itching as well. Dermatological conditions, cancerous lesions, and warts can cause itching, as can irritation by soaps, douching agents, or feminine-hygiene products.

Nontraumatic Vulvar Pain

Bartholin Abscess

Bartholin's glands lie in the 5 and 7 o'clock positions of the vagina. Infection of Bartholin's glands with gonorrhea, *E. coli*, or other bacteria can cause large, painful, reddened abscesses to develop. While some abscesses evolve slowly, others rapidly develop. If they are not surgically drained, these abscesses may spontaneously rupture within 3 days.

Trauma

A woman's vulva is very vascular, and even superficial injuries to it may bleed copiously. Vulvar trauma, most frequently seen in young girls and adolescents, may include hematomas, linear lacerations, and abrasions. Straddle injuries may result from falls onto bicycle frames, fences, or the wall of an above-ground pool. Vulvar hematomas can be excruciating and may obstruct urination, causing bladder distention and necessitating catheter placement at the hospital.

Sexual intercourse, sexual assault, and penetration with a foreign object can cause vaginal or rectal trauma, especially in those who have fragile vaginal walls, such as children, postmenopausal women, or women with vaginal abnormalities. A fall onto a pointed object can cause a penetrating injury to the vagina. Inserting a tampon with a plastic applicator can occasionally lacerate the vagina, especially in a virginal adolescent.

Other vaginal injuries may have less obvious etiologies. Pelvic fractures from falls and motor vehicle accidents can cause sharp bone fragments to penetrate the vagina and lower urinary tract. High-pressure water forced into the vagina can cause the walls to distend and tear. Such injuries are sometimes encountered in waterskiing and motorized personal watercraft accidents, or when a woman straddles a pool or spa water jet. Women have been known to attempt abortion, contraception, or to cure STIs with a vaginal infusion of carbolic acid, formaldehyde, sulfuric acid, iodine, or ammonia—any of which cause chemical burns. Occasionally a woman will attempt suicide by inserting poisonous or caustic substances into the vagina.

PEDIATRIC

NOTES

Many genital injuries described as "accidents" in the pediatric patient are actually due to sexual assault. Conversely, accidental trauma to the genitals may be erroneously ascribed to sexual assault.

As always, obtain a detailed history from the patient or bystanders to determine the mechanism of injury. The patient may be embarrassed or evasive when questioned about her injury, so it is important that the EMS provider remain comforting, objective, and nonjudgmental. Always consider the possibility of physical or sexual assault. Manage the patient with vulvar trauma with immediate application of ice packs and thick external dressings. If possible, have the woman hold pressure on her own wound. If blood loss is significant or shock is apparent, treat with oxygen and intravenous fluids.

Violence Against Women

Violence against women is common worldwide, and some cultures sanction the maltreatment and domination of women. Perpetrators of abuse and their victims can be men, women, or children. Because this book concerns girls' and women's health, and most abusers of women are men, it presents the abuser as male and the victim as female. The EMS provider may encounter abusive women or children and male victims in other circumstances.

Domestic violence affects one out of four North American women. It affects women of every nationality, race, income level, educational level, sexual orientation, religion, and age. Statistics suggest that one-quarter of all women will be abused by a current or former partner sometime in their lives. Battered women represent 22–35% of women seeking care for any reason in the emergency room and 30% of all injured women in the ER. Most domestic-violence victims seeking health care do not volunteer information about their abuse, and most do not report it to police, shelters, social service organizations, or the judicial system. Some abuse victims do not want help, and some fear that seeking help will increase the abuse and risk to their lives.

Battering, sexual assault, rape, and incest can physically or psychologically damage a woman for life. Abuse can take the form of physical, emotional, or sexual harm; it includes verbal attack, aggressive behavior, and threats. Often the EMS responder is the first person to encounter the victim after the incident, and may be the only professional with first-hand knowledge of the details of the abuse. Clues at the scene and the behavior of other persons present may provide details that the victim is hesitant to disclose. The EMS report, in turn, can be valuable to other professionals who attend the injured woman.

Physical Abuse

Not all abuse involves partners of either sex. A woman may abuse or be abused by roommates, coworkers, or others in her life. This book will concentrate on one of the most common kinds of maltreatment: partner abuse of a woman by her male partner.

When responding to the same address yet another time to find a woman who has been clearly abused, it is easy for the provider to wonder, "Why doesn't she just leave?" The answers are complex. Most abusers are very skilled at manipulation and can keep the woman in a state of constant fear. In the classic model, the abuser's need for power and control leads him to employ many tactics to create a feeling of helplessness in the victim, causing her to believe that escape is impossible or likely to cause her or others great harm.

The Abuser

Abusers are often charismatic people loved by the people they work and socialize with. Their violent natures are often kept secret from the world at large. Alcohol consumption often initiates the cycle of abuse. During courtship, abusive men often attach quickly and powerfully to the chosen woman, professing love early in the relationship and showering her with gifts and attention. In a culture in which meeting Prince Charming is prized, an attentive, devoted, compelling man often seems to the woman and her circle the optimal choice for a mate. Abuse begins later, although most women report that warning signs were present in the early stages, identifiable only in retrospect. Abuse usually proceeds in cycles: a tension-building phase; a large blowup; and a "honeymoon" phase, in which the abuser is loving, contrite, and apologetic, luring the woman back for another round of abuse.

The Abuser's Tactics

The violent partner typically controls his victim through manipulative or menacing behaviors:

- **Threats.** The abuser may threaten to commit suicide or homicide, to kidnap or harm the children, to report the victim as an unfit mother, or to leave her destitute.

- **Intimidation.** The abuser may convince the woman of his ability to harm her or the children by destroying her property, injuring pets, or displaying weapons.

- **Creating dependence.** The abuser often assumes the role as sole head of household, makes all major decisions, controls the money, and may prevent the woman from working.

- **Creating helplessness.** Abusers often insult and belittle the victim until she internalizes the criticism and blames herself for the abuse and her situation. She becomes convinced that she is a bad wife, a bad mother, and a bad person; and the abuser often socially isolates her so that outsiders cannot refute these assumptions.

- **Blaming the victim.** The abuser often denies that the abuse has occurred or blames the victim ("See what you made me do?"), plays mind games, or tells the woman that she is crazy.

The Victim

Women who remain in abusive relationships have often been raised to be passive and submissive and accept female sex-role stereotypes. They have sometimes been abused as children and have often been trained from an early age to believe that they are to blame when things go wrong. They often have deep-seated feelings of worthlessness and tend to be critical, aloof, and emotional. The abuser manipulates these long-standing patterns of self-doubt and insecurity. When the abuser tells her that she is stupid, worthless, or ugly, he reinforces her own deepest fears about herself and lends credibility to the abuse.

Seeking Help

Women are often fearful or reluctant to disclose abuse or seek help in leaving the relationship. Women who believe that abuse is their lot in life and that the situation is inescapable are more likely to stay in an abusive relationship. Women who have jobs and have never before been in abusive relationships are more likely to realize that escape is possible. Women who are frequently and severely beaten are also more likely to seek help.

Escape is also complicated by the fact that the woman often genuinely loves her abuser and is emotionally hesitant to leave. Most abusers can be charming and pleasant between abusive episodes. Many women believe that leaving the relationship would harm the children or would bring social disfavor or economic catastrophe. Women with no job skills and many children may be reluctant to leave economic security and struggle for essentials or rely on public assistance.

Abuse in Pregnancy

Abuse becomes more common during pregnancy, as new roles and dramatic maturational changes are thrust upon both partners. Studies suggest that 7–26% of pregnant women and 19–24% of postpartum women are abused. Domestic violence often escalates with increasing emotional stress or with anger over an unwanted pregnancy or jealousy of the attention given to the woman and the fetus.

Abuse during pregnancy frequently results in premature labor, preterm deliveries, low birth weight, injury, child abuse, and death of the fetus or the woman. Abused pregnant women frequently present with abdomen, genital, and breast injuries and are more likely to suffer placental abruption, preterm premature rupture of membranes, fetal growth retardation, miscarriage, and chorioamnionitis.

Victims often suffer anxiety and depression as they struggle with psychosocial stressors, including divorce, legal problems, financial and housing problems, and lack of social support. Many turn to alcohol or drugs to self-medicate and cope. Abused pregnant women may be inclined to make changes in their domestic environment for the safety of their children that they would not make for themselves, but such changes do not always end the abuse or its effects.

The EMS Provider and the Abused Woman

Health care providers are often the only outsiders that the severely isolated abuse victim may be allowed to see. Care providers often avoid discussing

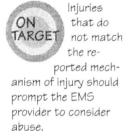

ON TARGET Injuries that do not match the reported mechanism of injury should prompt the EMS provider to consider abuse.

abuse because they are afraid or untrained, or they feel powerless to intervene constructively. Oftentimes, the woman will call for EMS for an unrelated somatic complaint as a ruse to get help and give her an escape route from the situation.

Injuries that do not match the reported mechanism of injury should prompt the EMS provider to consider abuse. Injuries to breasts, abdomen, face, or buttocks can suggest abuse, as does a socially isolated woman with poor eye contact, vague explanations of injuries, substance abuse, or a partner who refuses to leave the woman alone with providers.

Be polite and respectful to the woman's partner, even if your emotions are churning. She often loves him and may be very loyal to him, preferring to come to his defense rather than support her rescuer or save herself. Handle him with firm assertiveness and clearly state what he may or may not do.

Suspected abuse victims should be transported alone if at all possible. Some providers require the partner to take his own vehicle to the hospital to provide a safe environment in which to assess and question the suspected victim. Often the abused woman feels safer confiding in a woman provider.

When a woman discusses abuse, it is important to convey that you believe what she is telling you. Often women fail to discuss abuse for fear that they will not be believed or that the provider will accept their partners' stories over theirs. Women may hesitate to discuss abuse if they believe that their own inadequacies have caused the abuse. See Figure 11-2.

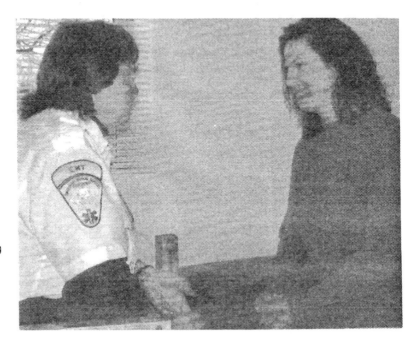

FIGURE 11-2
Listening without Judgment.
An attentive and caring prehospital provider can make a significant difference in the life of an abuse victim.
Photographed by Bonnie U. Gruenberg

The EMS provider can open the door to disclosure of abuse by pointing out that similar injuries are often seen in women who have been abused and that the victim is never responsible for the violent behavior of another. Ask the woman whether someone is hurting her. If she replies in the affirmative, ask what kinds of abuse she has suffered. Make it clear that you believe her description. Affirm that she does not deserve the abuse.

Let her talk if she will, and listen without judgment or blame. Do not advise her or tell her what she should do or what you would do in her circumstances. Do not encourage her to leave home—she is the only one who can make that decision, and if she leaves before she is ready, it is likely that she will return. Sometimes staying makes more sense than leaving abruptly—some abusers will kill a partner who leaves. Let her know that you will put her in contact with professionals who will listen to her and help her, whether or not she wants to leave the relationship.

Remember that her life has been about relinquishing control to others. It is most helpful to assist her in taking control of her own life and empowering her to make healthy decisions. Reassure her that hope exists and that trust in health care providers can help her improve her situation.

Sexual Abuse

Childhood sexual abuse occurs when a child is under 18, the abuser is at least 3 years older, and physical sexual contact occurs, although sexual abuse can also be emotional. Much sexual abuse goes unreported. A child who denies abuse may be unwilling to expose her abuser, afraid of the consequences, or unconsciously blocking the act from her memory. It is common for victims to remain unaware of the trauma until it surfaces many years later.

 PEARLS Many women who cut or injure themselves have a history of sexual abuse.

The sexually abused child frequently develops posttraumatic stress disorder, manifested by maladaptive behaviors that persist into adult life. Many women who cut or injure themselves have a history of sexual abuse. Often the trauma manifests as recurrent nightmares, sexual dysfunction, inability to trust others, resistance to intimacy, depression, anxiety, suicidal tendencies, or substance abuse.

The EMS provider may encounter an abused child or a woman with a history of childhood abuse, perhaps in a suicide attempt or depressive episode. Use tact and sensitivity in this situation, and at all times provide a safe and affirming environment.

Boundary issues are very important to the sexually abused woman. She often does not feel comfortable being touched by others and may have trouble setting limits and expressing her discomfort when her boundaries are violated. If you must examine her body, ask permission and explain why the exam is necessary. Without compromising care, give her as much control as possible over her treatment.

Women who have been abused as children may be phobic about being injured by others and may express high anxiety over needle sticks and other invasive procedures. Enlist the woman's cooperation with a clear explanation of its necessity, and if possible allow her to help choose the IV site. Show concern if she expresses pain.

Rape

Rape is a legal term rather than a medical one, and its definition varies from state to state. Definitions of rape of a woman include intercourse without consent; intercourse with someone incapable of giving consent, such as a child or mentally handicapped person; and intercourse when a woman is coerced by threats or incapacitated by drugs. Sexual assault is any sexual act performed by one person on another without that person's consent. Twenty-five percent of women will be sexually assaulted in their lifetimes. Forty percent of rapes involve physical injury to the victim.

Rape is an act of aggression, not lust, typically motivated by anger and a desire to hurt, humiliate, and control. Rape victims can be infants, elderly, or severely disabled. The victim is never at fault, even if she wears suggestive clothing or displays risk-taking behaviors. It is every person's right to say no to unwanted intercourse. Any violation of that boundary is rape. This is true even within a marriage or a dating relationship, yet women who have been assaulted by a partner or family member are much less likely to file a police report or seek treatment.

The media often portray women as secretly desiring rape, and some women report fantasies of "rape." But within a fantasy, a woman is able to control all aspects of the encounter. She has no control over an actual rape and is often traumatized, injured, infected, or impregnated during the attack. Most rape victims are affected by the act for the rest of their lives.

Many women fail to report rape. It is common for a woman to feel guilty and embarrassed about the assault, as if she were in some way responsible. Prosecuting the rapist can subject the woman to invasions of privacy as evidence and testimony are collected. Rape is often perpetrated by someone known and trusted by the victim. The victim may fear social repercussions if she prosecutes. The rapist may threaten dire consequences if the woman reports the crime.

Rape may be physically damaging and psychologically devastating. The woman's trust in the world may be eroded, and she may experience sexual dysfunction and fear of intimacy within her relationships.

Immediately after rape, most women experience rape trauma syndrome, exhibiting shock, confusion, and disorientation, followed by denial, anger, guilt, and withdrawal. PTSD is common, with nightmares, flashbacks, phobias, anxiety attacks, emotional lability, and depression. Many traumatized women develop vague physical symptoms, such as chronic abdominal pain, irritable bowel syndrome, muscular pain, or hyperventilation. A rape victim may feel permanently damaged and unclean. A sense of control over herself and her life becomes paramount.

Transporting the Sexual Assault Victim

The compassion of EMS personnel can be of lasting benefit to the sexual assault survivor. Do not attempt to extract details of the assault beyond those that may affect the care you give. Do not ask her what acts were committed. Ask where she hurts, whether she is bleeding, and whether she lost consciousness. Tend to her physical injuries as indicated, and reassure her that she is safe. Avoid asking questions that will create guilt or defensiveness in the victim, such as "Why did you let him take you home?" Remain objective and provide comfort without interjecting your opinions. See Figure 11-3.

There is no "correct" way to behave after a rape. Some women become very logical and unemotional as a means of regaining control.

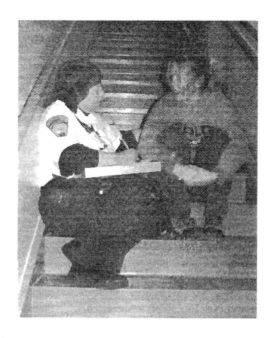

FIGURE 11-3
Comforting the Victim.
Honesty, compassion, and professionalism are paramount when treating the victim of sexual violence.
Photographed by Bonnie U. Gruenberg

Others are hysterical and difficult to comfort. Any of Elisabeth Kübler-Ross's stages of grief—anger, denial, bargaining, depression, and acceptance—can be seen at any time following a rape. A provider cannot judge the degree of trauma the woman has suffered by her outward behavior. The composed, rational woman may quietly commit suicide to escape her pain. The uncooperative, highly emotional woman may regain her balance after she vents her devastation. The provider should remain supportive and nonjudgmental no matter the victim's response.

PEARLS There is no "correct" way to behave after a rape. Anger, denial, bargaining, depression, and acceptance are all common responses, and these reactions may continue to surface for years or even decades after the assault. A provider cannot judge the degree of trauma the woman has suffered by her outward behavior.

Most sexual assault victims prefer a female provider. Protect the victim's modesty and her privacy. Separate her from curious onlookers and get her to a safe setting.

Be scrupulously honest with her. She needs to be able to trust you. Avoid empty reassurances such as "It will be okay," because it may not. Explain the rationale for everything you do, and ask her permission before touching her. Do not remove her clothing and do not examine her genitals unless she is hemorrhaging.

The Evidence

Rape is a crime. Evidence should be collected from the victim systematically and preserved. Most sexual assault treatment centers have kits designed for preserving evidence and personnel trained to collect materials in a sensitive and legal manner.

Prehospital providers are instrumental in preserving this evidence for collection by experts at the hospital. Avoid disturbing the crime scene when making initial contact with the patient. Touching the patient or irrigating wounds may disturb important evidence, so use caution. If you must remove clothing, carefully bag and label each item separately with minimal handling. If clothing must be cut from the victim, try not to cut through rips or tears. Cover her with a sheet if her skin is exposed, then give the sheet to the hospital personnel as evidence. Strongly discourage the woman from washing, urinating, defecating, douching, cleaning her fingernails, brushing her teeth or hair, or changing her clothing. Semen, skin, hair, and other substances may be taken from her clothing, vagina or other orifices, pubic hair, and from beneath her fingernails. Document objectively and thoroughly, including only known facts, injuries, and descriptions and avoiding speculation.

The hospital examiner will record physical injuries. She will also be tested for sexually transmitted diseases and perhaps given medications to prevent pregnancy. A counselor should attend to her emotional needs.

Sexual assault response teams (SART) or suspected abuse response teams include a nurse examiner, rape crisis advocate, and law enforcement personnel. The sexual assault/abuse nurse examiners (SANE) program provides specialized, standardized training for nurses who work with rape victims. The EMS provider should become familiar with relevant state laws pertaining to sexual assault.

Female Genital Mutilation

Female genital mutilation, also known as female circumcision, is practiced in some cultures. This procedure can include removal of the top of the clitoris and the skin surrounding it, or may be more extensive. Infibulation, the most common procedure, involves excision of the labia minora and clitoris and suturing together the external genitals, leaving only a single tiny hole for urination and escape of menstrual blood.

This practice is sometimes incorrectly associated solely with Islam, but female genital mutilation is a social custom that is performed on girls of many faiths, including Christians and animists. It is most commonly practiced in parts of Africa, but also occurs in some groups in Saudi Arabia, Indonesia, India, South America, and other locations. The procedure is illegal in the United States, but EMS providers may encounter genital mutilation in immigrant women.

Somalia is a country in which genital mutilation is a popular practice. In 1995, it was estimated that 98% of Somali women had suffered this procedure. Although it sometimes is done in hospitals, genital mutilation is typically performed by female relatives before Somali girls reach their fifth birthday. Traditionally, the unanesthetized child was held down by female family members while the operator excised her genitals with bits of glass or sharp knives, a practice still in use today. Afterward, the girl's legs were bound to allow the wound to close; often the bandage was not changed. Modern procedures may or may not incorporate scalpels, antiseptics, and cleaner technique. Hemorrhage, shock, painful scars, keloid formation, urethral stenosis, labial adherences, fistulas, incontinence, cysts, chronic infections, and depression are common after the procedure. Menstrual disorders, infertility, or even sterility may also occur.

Women of the cultures that practice female genital mutilation often strongly support the practice. Within their traditions, marriage is seen as the only honorable lifestyle for a woman, and in these cultures a female child is unlikely to marry if she does not undergo the procedure. Uncircumcised women are seen as unclean, and the clitoris is viewed as a dangerous organ that can cause uncontrolled lust, lesbianism, or injury to an infant during childbirth.

Female genital mutilation is considered a rite of passage, and it ensures virginity by creating a chastity belt made of the woman's own tissues. Proponents believe that a wife will be more faithful after removal of her organs of sexual pleasure. Mutilation is also thought to "purify" female sexuality by eliminating the lustful aspect of a woman's constitution and allowing her sexual function to center on procreation and gratifying male sexual needs. Genital mutilation may also increase the bride price a father can get for his daughters. When the woman marries, the scar is cut to allow intercourse, and cut wider still to allow childbirth.

EMS providers may encounter patients who have undergone genital mutilation. Urinary tract and vaginal infections are much more common in this population, and childbirth may be complicated by tissue that resists both stretching and tearing. In some cases, birth cannot occur until the patient arrives at the hospital and the physician or midwife incises the perineum to allow delivery.

SUMMARY

The EMS provider who is familiar with gynecological issues is best able to appropriately treat and transport. The EMS responder must bear in mind

- Chronic or acute vaginal bleeding can pose significant risks to a woman's health and well-being.
- Pelvic pain can be incapacitating and may be caused by life-threatening conditions
- Pregnancy and abuse can account for a wide range of clinical observations; keep both in mind during diagnosis.
- Treat known or suspected victims of sexual assault and other abuse attentively, with the highest possible regard for their personal space and the integrity of physical evidence.

REVIEW QUESTIONS

1. What are some possible etiologies for vaginal bleeding in a woman of childbearing age who states that she is not pregnant?

2. List the signs and symptoms of toxic shock syndrome (TSS).

3. Annie, age 68, complains of vaginal bleeding. What conditions can cause bleeding in a woman of her age?

4. When a woman has been raped, evidence should be collected from the victim systematically and preserved. When transporting the rape victim, what measures might you take to help preserve the evidence?

5. What are some common symptoms of childhood sexual abuse?

CHAPTER

12

Professional Issues

Objectives

By the end of this chapter you should be able to

- Accurately and objectively document your findings and treatment

- Describe the recommended activity restrictions for a low-risk pregnancy

- Identify professional obstetrical care providers and understand how they differ from one another

- Maintain a caring, patient-centered attitude while providing skilled and appropriate care

CASE Study

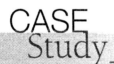

Emily returned from her midwife's office overjoyed after learning that she was 8 weeks pregnant. Emily had been a paramedic for 7 years and had been on countless ambulance calls involving pregnant women. She had even delivered four healthy babies in the field. Yet somehow the miracle of pregnancy seemed all the more wondrous now that there was a fetus growing in *her* body.

Emily found herself increasingly aware of the fragility of the growing life inside of her and worried that she might harm her unborn child. She looked critically at her habits and committed herself to a more healthy lifestyle. She gave up smoking, chose wholesome foods with minimal fats, sweets, and preservatives, and she eliminated raw meat and swordfish from her diet. She enrolled in a prenatal yoga class for stress reduction and conditioning. She even started wearing her seat belt consistently.

Emily looked at the demands of her occupation and realized that certain aspects of working as an EMS provider could pose a threat to her

315

pregnancy. Her work was physically demanding, and at any time an emergency call could expose her to chemicals or disease. Was she jeopardizing her pregnancy if she continued to work as a paramedic? Emily's anxieties flared the next day at work, when she transported a child with chicken pox (varicella) lesions, along with two siblings who were probably in the prodromal phase of the disease. Emily herself had suffered from chicken pox as a child, but she was afraid her unborn child was put at risk by the disease exposure.

Questions

1. Was Emily's fetus at risk from this first-trimester chicken pox exposure? What should she do?
2. How many pounds should Emily be allowed to lift if she continues to work full-time through her pregnancy?
3. Emily realized that the week before she learned she was pregnant (at 7 weeks' gestation) she was in the room with a patient when an X ray was taken. Will this exposure harm her unborn baby?
4. Later, in the 26th week of her pregnancy, Emily was struck hard in the abdomen by a combative patient. She said that she was "fine," but her supervisor insisted that she head to the hospital for evaluation. What tests might her midwife order to evaluate her?

Introduction

A holistic focus in patient care is important both in obstetrics and in an emergency setting, in which a patient's needs and emotions are at their most intense and immediate. The effective prehospital provider considers the patient's lifestyle, preferences, social bonds, spirituality, culture, developmental stage, occupation, and environmental influences when providing care and responds with compassion even in the chaos of an emergency situation.

But the commitment to holism should hold true in the EMS provider's own life as well. When any aspect of one's life slips out of equilibrium, the result may be illness, anxiety, fatigue, and despair, which can reciprocally affect other aspects of life. Occupational stress can drain an EMS professional of the creativity and energy necessary to give each patient and each situation the best effort. This holds especially true for the EMS provider who is herself pregnant and must reorder her life to accommodate both career and child. Social interactions, leisure activities, sleep, exercise, and proper nutrition can effectively balance the demands of the EMS career and make most stressors more bearable.

KEY TERMS

certified nurse-midwife, p. 329

colposcopy, p. 329

doula, p. 331

family-practice physician, p. 328

fetal phenytoin syndrome, p. 321

microcephaly, p. 321

perinatologist (maternal–fetal medicine specialist), p. 328

toxoplasmosis, p. 324

Documentation

Obstetrics is unique in the field of health care. Pregnancy and childbirth are natural processes that sometimes go awry, and an obstetrical crisis has the potential of directly harming not one person, but two. If damage occurs, providers involved in the care of the patient often end up in court. The parents of a child injured at birth may file a lawsuit two decades after the delivery. Awards granted to children who were injured at birth are often astoundingly large. After providing good care, an EMS professional's best protection against legal action is thorough and accurate documentation.

The EMS run report provides a record of the response to the call and care rendered, and it should be accurate enough to guide other health care professionals in providing subsequent care. Accurate records are essential when obtaining third-party reimbursement, especially from Medicare, Medicaid, HMOs, and insurance companies. EMS reports may be vital to legal action in accidents and in cases of sexual assault, domestic violence, child abuse, and other crimes. The EMS run report is often subject to painstaking scrutiny by doctors, nurses, supervisors, patients, patients' friends and relatives, law enforcement personnel, legal counsel, judges, juries, claims adjustors, journalists. . . . An inadequate run report may paint an inaccurate picture of what took place on a call, and it implies lack of professionalism in its creator.

When writing a run report, keep in mind that reimbursement usually hinges on whether the transport was necessary and the treatment reasonable. Ambulance transport is considered medically necessary in an emergency or if any other mode of transport would be harmful to the patient. The run sheet should clearly illustrate that the care was appropriate and performed competently. If transport or emergency care was necessary, *show* that it was necessary. Demonstrate that the emergency call truly was an emergent situation. Third-party payers may deny reimbursement if the EMS provider does not meticulously document medical history, physical findings, and treatment rendered in a way that proves treatment and transport were necessary. Third-party payers often apply other limitations and indications for reimbursement, and the EMS provider should become familiar with relevant guidelines.

Attention to detail is paramount in documentation. Juries often equate sloppy charting with a lack of professionalism, and verdicts in civil and criminal proceedings may turn on the accuracy and completeness of a run report. Further, a lucid, legible, objective, detailed account of the call speaks well for the provider's competency.

One goal of documentation is to record details that will aid memory if it ever becomes necessary to re-create events in an internal inquiry, a criminal investigation, a deposition, or a trial. Supervisors, law enforcement personnel, judges, and jurors tend to view run reports as more credible than the witness's memory. If your actions on a call are in question, the run report can be your best defense. If your assertions in court are different from what is documented on your run form, it may be hard to explain why your memory of events is more accurate than the written record. Details should clearly show that the care rendered was appropriate and properly provided.

Take care to ensure that all copies on a carbonless multipage form are legible. Black ink is favored for legal records because it tends to be easier to read, copy, and scan. Handwriting must be easily read, so that the meaning is not in question. Medical terms must be used and spelled correctly. Consider carrying a dictionary on the ambulance if crew members are weak in spelling.

The EMS run report should be an objective account of what the provider saw and did on the scene, including assessment findings, care provided, and response to treatments. Use only standard abbreviations, and avoid interjecting opinions, slang, or irrelevant judgments. Derogatory comments or sarcasm will appear unprofessional and inappropriate if the patient or others read the record. If a patient is abusive or resistant to care, his or her remarks and behaviors should be recorded as facts.

Ensure that you accurately describe the patient's condition, treatments, and response to treatments. When trying to capture a scene accurately and objectively, it is helpful to quote the patient's actual words whenever possible. A quotation can accurately convey the patient's state of mind, competency, and intentions:

Patient found in the bathroom sitting in a pool of about 300 cc of blood with steady trickle issuing from between legs. Patient stated, "I was past my due date so I tried to break my water with a coat hanger." Describes inserting straightened coat hanger into vagina. Bleeding began almost immediately after insertion. Reports no gush of fluid. Patient states, "I haven't felt the baby move since I stuck the hanger up there." Patient states, "I was alone when I did it—nobody helped me."

Document when patients fail to comply with recommendations:

Patient pulled IV catheter from arm, stating, "You people are trying to poison me." Patient had been advised prior to removing catheter that IV placement was necessary to raise her low blood pressure, a condition that could lead to fainting or even death.

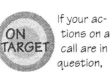
If your actions on a call are in question, the run report can be your best defense.

Run reports must not only be factual but also appear factual, especially when documenting the many unusual and improbable situations that prompt an ambulance call. In court, the provider may be questioned about every phrase and comment appearing on the report, including references to time and sequence. If the provider's accuracy in documenting is questioned, his or her performance may be questioned as well. A strong run report includes the timing of any intervention, including vital signs, rhythm interpretations, assessments, and treatments.

If you did make an error or misjudgment, it is always better to be forthright about it than to attempt to cover it up. Errors do not always imply negligence, but deceit always throws the provider's credibility into question. Consult your company's lawyer promptly if you make a serious error. In many cases a confession and apology to the patient are appropriate and may reduce the chances of the patient's filing suit.

A run report may include

- Call date and time
- Identification of the EMS agency and vehicle
- Presence of other agencies on scene as relevant to situation
- Patient identification: name, birthdate, age, sex, address, and so on
- Gravida, parity, and so on
- Chief and associated complaints; history of present illness or injury
- Significant medical history and preexisting conditions
- Description of symptoms as assessed with OLDCART or similar method
- Physical assessment findings, vital signs, and relevant observations
- Relevant details of scene and care given before arrival
- EKG rhythm, glucose test results, or results of other diagnostic measures
- Treatments and medications given with times, routes, dosages, and so on

- Responses to treatment
- For trauma patients: mechanisms of injury, Glasgow Coma Scale score, and trauma scores; rescue/extrication information; description of injuries
- Signatures, names of medical control personnel

The Pregnant Provider

EMS is a demanding career and presents many challenges to the provider who becomes pregnant. Strenuous physical activity, such as carrying a patient down from the third floor or carrying an airway bag and cardiac monitor up several flights of stairs, can be uncomfortable or dangerous to the pregnant provider and her fetus. Patients may harbor microorganisms that can endanger the fetus, and chemicals spilled at the scene may also put the pregnancy at risk.

Teratogen Exposure

Radiation, some chemicals, and certain drugs and microorganisms are potentially detrimental to a woman's reproductive capacity. Some, such as lead, have been clearly shown to cause infertility, spontaneous abortion, and stillbirths. Other hazards have been shown to cause damage in animals, so pregnant women are advised to avoid them. Not all birth defects are caused by teratogens, however; most are caused by chromosomal abnormalities.

The timing of exposure is important. The unborn child has intervals when he is particularly sensitive to the affects of a teratogen. A drinking binge on one day may cause significant harm to the fetus. On a different day, it may be less harmful. Some hazards are extremely damaging in the first trimester, but inconsequential later in pregnancy. Other hazards, such as ibuprofen and tetracycline, are most dangerous near term.

Exposures in the first 2 weeks after conception may prevent implantation, but are unlikely to harm the embryo. Because its circulation is not fully linked with the mother's, teratogens cannot yet pass from woman to embryo. At other times during the first trimester, the embryo is especially vulnerable to teratogens. The first trimester is when the developing fetus organizes body systems, so a toxic exposure at that time can throw the process awry and cause significant anomalies. Exposures during the last trimester are more likely to cause growth restriction, preterm labor, stillbirth, or problems with brain development.

Exposure to a teratogen at a critical time in the development of a structure or organ may produce abnormalities there, but not elsewhere.

For example, the critical period for limb development is 24–36 days after conception. If exposed during that interval to a substance that skews limb development (such as thalidomide), limbs will not develop normally. Exposure to the same substance weeks later will cause no visible harm to the limbs because they have already formed.

PEDIATRIC
NOTES

Thalidomide was prescribed in the 1950s in Europe, Japan, Canada, and elsewhere to treat anxiety, insomnia, and morning sickness. It was withdrawn from the market after more than 10,000 children were born with severe malformations, including flipper-like limbs or almost no limbs at all. The FDA had refused to approve thalidomide for use in the United states, sparing American babies from the tragic consequences of the drug.

ON TARGET Radiation, some chemicals, and certain drugs and microorganisms are potentially detrimental to the fetus.

fetal phenytoin syndrome
A disorder caused by exposure of an embryo to the anticonvulsant drug phenytoin (Dilantin), characterized by mental retardation, microcephaly, abnormal facial features, and other anomalies.

microcephaly
Abnormally small head.

One cannot often conclude, however, that any congenital anomaly results from exposure on a particular day to a particular substance. Women are frequently exposed to known teratogens without obvious ill effects to the embryo or fetus. A good example is **fetal phenytoin syndrome**. Prenatal exposure to the anticonvulsant phenytoin (Dilantin) causes multiple abnormalities in infants: facial abnormalities such as drooping eyelids, epicanthal folds, and broad, depressed nasal bridge; low-set ears; neck webbing; IUGR, **microcephaly**, hernias; mental retardation; short fingers and poorly formed nails; cardiovascular abnormalities; and other problems. Yet more than half of all embryos exposed to phenytoin are unaffected. It appears that the degree of vulnerability is determined in part by the genes of the embryo.

Chemical Exposure

The pregnant EMS provider may be exposed to chemicals at the base or at the scene of an emergency. Chemical exposure can cause menstrual or other gynecological problems, infertility, spontaneous abortion or stillbirth, IUGR, prematurity, and maternal health problems. Common hazardous chemicals include mercury and its compounds, carbon monoxide, and lead. Some pesticides and fertilizers can be harmful, and solvents should be generally avoided during pregnancy.

Radiation

Radiation can cause abnormalities in development or loss of the pregnancy. The amount of radiation exposure depends on the exposure dose, the timing of exposure, and how frequently the patient has been exposed. If the embryo has not implanted at the time of the exposure, it will generally be killed outright or suffer no obvious ill effects. The greatest risk of damage accompanies exposure late in the first trimester and early in the second. Exposure to low doses of radiation from being in the room while a patient is X-rayed; from receiving routine dental X rays; from plain films of the head, extremities, and chest (including mammograms); or from computerized tomography (CT) of the head or chest is unlikely to harm the fetus, but caution is still advisable.

The pregnant EMS provider who has been exposed to radiation must work with her physician to calculate the dose, frequency, and timing of exposure. Radiation work sites generally employ radiation-safety personnel and can consult experts to supply estimates of the dose to the fetus.

The electromagnetic fields of video display terminals have been extensively studied and have not been proven harmful to pregnant women. Women who work at computers, however, may suffer carpal tunnel syndrome, which may be exacerbated by fluid retention and postural changes due to pregnancy.

Disease Exposure

The pregnant prehospital provider may come in contact with infectious diseases that can damage her fetus or jeopardize her pregnancy.

Varicella (Chicken Pox)

Varicella and herpes zoster (shingles) are caused by the same herpes virus, varicella-zoster virus (VSV). It is spread via respiratory transmission and direct contact. Clinical signs and symptoms include malaise, chills, fever, and muscle and joint aches, followed in a few days by the eruption of the characteristic chicken pox lesions. Vesicles appear first on the face and neck, then the trunk and extremities. In time they break open and crust over. Varicella infection in adults can be dangerous, sometimes leading to varicella pneumonia, which carries a high mortality if untreated. Maternal varicella infection during the first half of pregnancy can cause serious injury to the developing child, including skin scarring, muscle atrophy, limb deformities, eye and brain damage, and mental retardation. After 20 weeks' gestation, however, there is little risk of damage to the fetus. When maternal disease develops from 5 days before delivery up to 48 hours postpartum, babies can develop neonatal VZV, an illness with high mortality. The pregnant EMS worker who has had chicken pox as a child is probably immune; those who have never had the disease or been vaccinated are at risk. Serological tests can determine immunity status.

Cytomegalovirus

Cytomegalovirus (CMV) is a herpes virus that infects 60–85% of Americans by age 40. Like all herpes viruses, after infection, CMV remains in the body for life and may be reactivated at any time. It is commonly contracted by children and may spread through day-care centers and classrooms. Transmission is by urine, saliva, blood, tears, semen, or breast milk. Most infected women have minimal or no symptoms or have mononucleosis-like malaise, fever, sore throat, muscle aches, fatigue, diarrhea, rash, and swollen lymph nodes. If a woman who has never before suffered cytomegalovirus infection contracts the disease during pregnancy, the fetus may be at risk. Often the fetal infection is not identified until after birth. Complications include hearing loss, vision impairment, and mental retardation. Current or past infection can be detected by a blood test.

Rubella (German Measles)

Rubella used to be a common childhood disease in the United States, but now it is largely prevented by vaccination. Rubella infection may be asymptomatic or may include low-grade fever, drowsiness, sore throat, rash, and swollen glands over the course of 3–5 days. It is spread via droplets and direct contact with respiratory secretions. If a pregnant woman suffers rubella infection in the first trimester, it is likely that the baby will be born with congenital rubella syndrome, which is associated with cataracts, deafness, and cardiac defects. Spontaneous abortion and stillbirth are common. Infection after the 20th week seldom causes defects. Most American women of childbearing age have been immunized against rubella, and titers are customarily checked during prenatal assessment to determine vulnerability.

Fifth Disease (Parvovirus B19)

Fifth disease, or erythema infectiosum, is caused by parvovirus B19, a single-stranded DNA virus. Signs and symptoms include a lacy, often itchy rash that begins on the trunk and moves out to the extremities and a "slapped cheek" redness of the face. Over several days or weeks, the rash may reappear after exercise, warm baths, or sun exposure. It may be accompanied by nonspecific flu-like symptoms, fever, malaise, muscle and joint pain, and headaches. Parvovirus is transmitted mostly through contact with respiratory secretions but also through exposure to blood. Children commonly contract the virus at school or day care and spread it to family members. Fifth disease is caused by a human parvovirus and cannot be transmitted to or by dogs or cats. The disease is most contagious before the onset of symptoms. The fetus of a woman who is infected during pregnancy may develop hydrops (generalized swelling) and blood disorders or may die. Parvovirus is diagnosed by a blood test, and blood titers can be drawn to check for immunity.

Hepatitis B

Hepatitis B virus is a double-stranded DNA virus in the Hepadnaviridae family. HBV is transmitted by contact with blood, semen, vaginal secretions, or wound exudates. Roughly half of acute HBV infections are asymptomatic in adults; the others present with acute hepatitis, anorexia, nausea, vomiting, fever, abdominal pain, or jaundice. Pregnant women with hepatitis can transmit the disease to their fetuses, but transmission can be thwarted by administration of immunoglobulin and vaccinations at birth. These babies do not appear to develop defects from the disease. But they are at very high risk for developing chronic HBV infection, and they may become chronic hepatitis carriers and suffer higher risk of cirrhosis or liver cancer later in life. Hepatitis B vaccine is recommended for pregnant women if they are at risk of acquiring HBV infection. Infants born to mothers infected with hepatitis B receive hepatitis vaccine plus hepatitis B immunoglobulin (HB16) within the first 12 hours of life.

Toxoplasmosis

toxoplasmosis
Infection by a parasite (*Toxoplasma gondii,* found in raw and rare meat, garden soil, and cat feces) not usually harmful to nonpregnant adults, but potentially damaging and sometimes deadly to the fetus.

Toxoplasmosis is a protozoal infection caused by the parasite *Toxoplasma gondii.* Cats carry the organism and pass it in their feces, so people who clean litter boxes or garden where cats have defecated may contract the disease. The EMS worker may unexpectedly encounter cat feces in a patient's home or at the scene of an accident. Most people contract the disease by eating undercooked meat.

Symptoms are vague and resemble flu or mononucleosis; they may include malaise, muscle aches, fever, sore throat, and enlarged lymph nodes in the neck. Toxoplasmosis can severely damage the fetus if a pregnant woman contracts it. Affected newborns often seem normal at birth, but subsequently develop seizures and motor or cognitive defects. Some children are born with microcephaly, hydrocephalus, or anencephaly. Serum testing can identify toxoplasmosis infection or show immunity.

HIV/AIDS

Human immunodeficiency virus is an RNA retrovirus that attacks T-helper lymphocytes and other cells, crippling the immune system. It is incurable, but can be managed as a long-term chronic disease. Transmission is by contact with blood or body fluids, intercourse, or sharing contaminated needles. Infants born to HIV-infected mothers stand a 25% chance of contracting HIV, but this risk is lower in a woman with a low viral load and on an appropriate medication regime. HIV testing is available to pregnant women who seek prenatal care.

There are many other infectious diseases that can affect pregnancy, and the pregnant EMS provider should discuss possible exposures with her physician or midwife.

Vaccinations

The pregnant woman at risk for infection may be vaccinated against hepatitis B, influenza, and tetanus (if previously vaccinated). Any health care worker considering pregnancy who may be exposed to infectious diseases on the job should make sure her vaccinations are up to date before conceiving.

Stress

EMS can be an intellectually and emotionally taxing profession. Prehospital providers cope with crisis daily and often witness incidents that leave them indelibly affected. Burnout is common, as is posttraumatic stress disorder. It is always a challenge to balance emotional connection to the patients with emotional withdrawal for self-protection.

High stress levels may increase the risk of preterm labor and low birth weight by releasing increased levels of cortisol and prostaglandins. Stress may also prompt a woman to skip meals, eat "junk" foods, smoke, or comfort herself with drugs or alcohol, all of which can adversely affect her pregnancy and her fetus. Research suggests that women who feel stressed may be more likely to develop pregnancy-induced hypertension.

 PEARLS High stress levels during pregnancy may increase the likelihood of preterm labor and hypertension.

How much stress is too much? A woman's *perception* of her stress levels is far more significant than the amount or kind of stress present in her life. A situation that would be overwhelming and unnerving to one person may be stimulating and interesting to another. Stress triggers differ. A paramedic on bedrest might experience more anxiety from her inactivity than she would if allowed to return to work. Others find it difficult to cope with the frenetic pace of emergency responses and improve markedly when transferred to light duty or placed on maternity leave.

Pregnant women, like all other people, should strive for a healthy balance in their lives, finding time for sleep, relaxation and pleasurable activities, social and family bonds, spirituality, hobbies, and other meaningful pursuits. A good support system, including coworkers, family, friends and others, is effective in providing emotional support or helping with tasks at home.

The pregnant EMS provider can explore stress reduction techniques such as biofeedback, meditation, guided mental imagery, and pregnancy yoga. Childbirth classes teach relaxation techniques, promote healthy self-care practices, and alleviate fear by demystifying labor and delivery.

Physical Activity

EMS can be a physically demanding profession, requiring frequent lifting, stair climbing, twisting, turning, pushing, and pulling. The American Medical Association has made recommendations on the amount of lifting, standing, and so forth that a pregnant woman should perform. These guidelines should be modified to fit individual circumstances. A fit athlete may continue fairly strenuous work at the discretion of her obstetrical provider. A woman with threatened preterm labor may need strict bedrest. Other conditions require activity modifications. Always discuss employment demands with your doctor or midwife and follow his or her recommendations.

In general, light clerical and managerial work that requires less than 30 minutes of standing per hour can be performed throughout pregnancy. Tasks that require prolonged standing should be performed no more than 40 hours a week in early pregnancy. After 24 weeks, standing should be reduced to 4 hours at a time. Work that involves intermittent standing for 30-minute intervals may be performed until the 32nd week.

Many pregnant workers can perform repetitive lifting of up to 50 lb until the 24th week of pregnancy if they have been lifting such weights for at least a year before pregnancy and continue to use proper techniques. After 24 weeks the limit is 25 lb.

A pregnant woman can climb ladders and poles until the 28th week of gestation, but should not do this more than 4 times per shift between weeks 20 and 28. She may climb stairs throughout pregnancy, but should limit this to 4 times per shift after 28 weeks. A pregnant employee may stoop and bend below knee level up to 10 times per hour to week 28, then a maximum of 2 times per hour for the rest of the pregnancy.

Pregnant women should avoid overheating. Core-temperature elevations of 102°F (38.9°C) or higher for an extended period may increase the rate of spontaneous abortion or birth defects, especially neural tube defects such as spina bifida or anencephaly.

PEARLS Pregnant women should avoid prolonged exposure to hot environments and overheating through vigorous work or exercise, and they should call their providers promptly if they develop fever not responsive to acetaminophen.

Other Concerns

During early pregnancy, women are often affected by fatigue and nausea. Later in gestation, they are burdened by a growing fetus, lax joints, poor balance, and other physiological changes. The pregnant EMS professional should modify her workday to maximize her health and comfort.

For example, she should take a break every few hours and a longer meal break every 4 hours, and vary work positions frequently, from sitting to standing and walking. She should avoid situations in which her altered balance puts her at risk for a fall. The pregnant EMS professional should avoid contact with combative patients because a kick or punch to the abdomen could put the pregnancy at risk, and her lax joints place her at increased risk for dislocations. Seat belts, worn low on the pelvis and between the breasts, are essential on and off the job. She should not scuba dive or exert herself at high altitudes.

Pregnant women need small, frequent, nutritious meals and should have a snack approximately every 3 hours. Long intervals between meals can trigger headaches, tachycardia, irritability, dizziness, and syncope. Meals consisting of simple carbohydrates—for example, a doughnut and juice—often trigger reactive hypoglycemia, a steep increase in blood sugar followed by a precipitous drop. The pregnant woman should include protein with every meal or snack and choose healthy foods.

Pregnant women must remain well hydrated. If urine is clear and watery, fluid intake is probably adequate. If urine is dark and concentrated, she needs to drink more. Water is preferable to coffee, carbonated soft drinks, and other sweet or caffeinated beverages. Dehydration can cause uterine irritability and constipation and increase the chance of urinary tract infections.

Working with Obstetrical Care Providers

Health care is an industry marketed to increasingly savvy consumers who demand greater choices and participation in the decisions that affect them. In a small community, a pregnant woman may select her clinician by default—often there is only one practice in town, and the laboring patient will be delivered by whoever is on call. In many situations, the patient's financial situation or insurance plan decides who will provide care, and the patient can do little more than hope that the provider proves adequate. In urban areas, there is often a wider range of options for prenatal and well-woman care, allowing the client to shop around for a practitioner who conforms to her expectations and

family-practice physician
A physician (M.D. or D.O.) who provides medical care for men, women, and children, but usually manages only low-risk pregnancies and deliveries.

perinatologist (maternal–fetal medicine specialist)
An obstetrician who has done a fellowship of 2–3 years after residency to specialize in high-risk pregnancies and has become board certified in maternal–fetal medicine.

requirements. In other cases, the pregnant woman may select a provider from a phone book or act on a friend's recommendation.

In many places there is a variety of qualified health care providers who may provide care for a pregnant woman. Each specialty embraces a different philosophy, and each provider within a specialty has a unique style of practice. It is helpful for the EMS provider to understand which providers may be giving care to obstetrical and gynecological patients. Prehospital professionals may work with obstetrical care providers when called to office emergencies, when providing interfacility transports, when responding to home birth emergencies, and in other situations.

- The obstetrician-gynecologist is a physician, either an M.D. (doctor of medicine) or a D.O. (doctor of osteopathic medicine). The obstetrician-gynecologist has completed 4 years of medical school, followed by at least 4 years of residency training in obstetrics and other aspects of women's health care. He or she is often certified by the American Board of Obstetrics and Gynecology. Obstetricians can manage most obstetrical situations, including normal vaginal deliveries, operative vaginal deliveries (vacuum or forceps), and cesarean sections. Most deliver exclusively in hospitals. There is great philosophical variation among obstetricians, and practices vary. Some specialize in high-risk patients. Others handle mostly low-risk patients and natural deliveries.

- The **family-practice physician** may be either an M.D. or a D.O. and provides medical care for entire families—men, women, and children. He or she is often board certified in family practice medicine and usually manages only low-risk pregnancies and deliveries. Family-practice doctors can sometimes perform operative deliveries, but cannot usually perform cesarean sections. Most collaborate with an obstetrician if the pregnancy or the labor becomes complicated.

- A **perinatologist** or **maternal–fetal medicine specialist** is an obstetrician who has done a fellowship for 2 or 3 years after residency to specialize in medically complicated pregnancies and has become board certified in maternal–fetal medicine. Some maternal–fetal medicine specialists act as consultants to obstetricians, and some also practice obstetrics with a focus on very high-risk women, ultrasound, or prenatal diagnosis. Perinatologists usually practice in hospitals, often in large teaching hospitals with neonatal intensive care units that can care for the sickest of babies.

- **Certified nurse-midwives (CNMs)** are registered nurses with advanced training in obstetrics and gynecology. Most hold master's degrees. CNMs provide primary health care to women, including prenatal care, labor and delivery care, care after birth, gynecological exams, newborn care, assistance with family-planning decisions,

certified nurse-midwife
A registered nurse with specialized graduate education from an accredited institution, certified and licensed to provide antepartum, intrapartum, and postpartum care; gynecological exams; newborn care; family planning; menopausal management; and counseling in health maintenance and disease prevention.

colposcopy
Examination of the vagina and cervix by means of a colposcope (a device that magnifies and photographs).

preconception care, menopausal management, and counseling in health maintenance and disease prevention. CNMs are sometimes trained to perform ultrasonography, **colposcopy,** endometrial biopsy, infertility treatment, artificial insemination, abortion, circumcision, and function as surgical first assistant. CNMs are committed to empowering women to take an active role in their own health care and to helping clients make informed decisions. Some CNMs practice autonomously and consult or refer to obstetricians only for complicated patients. Other CNMs work collaboratively with obstetricians and may comanage high-risk patients. In 2001, 97% of CNM-attended births occurred in hospitals, almost 2% in freestanding birth centers, and less than 1% in patients' homes.

CNMs are licensed in all 50 states and the District of Columbia and can prescribe medication in every state except Pennsylvania and Georgia.

Midwives are held to the same standards of safe practice as obstetricians. If problems develop that are beyond midwives' scope of practice, they will consult with an obstetrician, who may make recommendations, provide expert assistance, or take over care. Midwives' tendency toward nonintervention in natural processes leads to outcomes comparable with or sometimes even better than those of physicians with low-risk patients.

• Direct-entry midwives are independent practitioners educated in midwifery through self-study or apprenticeship, at midwifery schools, or in college- or university-based programs distinct from the discipline of nursing. Direct-entry midwifery is illegal in at least 10 states and unregulated in many others. Licensing standards in the state of Washington allow that direct-entry midwives need not be certified and are reimbursed by both Medicaid and some HMOs for home births.

• A certified midwife (CM) has not been a nurse, but has training similar to that of CNMs and is certified by passing the same examinations. CM is a new designation, and few states recognize it. Practice options for CMs are still being defined.

• Certified professional midwives (CPMs) are knowledgeable, skilled professional midwives who may be educated through a variety of routes. Besides didactics, the CPM must complete at least 1,350 hours of precepted clinical experience in prenatal, intrapartal, postpartal, and newborn care before applying for certification through the North American Registry of Midwives (NARM). This qualifies her to provide the Midwives Model of Care, which asserts that pregnancy and birth are normal life events and minimizes technical interventions. CPMs are regulated on a state-by-state basis. High-risk women are usually referred to obstetricians for care or comanagement. CPMs usually deliver at home or in freestanding birth centers.

• Lay midwives or traditional midwives are usually experienced with childbirth and the care of pregnant women, but are not certified or regulated by the government in most states. They have no training or continuing education requirements, no standards to meet, and no supervision. Some are knowledgeable and conscientious, continually educating themselves and attending workshops to stay current and improve skills. Others may be inexperienced or unsafe. Lay midwives typically attend only home births and are not credentialed to attend deliveries in birth centers or hospitals. Many have a backup arrangement with physicians in case problems arise; but some do not, and they may "dump" obstetric catastrophes at the emergency department or summon EMS.

• Nurse practitioners (NPs) are registered nurses with advanced education and training enabling them to diagnose and treat many common medical conditions, including chronic illnesses. NPs' practice centers on health maintenance, disease prevention, counseling, and patient education in a wide variety of settings. NPs must be licensed by the state of practice, and many are certified in specialty areas. Some nurse practitioners focus on obstetrics and gynecology and can provide menopausal and perimenopausal care; contraceptives; treatment of vaginal infections, gynecological problems, and sexually transmitted infections; physical exams, including Pap smears; antepartum and postpartum care; health screening; and disease prevention. They do not usually deliver babies. Advanced skills may include assisting in surgery, diagnostic ultrasounds, cervical procedures and biopsy and endometrial biopsy, infertility treatment, artificial insemination, abortion, and circumcision.

An NP can serve as a patient's regular health care provider, and studies show that NP care is cost-effective and shows outcomes as good as those of physicians treating patients with similar complaints. NPs are trained to give holistic, individualized care and usually rate high in patient satisfaction. NPs have prescriptive authority in every state.

• Physician's assistants (PAs) receive a generalist education emphasizing primary care. Physician's assistant training is modeled after physician education, and PA students frequently share courses, facilities, and clinical rotations with medical students. After 2 years of science and other college prerequisites, the PA student completes a program roughly 26 months in length. Physician assistants are not independent practitioners, but deliver care in partnership with physicians; the level of supervision varies. Similar to a nurse practitioner, the PA who specializes in obstetrics and gynecology may perform annual exams, including Pap smears; evaluate and treat gynecological complaints; manage contraception; and manage prenatal care. Some PAs assist in surgery and perform ultrasounds, colposcopy, infertility treatment and artificial insemination, biopsies, pessary fitting, abortion, and circumcision. Most PAs do not deliver babies, but some PAs attend low-risk deliveries.

doula
A nonmedical person who provides physical, emotional, and logistical support to a woman in labor.

• A **doula** physically and emotionally supports the laboring woman. She is not trained to make clinical decisions and is not responsible for the woman's medical treatment. Pregnant women hire doulas to support and guide them through the rigors of labor. Some doulas are certified by Doulas of North America (DONA). Studies have shown that women attended by doulas have lower cesarean rates and use fewer epidurals than women with traditional labor support.

Patient-Centered Practice

Earning Trust

Because health care is paramount to the optimal functioning of our bodies, minds, and emotions, the people who provide our medical treatment impact us at a fundamental and personal level. Sexuality and reproduction are very personal and emotionally charged aspects of a woman's life, and childbirth is a life-changing event. An EMS provider may remove a woman's clothing and examine or palpate various parts of her body while asking very personal questions. Exposing one's genitals to strangers is embarrassing and difficult for most women, yet a woman is expected to surrender all modesty during the birthing experience. A woman who is copiously hemorrhaging is in a state of complete dependence and must passively trust that her health care professionals have the skills, knowledge, and good judgment to save her life without sacrificing anything else important to her.

What is trust? Trust involves risk taking, or putting oneself in a vulnerable position without full investigation or evidence in the hope of receiving some good. An individual's capacity for trust begins in infancy and is modified and shaped by life experiences. Levels of trust vary among and within individuals. People who experience betrayal may be reluctant to trust again. People who are untrustworthy themselves may be less likely to trust others.

Psychology theorist Erik Erickson's eight psychosocial stages begin with "trust versus mistrust" as the first stage of personality development. Infants are in a position of absolute dependence; without appropriate care, they will die. The intensity of a normal labor can cause elements of this dependence-based trust to resurface; childbirth complications can bring a woman to the brink of death. When a woman calls for an ambulance in active labor, fear, other emotions, and intense physical sensations trigger vulnerability and dependence. Because the patient is at the limit of her own coping resources and looks to emergency providers for desperately needed support and leadership, trust can build instantly if the provider is competent and kind.

Many patients have valuable insights into the workings of their own bodies, but the care provider cannot benefit from them unless the patient is comfortable revealing them. The woman who trusts her provider is more likely to disclose information about sensitive issues that could affect outcomes, such as a history of sexually transmitted infection or substance abuse.

Trust begins when the patient concludes that the provider is "good." What, from a patient's perspective, characterizes a "good" prehospital provider? Technical competence is important, but so is emotional commitment to giving care. Patients respond positively to providers who smile, maintain good eye contact, use the patient's name, and solicit response and collaboration. Self-disclosure—appropriate sharing of certain personal feelings and experiences—encourages the patient to share her own, enhancing the emotional connection and the flow of relevant information.

Honesty is a cornerstone of trust. The EMS provider who withholds information for fear of upsetting the patient has just moved the relationship from a collaborative to a controlling one. The inevitable result is erosion of the patient's trust, who must wonder, "What else is she not telling me?"

Patients need to feel that their caregivers are competent. An attitude of confidence and decisiveness can reassure the patient of her provider's capabilities. Patients value stability in a provider. The professional who snaps at colleagues or slams objects on the table irately does not inspire much confidence. The caregiver must shelve unrelated issues before entering the room, because the patient will perceive negativity and perhaps assume that she is the cause.

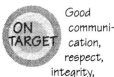

Good communication, respect, integrity, and an attitude of confidence can foster trust even in demanding circumstances.

Prehospital providers encourage the formation of trust by listening to what the patient has to say. The caregiver must note incongruities between verbal and nonverbal behaviors. Sometimes unspoken messages are the most significant ones. A woman who says, "I'm okay, I guess," while twisting her hands uncomfortably in her lap and averting her gaze is probably not "okay" at all. Such an occurrence should be taken as a cue for more communication and clarification and an opportunity to encourage the patient to express her true concerns.

Earning trust in an emergency setting has its challenges. EMS providers must make decisions and treat rapidly, often with incomplete information. The patient has no choice of providers, must accept whoever arrives, and often has never before met the provider. Some EMS patients are hostile, noncompliant, impaired by substance abuse, in police custody, or suffering injuries or illnesses related to illegal or risky activities. In addition, many people, especially the poor and disadvantaged, use EMS and the emergency department as a substitute for a relationship with a primary health care provider. Good communication, respect, integrity, and an attitude of confidence can foster trust even in demanding circumstances.

Excellence in Practice

If a primary goal of emergency medical care is to be of the greatest benefit to the patient, it is important for the EMS professional continually to develop techniques and attitudes that advance patient care and leave behind that which does not. This is especially true in women's health, wherein emergencies may place maternal and fetal lives on the line and involve body parts and personal information not generally shared with strangers.

In a woman's health crisis, as in other prehospital emergencies, the provider steps abruptly into the unvarnished truths of people's lives. EMS providers commonly encounter situations that stretch the bounds of credibility, from unlikely objects wedged deep within a vagina, gravid patients who deny pregnancy, and women who use cocaine to bring on labor.

Prehospital care providers must strive to free themselves of bias when encountering different races, customs, and mode of living. Every patient should be treated with an attitude of unconditional positive regard, even those with poor hygiene or unpleasant attitudes, and including those engaged in activities that clash with the provider's values. Troublesome patients should be handled with the same consideration as the cooperative, and the perpetrators of violent crime must be treated with the same respect as the victims. Although an appropriate sense of humor can help the provider, patient, and crew members through stressful times, "dark humor" must be kept in check if the patient or public is anywhere near.

Technical competence should be routinely assessed and sharpened. The most serious women's health emergencies often are once-in-a-career occurrences. Effective EMS professionals are committed to continually learning new techniques and reinforcing old ones, to building new knowledge and preserving skills from decay. It is helpful to debrief with a crew member after a call, discussing honestly how the situation could be handled better—how on-scene time could be shortened, how complications could be avoided, how patient comfort could be maximized, and how performance could be improved.

EMS professionals often let their work become the focal point of their lives. Its rewards are bountiful and obvious, and its adrenaline-pumping challenges can be habit forming. But rotating shifts and long hours can wreak havoc with circadian rhythms. Stress and burnout from the seemingly endless succession of crises can strike suddenly and can impair performance or prompt a career change. Stress can impair motor and cognitive function and has been associated with medical errors, interpersonal conflict, and absenteeism.

The prehospital provider must prioritize attending to his or her own needs, including eating well, getting adequate sleep, avoiding harmful habits, exercising, connecting with friends and family, and engaging in stress-relieving activities. A commitment to self-care fosters resilience and strengthens one's ability to weather change or misfortune.

Holism and Patient-Centered Practice

Emergency medicine is often fast paced and chaotic. Most patients require immediate assessment, stabilization and transport, and emergency medical personnel excel in meeting that need. Most of us enter the field of emergency medicine with a strong desire to alleviate suffering and give of ourselves to others in need. But in the turmoil of an emergency, it is easy to focus on symptoms, protocols, and procedures and thereby lose sight of the patient. Clearly, a patient who is in physical crisis needs medical stabilization above all. It is important to keep in mind, however, that behind the eyes of the critically ill patient dwells a fellow human who benefits from genuine compassion and caring. See Figure 12-1.

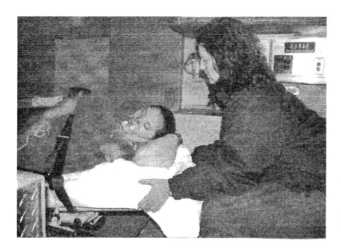

FIGURE 12-1
Holistic Prehospital Provider.
The holistic prehospital provider recognizes that the critically ill patient is also a fellow human being who benefits from genuine compassion and caring.
Photographed by Bonnie U Gruenberg

Caring is involvement, commitment, and concern that cannot be fabricated. Even in the throes of an emergency, when seconds count and interventions must be implemented rapidly, patients recognize and appreciate genuine thoughtfulness and concern. Nursing theorist Jean Watson asserts that a health care provider can influence the patient's capacity for healing just by walking into the room with a caring attitude.

It is often a challenge to balance technology with simple caring. In an era when treatment is often accompanied by tubes, wires, and beeping machines, humanistic, individualized care becomes all the more important. The woman with a pulmonary embolism needs her care providers to read her eyes almost as much as she needs them to read the cardiac monitor. Sometimes attending to the most basic of patient concerns is the most helpful and appreciated thing we can do to promote healing. A provider who thoughtfully assists the client to a position of comfort, supplies a bedpan, or listens to the individual's fears and concerns is often more appreciated than all that technology has to offer.

Modern Western medicine tends to remove symptoms from their context and divide them into soluble problems. Reductionism can be very effective in an emergency situation, but tends to address the effect instead of the cause. Lifestyle, emotions, social bonds, spirituality, culture, developmental stage, occupation, and environment influence an individual's level of wellness, and the effective prehospital provider takes these things into consideration whenever possible.

Besides managing medical, traumatic, and behavioral crises, emergency medical personnel help patients cope with catastrophe and change, with pain and fear. As they grow in experience, prehospital care providers become more skilled at seeing the big picture, knowing the right thing to say, remaining flexible, and solving complicated problems. Emergency care providers cannot always cure or ameliorate pain or suffering, but making a meaningful connection with the individuals they treat cultivates growth, healing, and transcendence in the provider as well.

ON TARGET A holistic focus is important precisely because the whole of a patient is greater than the sum of her parts or symptoms. We cannot achieve optimal outcomes when we separate an integrated body, mind, and soul into components.

Summary

A holistic focus is important because the patient is a whole person, greater than the sum of her parts, signs, symptoms, complaints, and laboratory results. It is not possible, even in an emergency, to divide a patient into neat, tractable parts or to separate her from her environment, family, beliefs—in short, her life. An EMS professional is also a whole person who benefits from professional conduct and modes of private living that reduce physical, emotional, and financial stress; meet basic needs; and balance the competing demands of a busy life.

1. How might lucid, objective, detailed documentation be of benefit in prehospital care?

2. What are the symptoms of toxoplasmosis, and what are the risks to the fetus?

3. Suzette, a pregnant paramedic, was exposed to chickenpox (varicella-zoster virus) on an ambulance call. What factors would determine whether her fetus is at risk?

4. According to the American Medical Association, what activity restrictions should a healthy woman observe during a normal pregnancy?

5. What vaccinations can a pregnant woman safely receive?

Introduction to Appendices

Appendix A, U.S. FDA Pregnancy-Risk Categories for Drugs, and related items in Appendix B, Drugs Commonly Seen or Administered in Obstetrical and Gynecological Emergencies, are provided for the reader's information although their relevance to EMS is often limited.

Many drugs, including common over-the-counter medications such as ibuprofen, are suspected to cause birth defects or problems with an unborn baby. Obstetrical care providers weigh the necessity of the medication against potential fetal harm. A pregnant woman with severe seizure disorders may continue to take teratogenic anticonvulsive medications because uncontrolled seizures are riskier to her and her fetus than are the medications. A woman with strong suicidal tendencies may remain on potentially harmful medications throughout pregnancy because without pharmacological stabilization her psychiatric disorder poses great danger to herself and her fetus.

The pregnant woman should generally avoid medications unless recommended or prescribed by her obstetric care provider; but in an emergent situation, drugs from any of the pregnancy categories may be indicated. The best thing that any emergency provider can do for the fetus is to keep the mother alive. In a life-threatening emergency, follow ACLS guidelines with modifications outlined elsewhere in this book. If in doubt whether it is advisable to use a medication on a pregnant woman, consult your medical control or local protocols.

It is useful for the EMS professional to have a working knowledge of both birth control methods and potential complications associated with use as well as of sexually transmitted infections. Appendix C, Overview of Contraceptive Methods, lists the risks, benefits, and efficacy of common contraceptive methods, as adapted from the FDA website. Appendix D, Sexually Transmitted Infections, lists important information on the microorganisms, symptoms, diagnosis, and treatment of sexually transmitted infections.

U.S. FDA Pregnancy-Risk Categories for Drugs

Please note that these categories (required by the U.S. Food and Drug Administration in drug labeling since 1975) do not necessarily constitute a ranking of risks or benefits. Some Category C drugs may be as safe and effective as those in Category A or B, but their safety or effectiveness has not yet been established by rigorous testing. Although they lack the compensatory benefits, certain Category X drugs may be no more toxic than some in Category D. Some drugs belong to multiple categories; ibuprofen, for example, is Category B during the first and second trimesters of pregnancy, but Category D in the third.

A   Adequate and well-controlled studies in pregnant women and in animals have failed to demonstrate a risk to the fetus. Example: Prenatal vitamins.

B   Animal studies failed to show damage to the fetus, but there are no adequate studies in pregnant women; OR animal studies have demonstrated fetal harm, but adequate and well-controlled human studies have not shown damage to the fetus.

C   Animal reproduction studies have shown an adverse effect on the fetus, and there are no adequate well-controlled human studies, but benefits of using the medication may outweigh the risks; OR there are no adequate animal or human studies.

D   Human studies demonstrate definite risk of harm to the fetus, but the benefits may outweigh the risk.

X   Studies in animals or humans have demonstrated fetal abnormalities or toxicity, and risks outweighs benefits.

Drugs Commonly Seen or Administered in Obstetrical and Gynecological Emergencies

Notes

- This appendix is not exhaustive and is not intended as a substitute for local protocols or standard pharmacological reference works. Including a drug or brand name in the following list does not imply endorsement, nor does omission imply disapproval.
- Known hypersensitivity to any drug is an implicit contraindication.
- Most of the following substances should be protected from direct sunlight and extremes of temperature.

Adenosine

Class

Antiarrhythmic

Trade Name

Adenocard

(Adenosine, *continued*)

Indication

Conversion of PSVT to sinus rhythm, including Wolff-Parkinson-White syndrome. Deemed equal in effectiveness to verapamil (see later) in converting PSVT, but less toxic.

Effects

Adenosine is a chemical that occurs naturally in the body. Given as a medication:

- Slows discharge of the SA node and conduction through the AV nodes; restores sinus rhythm.
- Onset (IV) is usually rapid, and half-life is less than 10 seconds; so effects and side effects are usually brief. Because of the short half-life of adenosine, PSVT may recur.

Possible Side Effects

- Central nervous system: lightheadedness, dizziness, headache, numbness, apprehension, blurred vision, burning sensation, heaviness or tingling in arms and neck, back pain
- Cardiovascular: dysrythmias (usually brief) including asystole, second- or third-degree heart block; PVCs, PACs, sinus bradycardia, or sinus tachycardia; palpitations; chest pain; hypotension
- Respiratory: dyspnea, chest pressure, hyperventilation, bronchoconstriction in patients with asthma and other respiratory diseases

Contraindications

- Second- or third-degree AV block.
- Sick sinus syndrome (except in patients with functioning artificial pacemakers).
- Do not give to patients who are taking dipyridamole (Persantin, Deplatol) or carbamazepine (Tegretol).

Considerations with Pregnant or Nursing Patients

Pregnancy Category C
Although adenosine occurs naturally throughout the body, its effects when administered to pregnant women have not been studied.

Other Precautions

- Arrhythmias, including blocks, are common at the time of cardioversion.
- Use cautiously in patients with asthma.
- Antagonized by caffeine, theophylline, and related compounds; potentiated by dipyridamole.
- Higher degrees of heart block may be produced if given in the presence of carbamazepine.
- Not effective for uncontrolled atrial fibrillation or flutter.
- When advisable, appropriate vagal maneuvers (e.g., Valsalva maneuver) should be attempted before adenosine administration.
- May crystallize if refrigerated.
- Make sure that the solution is clear.
- Contains no preservatives; discard the unused portion.

Route

IV—administer directly into a vein or into the medication port closest to the patient; follow with saline flush.

Adult Dosages

- 6 mg given as a rapid (that is, over 1–2 seconds) IV bolus and followed immediately by 20 mL saline flush; elevate extremity.
- If cardioversion does not occur after 1–2 minutes, 12-mg (maximum dose) rapid IV bolus. Do not administer if a high-level block occurs after the first dose.
- If cardioversion does not occur after another 1–2 minutes, the 12-mg dose may be repeated once.

Albuterol

Classes

Selective Beta-adrenergic sympathomimetic bronchodilator; smooth-muscle relaxant

Trade Names

Proventil, Ventolin

Indications

- Bronchial asthma
- Reversible bronchospasm associated with bronchitis, COPD, or exercise

Effects

- In low doses, causes bronchodilation and vasodilation
- At higher doses, causes typical sympathomimetic cardiac effects
- Onset 5–15 minutes

Possible Side Effects

- Central nervous system: tremors, dizziness, nervousness, headache, vertigo, hyperactivity, irritability, insomnia
- Cardiovascular: tachycardia, palpitations, peripheral vasodilation, angina, higher or lower blood pressure
- Respiratory: paradoxical bronchospasm (which may be fatal), cough, bronchitis, wheezing, hoarseness

Contraindication

Symptomatic tachycardia

Considerations with Pregnant or Nursing Patients

Pregnancy Category C

Other Precautions

- Use cautiously in patients with cardiovascular disorders, especially coronary insufficiency, dysrhythmias, and hypertension; in patients with convulsive disorders, hyperthyroidism, diabetes mellitus; and in patients being treated with MAO inhibitors or tricyclic antidepressants.
- Beta-blockers and albuterol inhibit each other's effects.
- Blood pressure, pulse, and EKG should be monitored.

Route

Inhalation

Adult Dosages

- Metered-dose inhaler 1–2 inhalations every 4–6 hours
- Small-volume nebulizer 0.5 mL of 0.5% solution (2.5 mg) in 2.5 mL normal saline over 5–15 minutes

Amiodarone

Class

Antiarrhythmic

Trade Name

Cordarone

Indications

- Ventricular fibrillation
- Hemodynamically unstable ventricular tachycardia

Effects

- Prolongs the QT interval, slows sinus rate and atrioventricular nodal conduction, slows intracardiac conduction
- Decreases peripheral vascular resistance

Possible Side Effects

- Central nervous system: malaise, fatigue
- Cardiovascular: hypotension, bradycardia, AV block, exacerbated or new arrhythmia

Contraindications

- Marked sinus bradycardia
- Second- or third-degree AV block (except in patients with functioning artificial pacemakers)

Considerations with Pregnant or Nursing Patients

Pregnancy Category D

Amiodarone may cause congenital defects, growth restriction, and neonatal arrythmias.

(Amiodarone, *continued*)

Other Precautions

- EKG should be monitored continuously.
- Amiodarone should not be confused with amrinone (Inocor, a cardiac inotrope, Pregnancy Category C). In order to prevent such mistakes, amrinone was officially renamed inamrinone lactate in 2000; but the old name is still in circulation.

Route

IV

Adult Dosage

Pulseless ventricular tachycardia or ventricular fibrillation: 300-mg IV push in 20–30 mL D_5W; may repeat at 150 mg in 3–5 minutes; maximum dose: 2.2 g/24 hr.

Calcium Chloride/Calcium Gluconate

Class

Electrolyte

Indications

- Reversal of magnesium sulfate
- Overdose of calcium-channel blocker, for example, nifedipine, verapamil (with bradycardia or cardiac arrest)
- Abdominal muscle spasm associated with black widow spider bites or scorpion or Portuguese man-of-war stings

Effects

- Replaces and maintains calcium.
- Reverses magnesium sulfate and calcium-channel blocker overdose

Possible Side Effects

- Cardiovascular: vasodilation, flushing, moderate hypotension, arrhythmias (bradycardia and asystole), cardiac arrest. When given too rapidly or to patients on digitalis, calcium chloride/calcium gluconate can cause ventricular fibrillation.

- Central nervous system: tingling sensations, drowsiness, syncope.
- Local: venous irritation during administration; extravasation may cause tissue necrosis.

Contraindications

- Ventricular fibrillation
- Patients receiving digitalis, especially those with digitalis toxicity

Considerations with Pregnant or Nursing Patients

Pregnancy Category C

Dietary calcium is a necessary nutrient, but calcium chloride and calcium gluconate have not been studied in pregnant women.

Other Precautions

- Rapid administration can produce bradycardia, sustained asystole, or cardiac arrest.
- Precipitates in the presence of sodium bicarbonate. Flush IV line well before and after administration of either substance.
- Antagonizes verapamil and other calcium-channel blockers.

Route

IV

Adult Dosage

Calcium chloride or calcium gluconate: 10 mL of a 10% solution, slowly IV

Dexamethasone

Classes

Steroid, anti-inflammatory

Trade Name

Decadron

(*Dexamethasone, continued*) # Indications

- Cerebral or tracheal edema.
- Anaphylaxis.
- Asthma.
- COPD.
- Obstetrical providers give dexamethasone to enhance lung maturation when premature delivery is expected and to decrease liver inflammation in HELLP syndrome.

Effects

- Reduces inflammation
- Suppresses immune response (especially in allergic reactions)
- Accelerates lung maturity and prevents brain hemorrhage in premature infants

Possible Side Effects

- Cardiovascular: hypertension, thromboembolism
- Central nervous system: convulsions, vertigo, headache, psychic disturbances
- Gastrointestinal: bleeding
- Hematological: fluid and electrolyte disturbances
- Skin: prolonged wound healing

Considerations with Pregnant or Nursing Patients

Pregnancy Category C

There are fetal benefits to dexamethasone in certain circumstances, but this drug has also been associated with intrauterine growth restriction.

Other Precaution

May exacerbate infections, especially fungal infections

Route

IM—inject deep into large muscle mass

Adult Dosage

To mature fetal lungs: 4 doses of 6 mg given intramuscularly 12 hours apart

Dextrose 50%

Classes

Carbohydrate, hypertonic solution

Indication

Hypoglycemia

Effect

Raises blood glucose level

Possible Side Effects

- Cardiovascular: thrombophlebitis
- Local: venous irritation
- Metabolic: hyperglycemia

Contraindications

- Intracranial or intraspinal hemorrhage
- Delirium tremens

Considerations with Pregnant or Nursing Patients

Pregnancy Category C
Dextrose has not been studied in pregnant women.

(Dextrose 50%, *continued*)

Other Precautions

- A blood sample should be drawn before administering.
- Use cautiously in thiamine-deficient patients (e.g., alcoholics); 100 mg of thiamine IV may prevent neurological problems.
- Make sure that the solution is clear.
- Discard the unused portion.

Route

IV

Adult Dosage

25-g slow IV; may be repeated once

Diazepam

Classes

Sedative-hypnotic (benzodiazepine), anticonvulsant, skeletal muscle relaxant

Trade Name

Valium

Indication

Status epilepticus

Effects

- Suppresses the spread of seizure activity in the cerebral cortex, thalamus, and limbic structures
- Depresses the limbic system, moderating emotional intensity, and the reticular activating system, reducing alertness
- Relaxes skeletal muscles

Possible Side Effects

- Central nervous system: drowsiness, lethargy, ataxia, depression, dizziness, syncope, headache, euphoria, fainting, slurred speech, tremor, confusion, vertigo
- Cardiovascular: transient hypotension, dysrhythmias, bradycardia, cardiovascular collapse
- Local: pain and phlebitis at injection site
- Respiratory: respiratory depression, apnea

Contraindications

- Respiratory depression
- Acute narrow-angle glaucoma

Considerations with Pregnant or Nursing Patients

Pregnancy Category D
Diazepam appears to cause cleft lip and palate, cardiac anomalies, craniofacial defects, inguinal hernia, and circulatory defects. When taken near term, it can cause growth restriction, lethargy, and feeding difficulties.

Other Precautions

- Administer only in normal saline IV; mixing with other substances will cause precipitation.
- Has a cumulative and potentiating effect with alcohol and other sedative drugs. Respiratory depression is generally caused by rapid IV administration. The rate of injection should not exceed 2 mg/min.
- Use cautiously with comatose patients, patients in shock, and victims of head injury.

Routes

IV (do not administer faster than 1 mL/min), IM, rectal

Adult Dosage

Status epilepticus: 5–10-mg IV

Diphenhydramine HCL

Class

Antihistamine

Trade Name

Benadryl

Indications

- Allergic reactions
- Anaphylactic shock
- Antidote for extrapyramidal (dystonic) side effects of phenothiazines (e.g., Compazine, Thorazine)

Effects

- Blocks histamine receptors
- Produces sedation

Possible Side Effects

- Cardiovascular: hypotension, palpitations, tachycardia
- Central nervous system: sedation, drowsiness, dizziness, fever, ataxia, excitement, confusion, headache
- Respiratory: thickening of bronchial secretions, chest tightness, wheezing

Contraindication

Acute asthma

Considerations with Pregnant or Nursing Patients

Pregnancy Category C first and second trimesters, B in third trimester

Other Precautions

- Incompatible with barbiturates, Dilantin, dexamethasone, methylprednisolone (Solu-Medrol), furosemide (Lasix).

- Do not inject into small veins.
- Potentiates action of atropine and other anticholinergics, alcohol, and CNS depressant drugs.
- Inhibits action of anticoagulants and some corticosteroids.
- Use cautiously in patients with a history of bronchial asthma and lower respiratory disease.

Routes

Slow IV push, deep IM

Adult Dosage

25–50 mg every 6–8 hours

Epinephrine

Classes

Sympathomimetic, synthetic adrenal hormone

Trade Name

Adrenalin

Indications

- Cardiac arrest
- Acute asthma attacks
- Severe allergic reactions and anaphylactic shock
- Profound symptomatic bradycardia (after atropine, dopamine, and external pacing)

Effects

- Cardiac stimulation
- Vasoconstriction
- Bronchodilation

Possible Side Effects

- Central nervous system: restlessness, euphoria, anxiety, vertigo, headache, cerebral hemorrhage
- Cardiovascular: palpitations, hypertension, tachycardia, syncope, EKG changes
- Respiratory: respiratory weakness, apnea, pulmonary edema, dyspnea
- Other: tremors

Contraindication

Hypovolemic shock (correct hypovolemia before administering)

Considerations with Pregnant or Nursing Patients

Pregnancy Category C

Other Precaution

Blood pressure, pulse, and EKG must be constantly monitored.

Routes

IV, endotracheal, subcutaneous

Adult Dosages

- Pulseless cardiac arrest: 1 mg (10 mL ephinephrine 1:10,000 IV push followed by 20-mL saline flush) or 2.0–2.5 mg in 10 mL normal saline endotracheal every 3–5 minutes during resuscitation
- Anaphylaxis or bronchoconstriction: 0.3–0.5 mL epinephrine 1:1,000 subcutaneously (mild); 1–2 mL epinephrine 1:10,000 slow IV (severe)

Furosemide

Class

Diuretic

Trade Name

Lasix

Indications

- Congestive heart failure
- Pulmonary edema

Effects

- Diuresis with excretion of sodium and potassium (When given IV, diuresis usually occurs within 30 minutes and lasts about 2 hours.)
- Inhibits sodium reabsorption in the kidneys
- Produces vasodilation

Possible Side Effects

- Cardiovascular: volume depletion, dehydration, orthostatic hypotension, EKG changes
- Central nervous system: dizziness, headache
- Metabolic: electrolyte imbalances
- Dehydration and significant electrolyte imbalance

Considerations with Pregnant or Nursing Patients

Pregnancy Category C

Other Precaution

Potentiates other antihypertensive drugs

Route

IV

(Furosemide, *continued*)

Adult Dosage

40 mg

Heparin

Class

Anticoagulant

Indications

- Acute deep venous thrombosis
- Pulmonary embolism
- To prevent the occurrence of thromboembolism

Effects

- Accelerates neutralization of activated clotting factors
- Does not break up existing clots

Possible Side Effects

- Cardiovascular: bruising, oozing of blood
- Central nervous system: dizziness, headache
- Gastrointestinal: abdominal pain or swelling; vomiting of blood; bloody or black, tarry stools; constipation
- Metabolic: electrolyte disturbances, hyperglycemia
- Respiratory: hemoptysis
- Skin: necrosis at site of subcutaneous injection

Contraindications

- Blood disorders, such as hemophilia and thrombocytopenia
- Recent neurosurgery
- Severe liver or kidney disease

Considerations with Pregnant or Nursing Patients

Pregnancy Category B
Heparin does not cross the placenta or cause congenital defects.

Routes

IV, subcutaneous

Adult Dosage

Loading dose: 5,000 sq every 8–12 hours for thrombus prevention

Hydroxyzine

Class

Antihistamine

Trade Name

Vistaril

Indications

- Nausea and vomiting
- To promote sleep
- Pruritus and other allergic reactions
- To potentiate the effects of natural and synthetic narcotics

Effects

- Antiemetic
- Reduces anxiety and promotes sleep
- Potentiates analgesic effects of narcotics and related agents

Possible Side Effects

- Central nervous system: drowsiness, dizziness, headache, confusion
- Cardiovascular: palpitations, hypotension
- Respiratory: thickening of bronchial secretions

Contraindication

Early pregnancy (safety has not been established)

Considerations with Pregnant or Nursing Patients

Pregnancy Category C

Manufacturer considers/hydroxyzine to be contraindicated in early pregnancy because of lack of clinical data. No evidence of harm when used after the first trimester.

Routes

Deep IM (gluteus maximus is the preferred administration site in adults), oral

Adult Dosage

50–100 mg

Insulin

Class

Hormone (Humulin, of which several varieties are marketed, and brands with similar names are synthetic human insulin. Other brands may come from cattle or pigs.)

Trade Name

Humulin

Indications

- Elevated blood glucose
- Diabetic ketoacidosis

Effects

- Increases uptake of glucose by cells
- Decreases blood glucose level
- Promotes glucose storage

Possible Side Effect

Skin: irritation at injection site

Contraindication

Hypoglycemia

Considerations with Pregnant or Nursing Patients

Pregnancy Category B

Other Precautions

- Overcompensation for blood glucose level may induce hypoglycemia.
- Illness, emotional disturbance, or administration of medications with hyperglycemic activity (e.g., oral contraceptives, epinephrine, corticosteroids) may increase the patient's insulin requirements.

Routes

IV, subcutaneous

Adult Dosage

Based on serum glucose levels

Isoetharine

Class

Sympathomimetic—predominantly beta 2—relaxes bronchial smooth muscle

Trade Name

Bronkosol

Indication

Asthma

Effects

- Bronchodilation
- Increased heart rate

Possible Side Effects

- Central nervous system: anxiety, headache
- Cardiovascular: palpitations, tachycardia
- Respiratory: possible paradoxical bronchospasm after excessive use
- Other: tremors

Contraindications

- Allergy to sodium bisulfite and related agents (e.g., sulfur dioxide, potassium metabisulfite).
- Use with caution with hypertension and tachyarrythmias.

Considerations with Pregnant or Nursing Patients

Pregnancy Category C

Other Precautions

- Blood pressure, pulse, and EKG must be constantly monitored.
- Do not use solution if it is pinkish or dark yellow or if it contains a precipitate.

Route

Inhalation only

Adult Dosages

- Metered-dose inhaler: 1–2 inhalations, preferably with spacer
- Nebulizer: 4 inhalations
- Small-volume nebulizer: 0.5 mL (diluted in 3 mL normal saline) given over 15–20 minutes

Labetalol

Classes

Alpha sympathetic blocker, beta blocker

Trade Names

Normodyne, Trandate

Indication

Severe hypertension

Effects

- Produces general vasodilation, lowers blood pressure, and reduces heart rate, cardiac output, and peripheral resistance
- Acts on the SA node, AV node, and ventricular tissue

Possible Side Effects

- Central nervous system: dizziness, headache, fatigue
- Cardiovascular: postural hypotension, angina, bradycardia, CHF, cold hands or feet, swelling of feet and lower legs
- Respiratory: wheezing, dyspnea, increased airway resistance, bronchospasm

(Labetalol, *continued*)

Contraindications

- Asthma
- Bradycardia
- CHF or cardiogenic shock
- Heart block

Considerations with Pregnant or Nursing Patients

Pregnancy Category C

Other Precautions

- Monitor vital signs, EKG, and lung sounds continuously. *Atropine* and transcutaneous pacing should be available.
- Be alert for signs of CHF, heart block, bradycardia, postural hypotension, or bronchospasm.
- Should not be administered to patients who have received IV verapamil.
- Use with caution in patients taking other antihypertensive agents.
- May enhance hypoglycemia.

Route

IV infusion

Adult Dosage

200 mg in 500 mL D_5W and infuse at 2 mg/min

Lidocaine

Classes

Antiarrhythmic, local anesthetic

Trade Name

Xylocaine

Indications

- To suppress premature ventricular contractions that occur more than 6 per minute or occur with myocardial infarction, in salvos, R on T, or are multifocal
- Ventricular fibrillation
- To prevent recurrence of ventricular fibrillation after defibrillation
- Ventricular tachycardia

Effects

- Suppresses ventricular ectopic activity
- Prevents recurrence of ventricular fibrillation after defibrillation
- Local anesthetic

Possible Side Effects

- Central nervous system: drowsiness, dizziness, lethargy, paresthesias, seizures
- Cardiovascular: myocardial depression, hypotension, bradycardia

Contraindications

- Allergy to local anesthetics
- Second- or third-degree heart blocks or idioventricular rhythm
- PVCs in conjunction with bradycardia
- Stokes-Adams syndrome (transient heart block with syncope)
- Wolff-Parkinson-White syndrome

Considerations with Pregnant or Nursing Patients

Pregnancy Category B

Routes

- IV bolus or infusion
- Injection into tissues for local anesthetic

Adult Dosages

For cardiac indications:

- IV bolus: Initial bolus of 1.0–1.5 mg/kg (70–100 mg); additional doses of 0.50–0.75 mg/kg can be repeated at 8–10-minute intervals until the arrhythmia has been suppressed or until 3 mg/kg has been given.
- IV drip: After the arrhythmia has been suppressed, a 1–4 mg/min infusion may be started for maintenance.

Magnesium sulfate ($MgSO_4$)

Class

Electrolyte

Indications

- Eclampsia, preeclampsia/PIH, HELLP syndrome
- Preterm labor contractions
- Ventricular fibrillation
- Refractory pulseless ventricular tachycardia
- Torsades de Pointes

Effects

- Antiarrhythmic
- Anticonvulsant
- CNS depressant
- Decreases likelihood of eclamptic seizures
- Relaxes smooth muscle—useful in stopping preterm labor contractions
- Causes peripheral vasodilation and bronchodilation

Possible Side Effects

- Central nervous system: drowsiness, depressed reflexes, malaise
- Cardiovascular: hypotension; flushing; circulatory collapse; depressed cardiac function or cardiac arrest, heart block
- Respiratory: respiratory depression or paralysis

- May cause respiratory depression in newborns if mother receives magnesium sulfate immediately before delivery
- May increase postpartum bleeding

Contraindications

- Heart block
- Respiratory depression

Considerations with Pregnant or Nursing Patients

Pregnancy Category B

Other Precautions

- Administration rate should be slowed or discontinued if respirations fall below 12 per minute or no patellar reflexes are observed.
- Calcium chloride should be available as an antidote for significant adverse reactions.
- Blood pressure, respirations, and level of consciousness should be monitored frequently during magnesium infusion, and the patient must be on a cardiac monitor.

Route

Intravenous infusion

Adult Dosages

Torsades de Pointes: 1–2-g IV diluted in 100 cc of normal saline.
Eclampsia:

- Initial: 4-g loading dose IV over 15–20 minutes if convulsion occurs after initial bolus, an additional 2-g IV over 3–5 minutes may be administered.
- Maintenance: 2–4-g/hr IV maintenance drip.

Morphine Sulfate

Classes

Analgesic, narcotic

Indications

- Pain and anxiety associated with acute MI
- Burns and isolated traumatic injuries
- CHF and acute pulmonary edema

Effects

- Depresses respiratory, cough, and vasomotor center in the medulla
- Relieves pain and raises pain threshold
- Reduces anxiety and produces euphoria and sedation
- Stimulates the vomiting center in the medulla and the parasympathetic nervous system
- Causes peripheral vasodilatation, which may lower heart rate and myocardial oxygen consumption

Possible Side Effects

- Central nervous system: sedation, confusion, headache, euphoria, altered consciousness
- Cardiovascular: bradycardia, asystole, hypotension
- Gastrointestinal: nausea, vomiting
- Respiratory: respiratory depression
- Skin: flushing, rashes, pruritus

Contraindications

- Respiratory depression
- Acute bronchial asthma or upper-airway obstruction
- Trauma to multiple systems
- Head injury
- Hypovolemia
- Undiagnosed abdominal pain
- Hypotension

Considerations with Pregnant or Nursing Patients

Pregnancy Category C

Other Precautions

- Closely monitor level of consciousness and airway patency.

- Effects are intensified by alcohol, barbiturates, other CNS depressants, and MAO inhibitors.
- Naloxone (see later) should be available as an antidote.

Routes

IV, IM

Adult Dosage

IV: 2–5 mg followed by 2 mg every 5 to 30 minutes until pain is relieved or respiratory depression ensues. Maximum 15 mg in the field.

Nalbuphine HCL

Class

Synthetic analgesic (a synthetic opiate agonist/antagonist chemically related to both naloxone—see next—and the potent narcotic analgesic oxymorphone)

Trade Name

Nubain

Indications

- Moderate or severe pain
- Used as an analgesic in labor and delivery

Effects

- Depresses CNS
- Decreases sensitivity to pain

Possible Side Effects

- Central nervous system: dizziness, drowsiness, restlessness, confusion, altered consciousness
- Cardiovascular: hypertension, hypotension, bradycardia, tachycardia, flushing
- Gastrointestinal: nausea, vomiting
- Respiratory: respiratory depression

Considerations with Pregnant or Nursing Patients

Pregnancy Category B

Other Precautions

- Occasionally causes severe fetal bradycaardia and breathing problems in the neonate if administered just before delivery.
- Use cautiously in patients with impaired respiratory function or hepatic or renal disease.
- Should not be given to patients receiving morphine (previous) or other opiates.
- Naloxone should be available as an antidote.

Routes

IV, IM

Adult Dosage

5–10 mg

Naloxone

Class

Narcotic antagonist

Trade Name

Narcan

Indications

- Overdose or undesirable side effects of narcotics
- To rule out narcotics in coma of unknown origin

Effects

- Competitive antagonist for certain opiate receptor sites; reverses some effects of narcotics and narcotic-like drugs (e.g., respiratory depression, sedation, hypotension), but not analgesia
- Reverses narcotic overdose

Possible Side Effects

- Gastrointestinal: (with higher than recommended doses or injected too fast) nausea, severe vomiting
- Other: withdrawal symptoms in patients dependent on narcotics

Contraindication

Do not give to neonates of narcotic-addicted or methadone-dependent mothers.

Considerations with Pregnant or Nursing Patients

Pregnancy Category B

Other Precautions

- Repeated doses may be required because most narcotics have longer durations of action.
- Be prepared to manage combative patients in narcotic withdrawal.

Routes

IV, IM, endotracheal

Adult Dosage

IV: 1–2 mg

Nifedipine

Classes

Calcium-channel blocker, tocolytic

Trade Name

Procardia

Indications

- Preterm labor contractions
- Severe hypertension
- Angina pectoris

Effects

- Relaxes smooth muscle, causing arteriolar vasodilation
- Relaxes smooth muscle, stopping uterine contractions

Possible Side Effects

- Cardiovascular: hypotension, tachycardia
- Central nervous system: dizziness, flushing, headache
- Gastrointestinal: nausea, heartburn

Contraindication

Hypotension

Considerations with Pregnant or Nursing Patients

Pregnancy Category C

Other Precautions

- Blood pressure should be constantly monitored.
- If given in field, cardiac monitoring must be used.

Routes

Oral, sublingual

Adult Dosage

10 mg sublingual; puncture the capsule several times with a needle; put it under the patient's tongue.

Procainamide

Class

Antiarrhythmic

Trade Name

Pronestyl

Indications

- Frequent PVCs
- Wide-complex tachycardia
- Ventricular fibrillation/tachycardia

Effects

- Slows conduction through myocardium by increasing electrical threshold of ventricle and HIS Purkinje system, and may raise the fibrillation threshold

Possible Side Effects

- Central nervous system: hallucinations, dizziness, confusion, convulsions, anxiety
- Cardiovascular: severe hypotension, bradycardia, AV block, ventricular fibrillation

(Procainamide, *continued*)

Contraindications

- High-degree heart blocks
- Torsades de Pointes
- Ventricular escape rhythms
- Prolonged Q-T interval

Considerations with Pregnant or Nursing Patients

Pregnancy Category C

Other Precautions

- Bolus administration of procainamide may result in hypotension and toxicity.
- Monitor vital signs, level of consciousness, and cardiac rhythm.

Routes

Slow IV bolus, IV drip

Adult Dosage

Infuse 20 mg/min until arrhythmia is controlled, hypotension occurs, QRS complex widens by 50% of its original width, or total of 17 mg/kg is given.

Promethazine

Classes

Antihistamine, antiemetic

Trade Name

Phenergan

Indications

- Nausea and vomiting
- Motion sickness
- Allergic reactions
- To potentiate the effects of analgesics or sedation

Effects

- Competes with histamine for H_1 receptor sites. Prevents but does not reverse histamine mediated responses.
- Potentiates effects of analgesics.

Possible Side Effects

- Central nervous system: drowsiness; sedation.
- Cardiovascular: hypotension, hypertension.
- Hematologic: blood abnormalities.
- Local: extravasation can cause severe irritation and gangrene.

Contraindication

Patients who have received other CNS depressants (including alcohol)

Considerations with Pregnant or Nursing Patients

Pregnancy Category C

Routes

IV, IM, oral

Adult Dosage

12.5–25.0 mg

Terbutaline

Class

Beta 2 sympathomimetic

Trade Name

Brethine

Indications

- Bronchial asthma
- Preterm labor or irritable uterus

Effects

- Relaxes uterine smooth muscle, inhibiting uterine contractions
- Bronchodilation
- Increased heart rate

Possible Side Effects

- Central nervous system: tremors, dizziness, headache, anxiety, restlessness, vertigo, drowsiness
- Cardiovascular: tachycardia, palpitations, dysrhythmias, hypotension, PVCs, angina

Contraindications

- Tachycardia.
- Do not give with other sympathomimetics, such as epinephrine.

Considerations with Pregnant or Nursing Patients

Pregnancy Category B

Other Precaution

Blood pressure, pulse, and EKG must be closely monitored.

Routes

Inhalation, subcutaneous injection, IV, oral

Adult Dosages

- Metered-dose inhaler: 2 inhalations, 1 minute apart
- Subcutaneous injection: 0.25 mg; may be repeated in 15–30 minutes
- Preterm labor: 0.25-mg IM or subcutaneous; may be repeated in 15–30 minutes as needed

Verapamil

Class

Calcium-channel blocker

Trade Names

Isoptin, Calan

Indications

- Stable narrow-complex PSVT refractory to adenosine
- Stable uncontrolled atrial flutter or fibrillation

Effects

- Slows discharge of SA node and conduction through AV node
- Relaxes coronary artery spasm
- Decreases myocardial contractility and oxygen demand
- Decreases systemic vascular resistance

Side Effects

- Central nervous system: dizziness, headache, and fatigue
- Cardiovascular: transient hypotension, heart failure, bradycardia, AV block, ventricular asystole, ventricular fibrillation

Contraindications

- Shock
- Hypotension
- Second- or third-degree heart block
- Sick sinus syndrome (except in patients with functioning artificial pacemakers)
- Wolff-Parkinson-White syndrome
- Severe heart failure
- Ventricular tachycardia (any wide complex tachycardia until proven not to be ventricular tachycardia)

Considerations with Pregnant or Nursing Patients

Pregnancy Category C

Other Precautions

- Monitor vital signs, level of consciousness, and cardiac rhythm.
- Can cause transient hypotension due to peripheral vasodilation; potentiates the effects of other antihypertensive agents.

Route

IV

Adult Dosages

- 2.5–5.0-mg slow IV push (over 2 minutes)
- If tachycardia is not resolved in 15–30 minutes: 5–10-mg slow IV push (repeated every 15–30 minutes to a maximum of 20 mg)

Overview of Contraceptive Methods

Male Condom

A polyurethane or latex sheath placed over the erect penis preventing sperm from entering the female reproductive tract

Failure rate: Typically 11–18 pregnancies per 100 women per year.

Risks: Irritation and allergic reactions in either partner may occur with latex or uncommonly with polyurethane.

Protection from STDs: After abstinence, condoms are the best protection against STDs such as chlamydia and including gonorrhea and HIV. Condoms provide incomplete protection against many viruses, such as those that cause genital warts and herpes, because these can be transmitted by other skin contact during intercourse.

Convenience: Applied immediately before intercourse; discarded after use.

Availability: Nonprescription, readily available in many locations.

Female Condom

A lubricated polyurethane sheath designed to line the vagina and prevent sperm from entering the female reproductive tract

Failure rate: Typically 21 pregnancies per 100 women per year

Risks: Irritation and allergic reactions

Protection from STDs: May give some STD protection; not as effective as male condom; does not fully protect against genital herpes or warts

Convenience: Applied immediately before intercourse; discarded after use

Availability: Nonprescription

Diaphragm with Spermicide

A dome-shaped latex disk with a flexible rim that covers the cervix so that sperm cannot reach the uterus. The diaphragm is filled with spermicide before use

Failure rate: Typically 17 pregnancies per 100 women per year

Risks: Irritation and allergic reactions, urinary tract infection, rarely toxic shock syndrome

Protection from STDs: Minimal if any protection

Convenience: Inserted before intercourse and left in place at least 8 hours after; can be left in place for 24 hours with additional spermicide for repeated intercourse

Availability: Prescription

Cervical Cap with Spermicide

A soft latex cup that covers the cervix

Failure rate: Typically 17–23 pregnancies per 100 women per year

Risks: Irritation and allergic reactions, rarely toxic shock syndrome

Protection from STDs: None

Convenience: May be challenging to insert; can remain in place for 48 hours without reapplying spermicide for repeated intercourse

Availability: Prescription

Spermicide Alone

A foam, cream, jelly, film, suppository, or tablet that contains nonoxynol-9, a sperm-killing chemical

Failure rate: Typically 20–50 pregnancies per 100 women per year

Risks: Irritation and allergic reactions, urinary tract infections

Protection from STDs: None

Convenience: Inserted 5–90 minutes before intercourse and usually left in place at least 6–8 hours after

Availability: Nonprescription

Oral Contraceptives—Combined Estrogen and Progesterone

A pill that suppresses ovulation by the combined actions of the hormones estrogen and progesterone

Failure rate: Typically 1–2 pregnancies per 100 women per year if pills are taken as directed—higher failure rate if pills are missed without using a backup method.

Risks: Dizziness; nausea; changes in menstruation, mood, and weight; rarely, cardiovascular disease, including hypertension, blood clots, heart attack, and strokes.

Possible benefits: Use of combined oral contraceptives may reduce endometrial, colorectal, and ovarian cancer; fibrocystic breast disease; pelvic inflammatory disease; osteoporosis; ovarian cysts; and acne. Oral contraceptives can also successfully treat menstrual cycle irregularities, iron deficiency anemia, menstrual cramps, and perimenopausal symptoms.

Protection from STDs: None.

Convenience: Must be taken on daily schedule, regardless of frequency of intercourse.

Availability: Prescription.

Oral Contraceptives— Progestin-only Minipill

A pill containing only the hormone progestin, which thickens cervical mucus to prevent the sperm from reaching the egg. May be used while breastfeeding.

Failure rate: Typically 2 pregnancies per 100 women per year if taken at exactly the same time every day

Risks: Irregular bleeding, weight gain, breast tenderness

Protection from STDs: None

Convenience: Must be taken at the same time every day, regardless of frequency of intercourse

Availability: Prescription

Oral Contraceptives—Estrogen and Progestin, 91-Day Regimen (Seasonale)

A pill containing estrogen and progestin, taken in 3-month cycles of 12 weeks of active pills followed by 1 week of inactive pills. Menstrual periods occur during the 13th week of the cycle.

Failure rate: Typically 1–2 pregnancies per 100 women per year.

Some risks and benefits: Similar to oral contraceptives—combined pill (see above). Woman only menstrate 4 times per year when on seasonale.

Protection from STDs: None.

Convenience: Must be taken on daily schedule, regardless of frequency of intercourse. May have spotting between periods.

Availability: Prescription.

Contraceptive Patch (Ortho Evra)

Skin patch worn on the lower abdomen, buttocks, or upper body that releases the hormones progestin and estrogen into the bloodstream

Failure rate: Typically 1–2 pregnancies per 100 women per year; failure rate is greater if woman weighs more than 198 pounds.

Some risks and benefits: Similar to oral contraceptives—combined pill (see above).

Protection from STDs: None.

Convenience: New patch is applied once a week for 3 weeks. Patch is not worn during the 4th week, and woman has a menstrual period.

Availability: Prescription.

Vaginal Contraceptive Ring (Nuvaring)

A flexible ring about 2 in. in diameter that is inserted into the vagina and releases the hormones progestin and estrogen

Failure rate: Typically 1–2 pregnancies per 100 women per year.

Some risks and benefits: Similar to oral contraceptives—combined pill (see above). Presence of the ring may cause vaginal discharge, vaginitis, or irritation.

Protection from STDs: None.

Convenience: Inserted by the woman; remains in the vagina for 3 weeks, then is removed for 1 week.

Availability: Prescription.

Postcoital ("Morning After") Contraceptives (Preven and Plan B)

Pills containing either progestin alone or progestin with estrogen—to be used after a contraceptive fails or after unprotected sex to prevent pregnancy by interfering with ovulation, fertilization, or implantation. Postcoital contraception will not interrupt an established pregnancy.

Failure rate: Almost 80% reduction in risk of pregnancy for a single act of unprotected sex.

Risks: Nausea, vomiting, abdominal pain, fatigue, headache.

Protection from STDs: None.

Convenience: Must be taken within 72 hours of having unprotected intercourse. Not to be used as routine birth control—typically side effects of postcoital pills make a woman feel very ill, and most women would not choose to use them on a regular basis.

Availability: Prescription; may soon be available over the counter.

Injection (Depo-Provera)

An injectable progestin that inhibits ovulation, prevents sperm from reaching the egg, and prevents the fertilized egg from implanting in the uterus for 3 months after administration

Failure rate: Typically less than 1 pregnancy per 100 women per year.

Risks: Irregular bleeding, weight gain, breast tenderness, headaches, exacerbation of preexisting depression.

Possible Benefits: After several injections, menstrual flow typically decreases or ceases; decreases menstrual cramping. Safe when breastfeeding.

Protection from STDs: None.
Convenience: One injection every 3 months.
Availability: Prescription.

Injection (Lunelle)

An injectable form of progestin and estrogen

Failure rate: Typically less than 1 pregnancy per 100 women per year.

Risks: Similar to oral contraceptives—combined pill (see above). May cause changes in menstrual cycle or weight gain.

Protection from STDs: None.

Convenience: Injection given once a month.

Availability: Prescription.

IUD (Intrauterine Device)

A T-shaped device inserted into the uterus by a health care professional

Failure rate: Typically less than 1 pregnancy per 100 women per year.

Risks: Cramps, bleeding, pelvic inflammatory disease, infertility, perforation of uterus.

Protection from STDs: None.

Convenience: One brand is a copper wire and can stay in the uterus for 10 years; the other contains progesterone and may remain in the uterus for 5 years.

Availability: Prescription.

Periodic Abstinence

To deliberately refrain from having sexual intercourse during times when pregnancy is more likely.

Failure rate: Typically 20 pregnancies per 100 women per year.

Risks: None.

Protection from STDs: None.

Convenience: Requires frequent monitoring of body functions (for example, body temperature or cervical mucus consistency). May be ineffective if cycles are irregular.

Availability: Instructions from health care provider or self-education from books or classes about fertility awareness.

Female Surgical Sterilization

The woman's fallopian tubes are blocked or removed to prevent sperm and egg from meeting.

Failure rate: Typically less than 1 pregnancy per 100 women per year

Risks: Pain, bleeding, infection, other postsurgical complications, ectopic pregnancy

Protection from STDs: None

Convenience: One-time surgical procedure that requires an abdominal incision

Availability: Surgery

Surgical Sterilization—Male

Sealing, tying, or cutting a man's vas deferens to prevent sperm from leaving the body

Failure rate: Typically less than 1 pregnancy per 100 women per year

Risks: Pain, bleeding, infection, other minor postsurgical complications

Protection from STDs: None

Convenience: One-time surgical procedure

Availability: Surgery

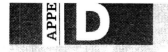

Sexually Transmitted Infections

Chlamydia

Chlamydia is the most common sexually transmitted bacterial infection in the United States.

Seventy-five percent of women and 50% of men with chlamydia are asymptomatic.

Microorganism *Chlamydia trachomatis*

Chlamydial infection can cause bladder infections, pelvic inflammatory disease, reactive arthritis, and sterility. Chlamydia transmitted to the infant at delivery can cause pneumonia, eye infections, and blindness.

Symptoms Symptoms, if any, appear in 7–21 days.

Most often no early symptoms; may have abnormal vaginal discharge or bleeding, pain or burning while urinating, painful intercourse, abdominal pain, nausea, fever.

Diagnosis Laboratory test, DNA probe; urine test also available.

Treatment Treatment based on clinical symptoms or partner's positive test.

Antibiotics: Doxycycline, Zithromax, Tetracycline.

Partners must be treated.

Gonorrhea ("Clap," "GC")

Eighty percent of women and 10% of men with gonorrhea are asymptomatic.

Gonorrhea and chlamydia often are found together—if a patient has one of the diseases, she may have the other.

Microorganism *Neisseria gonorrhoeae* bacteria (gonococci)

Gonorrhea can cause sterility, arthritis, and cardiac problems; pelvic inflammatory disease; or sterility. During pregnancy, gonorrhea can cause preterm labor, stillbirth, and severe eye infections in the infant.

Gonorrhea can infect the throat or the bladder as well as the reproductive tract.

Symptoms Often no symptoms—if present, usually occur within 10 days. Urinary burning or frequency, menstrual irregularities, pelvic or lower abdominal

	pain; pain with intercourse, yellow or yellow-green vaginal discharge swelling or tenderness of the vulva, or arthritis-like pain.
Diagnosis	Laboratory culture.
Treatment	Specific type and amount of penicillin or other antibiotic.
	Partners must be treated.

Trichomonas ("Tric")

Microorganism	*Trichomonas vaginalis*, a protozoan
Symptoms	Usually profuse, foamy yellow, green, or gray vaginal discharge with a strong odor. Pain with intercourse, irritation and itching of the genital area.
Diagnosis	Microscopic exam of vaginal discharge.
	May have asymptomatic infection long before acute episode.
Treatment	Oral or vaginal metronidazole (Flagyl).
	Partners must be treated.

Hepatitis B

Hepatitis B (HBV) is a common sexually transmitted virus that can be prevented with vaccination. Hepatitis A and hepatitis C can sometimes be spread through sexual contact.

Microorganism	Hepatitis B virus (HBV)
	Some 90–95% percent of adults with HBV recover completely; 5–10% become carriers and have chronic infection. Chronic HBV infection can cause liver failure and death. HBV testing is recommended for all pregnant women so that steps might be taken to prevent the infant from contracting the disease.
Symptoms	Initial symptoms: extreme fatigue, headache, fever, rash, body aches, anorexia, nausea and vomiting, abdominal pain.
	Later symptoms include dark urine, clay-colored stool, and jaundice.
	Hepatitis may be asymptomatic during its most contagious phases.
Diagnosis	Specialized blood test.
Treatment	No specific treatment; rest and good nutrition, avoidance of alcohol and other hepatotoxic drugs during convalescence.

Human Papilloma Virus

There are more than 100 different HPVs. Some strains cause genital warts, some cause cervical and vulvar cancer, and some remain asymptomatic indefinitely.

As many as 80% of sexually active adults harbor at least one strain of HPV.

Microorganism	Human papilloma virus
Symptoms	Genital warts grow more rapidly when the immune system is altered, as during pregnancy, or when infections or chronic health conditions are present.

Warts usually occur in clusters and have an irregular, cauliflower-like appearance. Warts appear on the genitals, anus, and, rarely, in the throat. Untreated genital warts can grow to block the openings of the vagina, anus, or throat and cause itching and discomfort.

Diagnosis Can be diagnosed by the warts' characteristic appearance. HPV lesions turn white when sprayed with acetic acid. Laboratory test confirms viral strain. Often discovered when an abnormal pap test indicates HPV-induced precancerous changes to the cervix.

Treatment There is no cure for HPV. Warts may be removed with medications or cryogenics.

HIV/AIDS

Microorganism Human immunodeficiency viruses (HIV-1 and HIV-2)

Symptoms HIV infection is often asymptomatic for many years, then may progress to acquired immunodeficiency syndrome (AIDS) with serious illnesses and opportunistic infections.

Diagnosis HIV antibody blood test shows exposure to HIV, but does not tell when or whether symptoms of AIDS will develop.

Treatment Antiviral medications; no cure.

Syphilis

Untreated, the syphilis spirochete can remain in the body for life and lead to disfigurement, neurologic disorder, or death.

Microorganism *Treponema pallidum* bacteria

Spread through kissing, vaginal, anal, and oral intercourse. The fetus of an infected woman risks stillbirth; damage to heart, nervous system, and skeleton; or blindness.

Symptoms *Primary phase:* Painless chancres often appear on the genitals, vagina, cervix, lips, mouth, or anus 21–90 days after infection. They are present for 3–6 weeks and often are accompanied by enlarged, tender lymph nodes.

Secondary phase: Body rashes (especially on the palms and soles), fever, fatigue, sore throat, hair loss, weight loss, swollen glands, headache, and muscle pains. May develop intermittently for years.

Latent phase: No symptoms. Latent phases occur between other phases.

Late phase: One-third of patients with untreated syphilis suffer serious damage to organ systems that may cause death.

Diagnosis Blood test (VDRL or RPR, FTA). The VDRL and RPR are initial tests; if positive then FTA is ordered.

Most pregnant women are screened for syphilis as part of routine prenatal bloodwork.

Treatment Specific type and amount of penicillin or other antibiotic.

Partners must be treated.

Answers to
Case Study Questions

Chapter 1

Julia has a unicornuate ("one-horned") uterus. This defect is one of a group of uterine defects known as Müllerian anomalies, most of which pose significant risk to pregnancy. Certain Müllerian anomalies respond well to surgical repair, but the unicornuate uterus does not, because no surgical procedure will enlarge the uterus.

1. A unicornuate uterus is a congenital defect in which the individual is born with a banana-shaped half uterus that may have a rudimentary uterine horn attached. A woman with a unicornuate uterus is at high risk for spontaneous abortion, ectopic pregnancy, preterm labor, fetal growth restriction, uterine rupture, and fetal malpresentations.

2. Yolanda and Victor guessed that the fetus was probably breech, knowing that space is limited in a unicornuate uterus and the fetus often adopts a breech position to conform to the shape of the uterine cavity. It is unlikely the paramedics could have determined a breech presentation by abdominal palpation—at 24 weeks it is difficult to differentiate a head from a rump using this method. Julia also probably knows her fetus's position from her weekly sonograms if he has been persistently breech.

3. The 24-week fetus is viable, but needs specialized neonatal intensive care for several months if he is to survive. Surviving infants are at high risk for long-term problems such as lung damage, brain damage, and blindness. He will need aggressive resuscitation at birth. He is thin skinned, delicate, red and wrinkled, with minimal subcutaneous fat. He usually has hair on his head and body, and his eyes may be sealed closed—eyes usually open at 25 weeks. Weight is about 820 g, about a pound and a half.

4. Yes, Julia may be in preterm labor. Yolanda and Victor took steps en route in anticipation of sudden delivery of a very immature infant—preparing OB and pediatric airway kits, heating the back of the ambulance, and arranging for backup if delivery occurred. Preterm labor can present subtly, with vague symptoms such as reports of abdominal tightness, cramps, changes in vaginal discharge, pelvic pressure, and bleeding. With Julia's history, the paramedics took her symptoms seriously and transported rapidly to a facility with a neonatal intensive care unit.

    Their efforts paid off in this case. En route, Julia's amniotic sac ruptured and at that point she went into rapid, obvious labor. The hospital was prepared for their arrival and neonatal specialists were there to attend the birth of Julia's 24-week premature infant, born footling breech shortly after their arrival at the hospital. The infant had a difficult first few weeks and suffered many setbacks and trials before finally turning the corner and thriving. He was discharged about 4 months later, and by the age of 3 he showed few deficits related to his early birth.

Chapter 2

A pregnant patient who has not had prenatal care may have an uncomplicated pregnancy or present to emergency providers in serious medical crisis. The EMS responder must carefully assess the patient, consider every possibility, and stand ready to manage any unexpected turn of events.

1. Laura formed the clinical impression of active labor upon discovering Tara's pregnant abdomen and intermittent contractions. If Tara's story about the conception date was correct, she was in labor with a premature or immature baby; but the size of her abdomen indicated a full-term pregnancy. Tara's fundal height of 2 fingers below the xyphoid process suggested a 38-week pregnancy, possibly more advanced. Laura considered the possibility of premature twins, but it seemed more likely that Tara's stated history was not reliable. With Tara's report of "urine" leakage, Laura surmised that the amniotic sac had been ruptured for 2 days, posing a risk of infection. Laura suspected fetal distress when she saw the mustard-colored and somewhat particulate amniotic fluid indicating meconium staining. Laura also considered the possibility of fetal compromise secondary to drug and alcohol use. Tara's report of "menses" 2 months ago indicated third-trimester bleeding of unknown etiology—Laura considered the possibility of placenta previa or abruption. The presence of fetal movement was a reassuring sign that the unborn child was still alive.

   Laura was alarmed by Tara's blood pressure. Coupled with the swelling, epigastric pain, and headache, Laura recognized that Tara had severe preeclampsia and was at high risk for seizures, cerebral bleeding, placental abruption, or other life-threatening sequelae. (Hypertension in pregnancy will be discussed in detail in chapter 3.)

2. Heidi and Laura's initial impression was that Tara probably had a urinary tract infection, although pelvic inflammatory disease was also a possibility. The EMS crew was not convinced that Tara had been forthright about her sexual history, and pelvic inflammatory disease (PID) secondary to a sexually transmitted infection would cause pain of the magnitude Tara was experiencing. Tara's history of migraines could have explained her severe headache. Laura would have assessed her further to determine whether this headache followed her usual migraine pattern, but the discovery of a gravid abdomen put these symptoms into an entirely different context. Tara could also have had a urinary tract or uterine infection while in labor.

3. Tara should be transported in the left lateral position, which maximizes placental perfusion and optimizes blood pressure. Laura initiated intravenous access,

started oxygen therapy, began maternal cardiac monitoring, and contacted medical control for medication orders.

At the hospital, the on-call obstetrician examined Tara and found her to be completely dilated, although Tara did not feel a pushing urge. The fetal monitor showed a reassuring pattern. The obstetrician started oxygen and ordered a complete blood count (CBC) with differential, blood type, antibody screen, rubella antibody titer, hepatitis test, an HIV antibody screen, hepatic-function panel, coagulation studies, uric acid, and basic metabolic panel. A urine dip showed +3 proteinuria. Tara's blood pressure reached 230/120, prompting her immediate treatment with apresoline to lower her blood pressure and magnesium sulfate to reduce the likelihood of seizures. The apresoline reduced Tara's blood pressure to 180/98, still seriously elevated.

Tara did not feel the urge to push and had to be persuaded to bear down with the contractions of second-stage labor. Two hours later, she delivered a 6-lb, 2-oz full-term boy with Apgars of 7 and 8. Tara remained on the magnesium sulfate for 24 hours after the delivery and was normotensive by the fourth postpartum day.

Chapter 3

An intensive search ensued to find Estella and bring her back to the hospital.

1. Low platelets are a red flag for a potentially life-threatening complication of pregnancy called HELLP syndrome (hemolysis, elevated liver enzymes, and low platelets). Estella's elevated liver enzymes confirmed the diagnosis. Some authorities consider HELLP a variant of preeclampsia; others deem it a distinct illness. Most cases develop between 22 and 36 gestational weeks, but some occur postpartum.

2. Many patients with HELLP do not look or feel ill despite alarming laboratory values. When signs and symptoms are apparent, the most common presentation is right upper quadrant, substernal, or epigastric pain, with or without nausea, vomiting, or malaise. Many patients are hypertensive. Symptoms of HELLP may be confused with those of hepatitis. Less commonly, the patient may exhibit pulmonary edema, jaundice, ascites, DIC, hemorrhage, or renal failure.

3. Estella could hemorrhage, experience hypertensive crisis or stroke, suffer placental abruption, or suffer liver failure or rupture. Her fetus could die *in utero*.

4. The ambulance crew was prepared to manage the possible complications that they might encounter, such as seizures, hypertensive crisis, hemorrhage, or cardiac arrest. An intravenous line of lactated Ringer's was in place, and Estella breathed low-flow oxygen via nasal cannula. Estella required a fetal monitor, so a labor and delivery nurse accompanied her en route. The crew was instructed to initiate a magnesium sulfate infusion if Estella showed signs of decompensation—visual disturbances, severe headache, epigastric pain, hyperreflexia, or hypertension. Cardiac monitoring would be instituted if magnesium were started or if the patient became symptomatic or unstable.

The obstetrician ordered betamethasone injections to accelerate fetal lung maturity because it was likely that Estella's baby would be delivered prematurely. The steroids also improved Estella's liver function; the next set of laboratory tests showed slightly improved values, and her chest pain was gone. She said that she felt fine and questioned why she needed to be in the hospital.

Delivery of the infant is the only definitive cure for antepartum HELLP syndrome, and a woman with this diagnosis is never truly stable. Dr. Presque, however, considered her stable enough to transport by ambulance to the tertiary-care hospital near her home.

Estella arrived safely at her local hospital none too soon. Twenty-four hours after admission, her blood pressure rose to 160/96, her chest pain returned, and her platelet count fell to 22,000. Her obstetrician infused magnesium sulfate, transfused platelets, and performed an emergency cesarean section to extract a 3-lb, 3-oz male infant. After 2 months of care in the neonatal intensive care unit, he was discharged. Estella remained on a magnesium sulfate infusion for 24 hours after delivery and under close observation for 3 days. Her platelets began to climb again, and she was asymptomatic and normotensive, so she was discharged on postoperative day four. Her recovery was uneventful.

Chapter 4

1. Mick and Sean used the FETAL mnemonic to assess Samantha's pregnant abdomen and fetal status:
   Fetal heart rate or presence of fetal movement
   Estimated gestational age
   Trauma such as bruising or broken skin
   Abdominal palpation for tenderness and presence of uterine contractions, and
   Loss of amniotic fluid or vaginal bleeding

2. Direct trauma or shearing forces can cause preterm labor, preterm rupture of the membranes, and placental abruption, even after minor accidents. Samantha should be transported to the hospital, evaluated in the emergency department for injury, and then sent to labor and delivery to monitor for presence of contractions, persistent uterine tenderness, nonreassuring fetal heart rate, vaginal bleeding, or rupture of the membranes.

3. Mick and Sean will immobilize Samantha on a backboard as with any trauma victim, but will avoid placing her supine. Placing a pregnant woman flat on a backboard can reduce her cardiac output by as much as 30%, which can endanger the fetus more than Samantha's actual injuries. Mick and Sean avoided maternal and fetal compromise by raising the right side of the backboard 4–6 in. to place it at a 15–30° angle.

4. Pregnant victims of trauma should generally be treated like other trauma victims, but with accommodations for the physiological and anatomic changes of pregnancy. Strapped to a backboard, Samantha may find that her gravid uterus

puts pressure on her full stomach and causes her to vomit. Airway management is a priority. High-flow oxygen by mask should be in initiated at the earliest opportunity, along with infusion of intravenous volume expanders such as lactated Ringer's or normal saline. Sean and Mick will watch for signs of internal hemorrhage, uterine tenderness, vaginal bleeding, contractions, and fetal movement and auscultate the fetal heartbeat if possible.

Chapter 5

1. Amanda had a history of a rapid, easy first labor and delivery. Second babies tend to come faster than the first. This baby was smaller than the first one, deep in the pelvis, and the cervix was very soft, thin, and dilated.

2. Amniotic fluid should be clear or straw colored, though white flecks of vernix caseosa may be present. Green or mustard-colored fluid, with or without particulate material, indicates the presence of meconium. A foul odor would indicate infection, and the odor of urine would indicate that her bladder had voided. When a multiparous woman experiences rupture of membranes in the presence of regular contractions, the baby is often soon to arrive. Rupture of amniotic membranes also carries a small risk of cord prolapse. The provider should assess for fetal movement or a reassuring fetal heart rate as soon as possible after membranes rupture.

3. If Amanda would not leave the toilet and the baby were emerging, Edward could have moved her forward to perch on the edge of the toilet seat, allowing the toilet to serve as a kind of birthing chair as he assisted delivery—or, in this case, caught the baby as it rapidly emerged.

4. The third stage is usually quick and easy, but there is an increased risk of immediate postpartum hemorrhage due to uterine atony following a precipitous delivery. Amanda did bleed heavily after her placenta delivered intact. Edward and Kim massaged her fundus vigorously while establishing a large-bore intravenous line and rapidly infusing lactated Ringer's or normal saline. Following local protocols, Kim injected 10 units of pitocin intramuscularly and infused another 10 units diluted in 1,000 cc of lactated Ringer's. She prepared 0.2 mg of methergine for intramuscular injection in case the pitocin was ineffective, but fortunately Amanda's bleeding stopped and her uterus stayed firm. (See chapter 7 for management of postpartum hemorrhage.)

Chapter 6

1. His priority is to clamp the cord somewhere between the torn end and the infant's abdomen. As soon as the baby is born, Chris should grasp the cord between his fingers and squeeze it to stop bleeding until a clamp or cord tape can be applied. Clamping the maternal end of the cord is not necessary unless there could be a twin remaining in utero (though it should be done to limit contamination of the

scene with blood). Blood lost from the placental end of the cord is fetal in origin, not part of the maternal circulatory system, and is hemodynamically unimportant to either mother or infant.

2. After the umbilical cord has been clamped, resuscitation can proceed as usual, with suctioning, positioning, stimulation, drying and warming, oxygen, bag mask ventilation, chest compressions, intubation, and medications as necessary. This baby may also require an intravenous fluid bolus if he has become hypovolemic from the cord breakage.

3. A thin, weak, or short cord may be related to malnutrition, maternal smoking or hypertension, IUGR, oligohydramnios, or genetic anomalies. A short cord may also be genetically determined or result from low fetal activity.

4. Chris should avoid any traction on the cord during third stage. If it broke again, the placenta might have to be manually removed at the hospital. He should also recognize the potential for placental abnormalities and be prepared to treat maternal hemorrhage if it occurs.

Chapter 7

1. Shoulder dystocia is a fairly common complication of labor and delivery involving impaction of the fetal shoulder above the maternal pubic symphysis after birth of the head, preventing delivery of the body. Risk factors include a long, slow second-stage labor, fetal macrosomia, gestational diabetes, prior shoulder dystocia, post-term pregnancy, short maternal stature, and abnormal pelvic structure.

2. Call for backup immediately. The first step in resolving a shoulder dystocia is McRobert's maneuver, flexing the maternal hips until her thighs are on her abdomen to open the pelvis. When the woman is in McRobert's position, an assistant should stand on the side of the baby's back and apply deep pressure straight down just above the mother's pubic bone. Have the mother push hard while you gently guide the head downward. In most cases, these two maneuvers will resolve the shoulder dystocia. If they do not, immediately flip the woman to her hands and knees, grasp the fetal head, and gently guide it downward, attempting to deliver the posterior shoulder (Gaskin maneuver). If none of these maneuvers is successful, rapid transport to the nearest facility is in order. Transport the mother either on hands and knees or in McRobert's position, and continue repeating the above maneuvers en route. Initiate high-flow oxygen for the mother, and start a large-bore intravenous line of crystalloid solution.

3. For the fetus, shoulder dystocia poses the risk of hypoxia or anoxia that can cause irreparable neurological damage, brachial plexus palsies, and fractures of the clavicle or humerus. The baby born after a shoulder dystocia will probably require resuscitation.

4. Uterine atony and subsequent hemorrhage are common after shoulder dystocia, and it is common for the woman to suffer third- or fourth-degree perineal lacerations.

Chapter 8

1. Following local protocols, Latitia should administer 10 units of IM pitocin intramuscularly and then rapidly establish a large-bore intravenous line of lactated Ringer's, run wide open. Protocols may recommend adding an additional 10–20 units of pitocin into the IV bag. Kayleigh should be treated for shock and started on high-flow oxygen by nonrebreather mask. Maki should continue to massage Kayleigh's fundus and reassess the bleeding. If Kayleigh has no history or evidence of hypertension, the EMS personnel may administer 0.2 mg of intramuscular methergine. Rapid transport is essential.

2. The EMS provider can expect atony in any birth involving an overstretched or overworked uterus, as with a long, difficult labor; a rapid, intense labor; multiple gestation; polyhydramnios; fetal macrosomia; or grand multiparity. A placenta may fragment if the woman has surgical scars on her uterus that interfere with placental implantation or has an unhealthy placenta secondary to malnutrition, hypertension, tobacco use, or other factors. However, hemorrhage can strike without warning after a very normal, easy delivery, as in this case study.

3. The most common etiologies are uterine atony, a uterus filled with blood clots, or retained placental fragments. Uterine atony is the failure of the uterus to contract following delivery of the placenta. A flaccid uterus may fill with blood that then clots, blocking the uterus's ability to contract. Sometimes fundal massage can dislodge these clots. Retained placental fragments occur when the placenta delivers incompletely, leaving pieces or perhaps a succenturiate lobe inside the uterus. The uterus is unable to contract and bleeding ensues.

4. Postpartum hemorrhage may occur anytime during the first 2 months after delivery, but is most likely immediately after delivery or within the first few days postpartum.

Chapter 9

Exact estimation of gestational age is beyond the scope of practice for the prehospital provider, but knowing physical features of maturity can help the EMS professional to rapidly assess and manage the newborn infant.

1. All the physical features of this infant point to prematurity. In addition, her lungs may be less developed than those of other babies of her gestational age because of her mother's diabetes.

2. This baby is premature. Preterm and small for gestational age (SGA) babies have smaller muscle mass, less brown fat, and less insulating fat, all of which contribute to less heat production and more heat loss. Premature and SGA infants may have smaller glycogen stores and may be especially vulnerable to hypoglycemia. Infants born to diabetic mothers are susceptible to hypoglycemia. Premature babies are also at greater risk for respiratory difficulty.

3. No more so than with any other infant. If Susan accurately reported her medical history, she had normal blood-sugar readings between her pregnancies. Diabetes causes birth defects only when the blood sugar is elevated during the first trimester. Gestational diabetes typically arises during the second half of pregnancy.

4. Yes, the vital signs for this infant are in the normal range.

Chapter 10

Effective resuscitation can make the difference between life and death for the compromised neonate.

1. Apgars at 1 minute would include 0 point for appearance or color, 1 point for pulse, 1 point for grimace, 0 for activity, and 0 for respirations, for a total Apgar of 2. By 5 minutes he was crying vigorously (which earned him 2 points each for respiration and grimace), was moving actively (2 points), and had a pulse of 120 (2 points). He still showed central cyanosis and scored 0 points for color. His 5-minute score was 8.

2. If meconium-stained fluid is noted, when the head emerges the birth attendant must suction the infant's mouth, oropharynx, hypopharynx, and nares. The body is then delivered. If the newborn is vigorous, defined as having a heart rate over 100, spontaneous crying or breathing, and flexed or flailing extremities, then care proceeds routinely unless the baby subsequently declines. If the infant is not vigorous, the EMS professional cuts the cord and moves the baby with minimal stimulation to a surface where resuscitation can be readily performed.

   The provider intubates the infant and performs suctioning through the endotracheal tube itself, using a meconium suction adapter, by occluding the suction control port on the aspirator and gradually withdrawing the tube. If suctioning yields meconium and the heart rate is not significantly bradycardic, the provider reintubates and repeats until little or no meconium is extracted or the heart rate begins to drop. Then the infant is ventilated and stimulated as usual.

3. The fetus who has suffered a shoulder dystocia may also suffer brachial plexus palsies or fractures of the clavicle or humerus. Observe the baby to assess whether he is moving his limbs and whether there is bruising or any other evidence of trauma. Document your findings carefully.

Chapter 11

1. Debbie should ask questions about Kaitlyn's physical condition, such as where she hurts and whether she lost consciousness. Debbie should avoid asking questions that may put Kaitlyn on the defensive, such as "Why didn't you lock your door?" and "Didn't you try to fight him off?" Debbie should remain supportive and objective, providing comfort without interjecting her personal feelings. She should not ask Kaitlyn for the details of the attack or what acts were committed.

2. Debbie's priority is to identify and treat all major and life-threatening injuries while disturbing evidence of the assault as little as possible and protecting Kaitlyn's privacy. If it became necessary for Debbie to remove clothing, she should carefully bag and label each item separately with minimal handling. If she needed to cut clothing from her patient, she should avoid cutting through rips or tears. Debbie should explain every procedure and ask Kaitlyn's permission before touching her, giving her as much control as possible over her treatment. She will need to examine Kaitlyn's genitals to evaluate her bleeding, but should carefully drape the patient with a sheet and shield her from onlookers. Debbie would then give the sheet to the hospital personnel as evidence.

3. Once Kaitlyn emerged from the cupboard, Louis and Debbie strove to keep on-scene time to a minimum. They did not allow Kaitlyn to walk to the stretcher and did not allow her to exert herself—for example, by walking or standing unassisted to transfer to the stretcher. Kaitlyn begged them to let her shower and brush her teeth, but Debbie emphasized that she should not wash, urinate, defecate, douche, clean her fingernails, change clothing, or even brush her teeth or hair until she had been thoroughly examined at the hospital, and it was essential to preserve all evidence of the attack until the hospital could systematically collect and document it.

4. Debbie must remember that her run form is a legal document that may provide essential evidence regarding the assault months or years later. Her report should be a thorough record of all findings, injuries, and treatments; the patient's complaints (this can be effectively charted as quotations); and objective observations. She should also include the name of the hospital staff member who received her report upon transfer of care.

   As Debbie had suspected, Kaitlyn had been sexually assaulted and beaten by a male attacker. The trauma haunted Kaitlyn for years to come; but with counseling and the support of her family, she was able to function again. Her attacker was caught, convicted, and sentenced to a prison term.

Chapter 12

1. Maternal varicella-zoster infection during the first half of pregnancy can cause serious injury to the developing child, including skin scarring, muscle atrophy, limb deformities, eye and brain damage, and mental retardation. Emily had had chicken pox when she was in kindergarten, however, and so probably has immunity to varicella. Emily should have her varicella-zoster titer drawn to make sure that she is still immune. If she had not had chicken pox previously and contracted the disease during early pregnancy, there would be a 25% risk her fetus would be infected and a 1–2% rate of congenital anomalies resulting from the exposure. Nonimmune women may take zoster immune globulin (ZIG) within 4 days of exposure to help prevent infection.

2. American Medical Association recommendations permit a pregnant EMS provider to perform repetitive lifting of up to 50 lb until the 24th week of pregnancy if the woman has been accustomed to this workload for at least 1 year before pregnancy and observes proper body mechanics. After 24 weeks of gestation, her limit is 25 lb.

3. Being in the room when one X ray is taken has not been shown to cause harm to the fetus, but Emily should avoid exposure to X rays for the duration of the pregnancy.

4. Emily needs to be treated the same as any other pregnant trauma victim. Her midwife sent her to labor and delivery for comprehensive evaluation. Emily must remain on a fetal monitor for a minimum of 4 hours, longer if she develops contractions, vaginal bleeding, or a nonreassuring fetal heart rate. Her midwife ordered a sonogram for fetal well-being and to assess for possible placental abruption. She ordered a Kleihauer-Betke test to look for the presence of fetal cells in the maternal circulation that could indicate abruption. If Emily were Rh-negative, she might have required RhoGam if fetal blood had entered her circulation. After all tests proved negative, Emily was reminded that abruption can occur as many as 5 days following the original trauma and can follow even relatively minor insults. She was told to call if she experienced contractions, bleeding, decreased fetal movement, pain, or leaking.

Answers to
Review Questions

Chapter 1

1. Ovulation. Release of an ovum is often accompanied by pain known as *mittelschmerz*, and heavy clear mucus discharge. Ovulation usually occurs midcycle, typically around day 14.

2. At birth
   - Fluid is squeezed out of the respiratory tract as the baby moves though the vagina.
   - Lungs fill with air at first breath; remaining lung fluid is absorbed.
   - Blood oxygen levels increase, causing vasodilation in the lungs.
   - Systemic blood pressure increases with cord clamping.
   - Blood flow to the newborn's lungs increases.
   - Blood moves into the pulmonary vessels instead of the ductus arteriosus, which begins to constrict.
   - The foramen ovale closes, and circulation begins to follow the usual route.

3. An overview of the first phase of the menstrual cycle, onset through ovulation:
   - Hypothalamus sends gonadotropin-releasing hormone (GNRH) to anterior pituitary and prompts it to release follicle-stimulating hormone (FSH) and luteinizing hormone (LH).
   - Ovary responds to FSH by producing about 18–20 follicles.
   - Follicles secrete increasing levels of estrogen, estrogen stimulates endometrium to thicken.
   - Rising estrogen levels tell the pituitary that FSH is no longer needed.
   - Follicles develop rapidly, and then one follicle becomes dominant. Dominant follicle produces more estrogen than the others and develops more FSH receptors to capture most of the available FSH.
   - Unable to secure adequate quantities of FSH, competing follicles degenerate.
   - Once estrogen levels high for 2–3 days, pituitary sends surge of LH and FSH.
   - 24–36 hours after the LH surge, ovulation occurs; ovum is drawn into fallopian tube.

4. Laurel's murmur is a normal part of pregnancy. In pregnancy, maternal blood volume increases 40–45%. Ninety percent of pregnant women have a systolic murmur, attributable to the increased intravascular volume. In pregnancy, cardiac

output increases 30–50% over nonpregnant levels as a result of lower systemic vascular resistance and higher heart rate. The paramedic may also notice a loud, exaggerated splitting of the first heart sound and a third heart sound.

5. The placenta is the life-support system that allows the fetus to obtain nutrients, oxygen, and other substances from the maternal bloodstream and allows the fetus to eliminate waste products. It is an important endocrine gland that manufactures hormones crucial to the pregnancy. It transfers maternal antibodies to the fetus to protect him from disease at birth. It synthesizes glycogen, cholesterol, and fatty acids.

Chapter 2

1. Probable signs of pregnancy and alternative explanations are as follows:
   - Positive pregnancy test—home pregnancy tests are very accurate, but false positive results do occur on occasion.
   - Braxton Hicks contractions—painless uterine contractions can be palpated during the third trimester. Abdominal muscle tightening can mimic a uterine contraction.
   - Abdominal enlargement—Tumors, ascites, and obesity can also cause abdominal enlargement. Abdominal enlargement of pregnancy can be hidden by obesity or strong muscle tone.
   - Palpation of fetus—sometime after the 20th week (but often not until 30 weeks or later), the examiner can palpate the fetal outline. Because uterine fibroid tumors or large ovarian masses can feel very similar to a fetus, this is considered only a probable sign.

2. Most complaints and pains, obstetric or not, can be evaluated using the OLD-CART mnemonic:
   - Onset—When did this begin? What were you doing? Was the onset gradual or rapid? In what order did the symptoms occur?
   - Location—Where does it hurt? Did the pain start there or has it moved? Is it localized or does it radiate?
   - Duration—How long have you had the symptoms? Do they come and go? Have you experienced them before?
   - Characteristics—Quality and quantity of the pain—sharp? Dull? Frequency? On a scale of 1–10, with 10 being the worst pain you ever had, what number would you give this pain?
   - Associated symptoms—What other symptoms are you experiencing?
   - Relieving/aggravating factors—What makes your symptoms better? What makes them worse?
   - Treatment—Have you treated the symptoms (with medications, herbs, remedies, hot soaks, etc.)? Did the treatment help or make things worse?

3. If a pregnant woman beyond about 20 weeks lies supine, the vena cava may become compressed between the spine and the gravid uterus, reducing cardiac

return and consequently cardiac output by up to 30%. The woman may experience supine hypotension syndrome, evidenced by pallor, anxiety, hypotension, tachycardia, fetal distress, or syncope. Supine positioning can also cause respiratory compromise by limiting lung expansion and diaphragm excursion.

4. If fetal heart rate is low, transport rapidly with mother in lateral recumbant position or on hands and knees or knee chest (whichever best improves fetal heart rate), with high-flow oxygen in place and an intravenous line of lactated Ringer's running briskly. Have advanced life support available for neonatal resuscitation if delivery is likely to occur en route.

5. If the mother has regular menses and is sure of her dates, subtract 3 months from the first day of her last period, then add 1 week and 1 year (Naegele's Rule). A gestational wheel (two paper discs that align to calculate the relationships among LMP, due date, and gestational age) can be helpful in calculating a due date. If the woman has early prenatal care, her due date may been determined very accurately by first trimester ultrasound scanning. Due date can be approximated by abdominal examination as well. Measuring from pubic bone to fundus, the number of centimeters measured should roughly equal the weeks of gestation after about 22–24 weeks. The fundal height may also be measured in relation to the pubic bone, umbilicus, and xyphoid.

Chapter 3

1. In placental abruption, shock may be disproportionate to visible blood loss. Abruption may be accompanied by DIC.

   Signs and symptoms of abruption include
   - Vaginal bleeding that is scant or profuse, dark or bright red
   - Boardlike, rigid abdomen
   - Change in uterine size and shape
   - Decreased fetal movement
   - Sharp, tearing pain—abruption may be excruciating, uncomfortable, or painless
   - Uterine contractions
   - Fetal bradycardia or tachycardia

Placenta previa involves painless bleeding that may be scanty or profuse. Typically, the first bleeding episode is slight, and each subsequent hemorrhage is more copious. A woman who has had regular prenatal care and a second or third trimester ultrasound has usually been told if her placenta is partial or complete previa.

2. Field management of first trimester bleeding:
   - Obtain complete history.
   - Monitor vital signs carefully; take orthostatic signs if bleeding is heavy.
   - Watch for signs of shock.

- If blood loss is significant, transport lateral recumbent or in shock position on high-flow oxygen, with at least one large-bore IV. Manage airway as needed. Consider cardiac monitoring.
- Draw blood if protocols permit.
- Count pads to measure bleeding.
- Save all material passed.
- Consider getting fetal heart tones with a Doppler if patient is beyond 12–14 weeks, but realize that failure to find them will upset the woman.
- Provide emotional support.

3. The hypertension of preeclampsia can result in cardiac failure, brain hemorrhage, placental abruption, or pulmonary edema. Liver and kidney damage may occur. Clotting processes may be altered and DIC can develop. Central-nervous-system involvement can cause convulsions, coma, altered mental status, and cortical blindness. The woman with PIH may experience significant third-spacing as fluid moves from her intravascular space to the interstitial space, causing edema and intravascular depletion. Fetal distress and growth restriction are common complications of preeclampsia.

4. Nonobstetric causes of abdominal or pelvic pain that may be experienced by the pregnant patient
   - Pelvic inflammatory disease (infection of the upper genital tract)
   - Chorioamnionitis
   - Hydronephrosis
   - Renal calculi
   - Urinary tract infection
   - Appendicitis
   - Ligament pain
   - Cholecystitis/cholelithiasis
   - Intestinal gas or diarrhea cramps
   - Uterine fibroids
   - Adhesions from uterine or abdominal surgery
   - Pancreatitis
   - Peptic ulcers
   - Gastric reflux
   - Ruptured or twisted ovarian cysts
   - Gas or diarrhea cramps
   - Fibroid tumors causing bleeding and pain
   - Adhesions from prior surgeries causing pain as uterus grows

5. A woman with the symptoms of ectopic pregnancy should be treated as such unless proven otherwise, but these conditions can present similarly:
   - Spontaneous abortion
   - Ruptured ovarian cyst

- Appendicitis
- Salpingitis
- Torsion (twisting) of the ovary
- Round ligament pain
- Uterine fibroid
- Kidney stone
- Abscess
- Urinary tract infection

Chapter 4

1. The three most common mechanisms of trauma in pregnant women are
   - Motor vehicle accidents
   - Domestic violence
   - Falls
2. The flared ribs, raised diaphragm, increased body fat, and breast enlargement of pregnancy interferes with proper hand placement for compressions. A pregnant woman is more likely to vomit.

   Third-trimester CPR may result in cardiac output that is 10% of normal due to pressure of the uterus and fetus on the vena cava and aorta. (In patients greater than 20 weeks' gestation, one rescuer should manually displace the uterus during CPR.) The pregnant woman and her fetus have poor oxygen reserves. In a hospital setting, if the pregnant woman cannot be resuscitated within 4 minutes, immediate perimortem cesarean delivery is usually performed, not only to save the fetus, but also to improve chances of maternal survival.
3. Risk factors include
   - Pregnant or postpartum patient
   - Varicose veins in the legs
   - Obesity
   - Hereditary tendency to clot excessively
   - Recent surgery
   - Injury to the leg
   - History of DVT
   - Smoking
   - Bedrest and prolonged periods of inactivity
4. Asthma is stable in about half of pregnancies, worsens in about one-quarter, improves in about one-quarter. Patients are usually managed on the same medications used before pregnancy—bronchodilators and steroids.

   Follow usual protocols for asthma with the pregnant patient:
   - Oxygen—high-flow for moderate or severe distress, low-flow for mild distress.
   - Intravenous line of D_5W or normal saline, cardiac monitoring.

- Albuterol (Proventil), metaproterenol (Alupent), and isoetharine (Bronkosol), administered in normal saline via nebulized inhaler, are all category B and considered safe for pregnant women.
- Terbutaline (Brethine)—effective, but slower acting.

5. Signs and symptoms of preterm labor may be vague:
   - Contractions
   - Generalized crampiness
   - Back pain
   - Half of all women in preterm labor feel no pain
   - Diarrhea
   - Change in vaginal discharge
   - Vaginal bleeding
   - Gush of fluid may indicate rupture of membranes
     Differential diagnoses that can both cause and mimic PTL:
   - Urinary tract infection
   - Appendicitis
   - Cholecystitis
   - Gastroenteritis
   - Hydronephrosis
   - Renal calculi
   - Musculoskeletal pain
   - Vaginal infection

Chapter 5

1. Signs of Impending Labor
   - Fetus descends into the pelvis, causing increased pelvic pressure and change in maternal abdominal contours.
   - Cervix shortens (effaces), dilates, and softens.
   - Labor starts with ROM in 12% of births.
   - Mucus plug may be lost during labor or up to several weeks before.
   - Blood-tinged mucus is often passed as the cervix dilates before or during labor.
   - Woman may experience runs of contractions which may or may not be painful.

2. **Passage**—The birth passage includes the bony pelvis and the overlying soft tissues. Does this baby fit though this pelvis?

   Passenger—The passenger is the fetus, who may slow labor or may thwart vaginal delivery if he grows too large or adopts an unfavorable position.

Powers—The powers of birth are uterine contractions and also maternal pushing effort. Strong, long, frequent, well-coordinated contractions hasten delivery. Maternal position influences the powers of labor.

Psyche—The psyche is the mother's psychological state at the time of labor. Tension and fear can inhibit normal labor progress, and fear of pushing can delay delivery for hours.

3. Factors that would influence your decision to stay and deliver on scene or initiate transport include

- How far are you from the hospital?
- Is she obviously in advanced labor or starting to crown? The time span between crowning and delivery is usually short, especially with a multiparous patient.
- Does she have an urge to push or rectal pressure? Is she involuntarily pushing? Delivery may be imminent.
- Does the woman tell you "the baby's coming"?
- Are her membranes ruptured? If so, when did they rupture? Often when membranes rupture spontaneously in a multiparous patient in advanced labor, the baby rapidly follows.
- Consider the expected length of labor—is this her first labor, or has she had other babies? If she has, how long were her other labors?
- Has she had a recent vaginal exam with her provider? If her cervix was 4 cm and thin and the fetus was at 0 station in the office yesterday, she is more likely to have a fast labor than someone who was long, thick and closed with a baby high in the pelvis—especially if this is not her first baby.
- Does she have any known complications, such as a breech presentation, preterm labor, multiple gestation; severe preeclampsia, chorioamnionitis, or suspected abruption? High-risk pregnancies benefit greatly from a hospital delivery, and rapid transport with the woman panting or blowing to avoid pushing may be the best course in some circumstances. If you must deliver a high-risk pregnancy in the field, call for ALS backup—extra hands and ALS capability may improve chances of a good outcome for mother and infant.

4. The prehospital provider may consider using the following comfort measures for pain relief in the laboring patient:

- Provide emotional and social support by listening, caring, attending to her needs, and involving the people important to her.
- If possible, allow her to choose a position of comfort.
- If the patient is experiencing back pain, position her on hands and knees or side and massage sacrum firmly.
- Apply hot or cold packs to back or lower abdomen.
- If she feels hot, place a damp washcloth on her forehead or fan her with a glove packet or similar object.
- Coach her in controlled breathing and relaxation.

- Employ distraction techniques.
- Ensure that she stays clean and dry.

5. The contractions of false labor
   - Often occur an irregular pattern but may mimic labor
   - Do not grow progressively longer; stronger and closer together
   - May disappear with change in activity or fluid bolus

   In addition
   - Bloody show is not usually present.
   - On palpation, uterus will feel as hard as the tip of the nose.
   - Woman is usually still sociable and able to walk or talk though contractions
   - Woman does not usually show associated signs of advanced labor, such as flushing, sweating, vomiting or tremors.
   - False labor can be very painful, but does not progressively dilate the cervix.

   The contractions of true, active labor
   - Grow longer, stronger, and more frequent with time.
   - Usually start in the lower back, curl around her hips, and knot above the pubic bone
   - May be accompanied by nausea and vomiting, sweating, flushed cheeks, trembling, increasing pelvic pressure.
   - Increase to every 2–3 minutes and last up to 90 seconds, sometimes peaking twice before returning to baseline.

   Further
   - Fundus palpates firm with contraction.
   - Bloody show may be present.
   - Woman develops internal focus and is usually unable to walk or talk though contractions of advanced labor.
   - Rarely, true labor can be virtually painless and subtle until delivery is imminent, especially if preterm.

Chapter 6

1. Forward-leaning positions (hands and knees, side-lying) and asymmetrical positions (one leg elevated) tend to reduce back pain and encourage fetal rotation. Upright birth positions (sitting, squatting, birth stools) shorten the second stage and improve fetal heart rate patterns over dorsal positions. Upright positions also result in less discomfort, easier pushing, and a more normal delivery; but studies suggest that they cause almost as much perineal trauma as dorsal positions.

Supine (Dorsal, lithotomy)

- Can reduce cardiac output to its lowest, and blood pressure can decrease (or increase in the case of PIH)
- Fetal hypoxia may develop more rapidly
- Limits pelvic expansion
- Can lengthen the second stage of labor and increase the likelihood of perineal lacerations
- Convenient for the provider to visualize perineum and control delivery

Squatting

- Physiologically beneficial—allows pelvis to expand and gravity augments maternal pushing
- Many women find squatting posture difficult to maintain
- Contraindicated for women with severe varicosities of the legs
- Perineal swelling and laceration may be increased
- Generally impractical for prehospital provider and awkward for the inexperienced birth attendant

Semi-Fowler's Position

- Works very well in the field
- Uses gravity and abdominal muscles to advantage
- Improves cardiac output
- Convenient for birth attendant

Lateral Recumbent

- Excellent position for field deliveries
- Maximizes cardiac output
- Normalizes blood pressure of hypertensive patients
- May improve condition of distressed fetus and reduce stress on preterm infants
- May slow precipitous deliveries
- Minimizes tearing of the perineum
- Convenient for birth attendant

Hands and Knees

- Difficult for inexperienced birth attendant
- Useful for woman with back pain
- Can improve fetal distress
- Helpful in case of shoulder dystocia

2. • Tell the mother not to push.
  - If cord is around the neck, gently grasp cord in hooking motion and slip it over the head.

- If unsuccessful, loosen cord and slip over shoulders.
- If still unsuccessful, you may clamp the cord in two places, cut between the clamps carefully with scissors, then unwind cord from the neck. Alternatively, consider somersault maneuver—flex the baby's head toward the mother's thigh and hold it there while the body slips out, then unwind the cord from neck.
- Babies with tight nuchal cords are often born hypovolemic, pale, and stunned. Keep cord intact while starting resuscitation if possible, but never delay resuscitation.

3. To reduce the chance of a perineal laceration
   - As the head distends the perineum, discourage forceful pushing and allow the baby to emerge gradually.
   - Control the emergence of the head by keeping counter pressure on the skull bones as the head emerges.
   - Encourage the woman to relax her bottom and tolerate the stretching rather than tensing against the pain.
   - Side-lying positioning decreases the likelihood of tearing by allowing baby to emerge slowly and gently.
   - If the fetus is in distress, the emphasis shifts to getting the baby out quickly rather than preventing lacerations—a bad laceration is preferable to a depressed infant.

4. Contractions begin 3–5 minutes after delivery of the infant, and normally the placenta will be expelled within 5–20 minutes.

   Signs of placental detachment:
   - A sudden trickle or small gush of blood. Often there is little or no bleeding before the placenta separates.
   - The umbilical cord protruding from the vagina lengthens.
   - The uterus, as felt though the abdominal wall, contracts into a globular grapefruit-like mass and rises in the abdomen.

5. - It is not truly necessary to cut cord before transport.
   - Cord pulsations stop first near the mother's vulva.
   - Place two clamps on the cord about 2 inches apart, 6 inches from the infant's abdomen.
   - Apply clamp nearest baby, squeeze cord flat, and strip an inch or two of cord before applying the second clamp. This prevents blood from spurting.
   - Do not milk or strip the entire length.
   - Cut between the two clamps with sterile scissors or a scalpel.
   - Cord clamps can be improvised from gauze bandage, new shoestrings, etc.
   - Monitor the infant's cord stump and reclamp immediately if the clamp loosens.

Chapter 7

1. • Anticipate. If your laboring patient has risk factors for postpartum hemorrhage, establish intravenous access.

   • Act quickly.

   • Grasp the uterus through the abdominal wall with your two hands and knead firmly. If the uterus feels soft and doughy, massage it vigorously until it firms.

   If bleeding does not slow immediately

   • While you rub her uterus, have a crew member establish at least one large-bore intravenous line and rapidly infuse lactated Ringer's or normal saline.

   • If local protocols allow, administer either 10 units of pitocin IM or 10–20 units diluted in 1,000 cc of lactated Ringer's, run wide.

   • If the uterus does not respond, follow with 0.2 mg of IM methergine. (**Note:** methergine is contraindicated in patients with preeclampsia or high blood pressure.)

   • Treat for shock

   • Administer high-flow oxygen and consider cardiac monitoring.

   • Monitor vital signs closely.

2. • Premature delivery

   • Grand multiparity

   • Polyhydramnios

   • Oligohydramnios

   • Certain fetal anomalies

   • Uterine abnormalities

   • Fibroid tumors

   • Multiple gestation

   • Previous breech

3. To deliver a frank breech in the field

   • Avoid handling the infant as it delivers. "Helping" the baby can cause trauma.

   • Remember that the frank breech usually delivers with one hip toward the pubic bone and the other toward the mother's sacrum. First the anterior hip delivers, then posterior hip with lateral flexion.

   • Let the body emerge to the umbilicus.

   • Encourage mother to push hard with contractions.

   • The back should then face up; gently guide the back to the anterior if it doesn't spontaneously rotate.

   • You may gently pull down slack in the cord when the umbilicus is seen.

   • The feet should spring free as the body descends.

   • Wrap the emerging infant in a warm towel or blanket.

   • Do not attempt to pull the baby out.

- To deliver the head, lift the fetal body slightly.
- Anticipate possible need for neonatal resuscitation with any breech delivery.

  If head does not deliver
- Rapid transport is critical.
- Insert hand into vagina and make an airway for the baby.
- Supply blowby oxygen to the baby
- If umbilical cord is pulsing, keep it warm and moist and avoid handling it.
- Keep the fetal body wrapped in dry, warm towels.
- Establish intravenous access in the mother.
- Put the mother on high-flow oxygen.
- Have the mother continue to push hard with contractions while you lift the fetal body parallel to the floor and have an assistant apply suprapubic pressure

4. Managing a cord prolapse in the field:
   - Immediately place the mother in knee-chest position or lay her on her back with hips elevated.
   - Don sterile gloves and insert entire hand, if possible, into the woman's vagina.
   - Push the fetal presenting part up and off cord.
   - Hold the fetus back and prevent compression of the cord.
   - Keep hand in place until baby is delivered by cesarean section.
   - Do not compress the cord to check the pulse.
   - If segment of cord protrudes outside the vagina, keep it moist and warm.
   - Transport immediately.
   - Initiate high-flow oxygen.
   - Establish intravenous access.
   - If possible, do all the above en route.
5. In the shoulder or transverse presentation, the fetus lies obliquely across the uterus.
   - Rapid transport to the hospital is essential.
   - Arm may hang out of the cervix.
   - Cord may prolapse.
   - Put mother in knee-chest position.
   - Start high-flow oxygen.
   - Administer IV crystalloid solution.
   - Transport to facility with capacity for immediate cesearean section.

Chapter 8

1. If fundus is palpated in the right upper quadrant, the woman probably has a full bladder displacing the uterus and preventing adequate uterine contraction. The

woman may be unaware of her need to urinate. Have her void and then reassess. If fundus is midline, below the umbilicus and firm after voiding, and her bleeding has stopped, she may not need transport.

2. Endometritis, or infection of the uterine lining, is most likely to develop during the first 10 days after delivery. Prehospital care of the postpartum patient with endometritis includes

- Intravenous line of lactated Ringer's or normal saline run at a rate consistent with vital signs
- Oxygen by nasal cannula
- Monitoring blood loss and saving any material passed.

Sepsis and shock are uncommon, but if the patient becomes unstable, cardiac monitoring is in order.

3. Postpartum bloody discharge is called lochia. Normal lochia may include small clots and should smell similar to a normal menstrual flow.

Lochia rubra begins shortly after delivery, and consists of a dark-red flow like a heavy menstrual period.

Lochia serosa begins by the second or third day postpartum and continues until about day 10, consisting of lighter, pinkish, serous flow.

Lochia alba, a whitish or brownish discharge, continues for the next week or two.

4. Thrombophlebitis may occur in a superficial or deep vessel. Superficial thrombophlebitis presents with swelling, local heat, redness, pain, and swelling. Deep-vein thrombosis may present with swelling of the distal extremity, purple hue or redness to the affected leg, fever, and pain. Thromboses can also form in the iliac arteries.

Homan's sign may or may not be positive.

5. Postpartum psychiatric illness is indistinguishable from major depression that occurs at other times. The condition typically develops gradually over the first 3 postpartum months, although symptoms can occur with unexpected suddenness anytime during first year. Signs and symptoms include

- Persistent and intense sadness
- Anxiety and despair
- Tearfulness
- Inability to enjoy pleasurable activities
- Insomnia
- Fatigue
- Appetite disturbance
- Suicidal thoughts
- Recurrent thoughts of death
- Obsessive worry about baby
- Negative feelings toward infant or lack of attachment
- Trouble coping with daily tasks

Chapter 9

1. Signs and symptoms of hypoglycemia in the neonate include jitteriness, lethargy, hypotonicity, weak or high-pitched cry, poor feeding, respiratory distress, apnea, and seizures.

2. • Heart rate: 120–160 beats per minute
   • Respiration: 30–60 respirations per minute
   • Axillary temperature: 36.4–37.2° C (97.5–99° F)
   • Rectal temperature: 36.6–37.2° C (97.8–99° F)
   • Blood pressure at birth: 80–60 mm Hg systolic over 45–40 mm Hg diastolic

3. • The body produces norepinephrine when stressed by cold.
   • Norepinepheine stimulates metabolism of brown fat.
   • Metabolic rate and oxygen consumption increase.
   • If unable to meet the demand for additional oxygen, the baby may become hypoxic.
   • Norepinephrine also causes pulmonary vasoconstriction, which leads to hypoxemia and pulmonary hypertension.
   • When the baby is hypoxic, glucose is broken down by an alternative hypoxic pathway (anaerobic glycolysis), which forms lactic acid.
   • The baby develops metabolic acidosis.
   • Anaerobic metabolism metabolizes more glycogen, eventually causing hypoglycemia.
   • If the baby is not feeding well, there is no caloric intake to offset this energy depletion.

4. Seizures in a neonate seldom present as tonic-clonic activity, but may include sucking or grimacing, abnormal rhythmic movements; alterations in tone, swimming, or bicycling movements; abnormal facial, tongue, or eye movements; and alterations in breathing pattern. Some neonatal seizures occur with few or no observable signs.

   Jitteriness occurs with no associated ocular movement and may be triggered by stimulation. Tremors can usually be stopped by flexion of the affected extremities.

   Jitteriness may indicate an abnormality if it persists longer than 4 days or if episodes are prolonged or very easily elicited. Jitteriness can also indicate hypoglycemia

5. It is normal for a breastfed baby to have as many as 6–10 moist, semiliquid, yellow, often large stools every day. Formula-fed babies may have only one or two (but as many as 5) semisolid stools per day. Infants with diarrhea have very frequent stools, usually watery, green, and full of mucus (or specks of blood). Diarrhea is usually foul-smelling. Diarrhea be accompanied by fever and irritability. Excessive fluid loss may lead to dehydration, which is evidenced by decreased urination, dry mouth, lethargy, sunken eyes and fontanelles, or shock.

Chapter 10

1. • Prematurity or postmaturity
   • Prolonged rupture of membranes
   • Lack of prenatal care
   • Fetal distress during labor
   • Malpresentations
   • Multiple gestation
   • Substance abuse
   • Fetal heart-rate abnormalities
   • Meconium in the amniotic fluid
   • Maternal problems such as diabetes and preeclampsia
   • Tight nuchal cord at delivery or shoulder dystocia
   • Birth injury
   • Congenital anomalies may also be at greater risk
      About 40% of babies that require resuscitation have no risk factors.

2. Sometimes the fetus moves his bowels into the amniotic fluid, then gasps and aspirates it into his lungs. Meconium aspiration syndrome (MAS) may result, causing severe respiratory distress. About 20% of infants with moderate to thick meconium-stained amniotic fluid will develop MAS. In MAS, meconium creates a partial airway obstruction that allows air to flow into the lungs on in-spiration but blocks exhalation, causing hyperinflation of the lungs distal to the blockage. Babies with MAS are often hypoxic and depressed at birth, showing floppy "rag doll" tone, retractions, grunting, tachypnea or apnea, cyanosis or pallor, and nasal flaring similar to that seen in infants with respiratory distress syndrome.

3. Omphalocele is the herniation of the intestines and sometimes other abdominal organs into the umbilical cord. It is frequently associated with other malforma-tions and lethal chromosomal anomalies.

   With gastroschisis, the abdominal wall is incompletely formed and the in-testines protrude through the defect, without a protective membrane surround-ing them. The incidence of associated malformations is low, and the prognosis is generally good after surgery.

   EMS management includes

   • Thermoregulation
   • Protecting the defect from trauma, infection, and fluid loss with a moist dressing

      Consider intravenous fluids to counteract fluid loss. If possible, reduce the infant's crying. Do not allow him to feed. If possible, transport to a tertiary-care facility with a neonatal intensive-care unit.

4. Cerebral palsy is a nonprogressive disorder that involves damage to parts of the brain that control movement and posture. This condition may be accompanied

by other abnormalities of brain function, such as mental retardation, learning disabilities, seizures, and sensory impairment. Most cases result from

- Antepartal insults, such as infections
- Premature birth
- Severe hyperbilirubinemia
- Rh disease or blood-clotting disorders
- Genetic diseases
- Brain injuries in early childhood

Fewer than 10% of cases result from intrapartum hypoxia or anoxia. Often the cause is unknown.

5. Gestational dating is not always accurate, even if the woman has had prenatal care, and the infant may prove more or less mature than expected. Most premature babies under 35–36 weeks will need resuscitation or specialized supportive care after birth, so advanced life support should be available at delivery. Ideally the baby should be directly transported to a hospital with a neonatal intensive-care unit. Preterm birth may be rapid and unexpected, and the fetus is often delivered in a non-vertex presentation. Premature babies are extremely delicate and susceptible to birth trauma. The birth attendant can position the mother on her side to reduce pressure on the fetal head.

The premature infant may respond to noise or rough handling with apnea or bradycardia. Premature infants require warmth and can rapidly decompensate if chilled. They may have immature lungs and may require respiratory support. Delicate blood vessels in the brain may break during delivery and cause intracranial hemorrhage. Hypoxia, rapid changes in intravascular volume, and rough handling can also cause bleeding in the brain. Preterm infants are more likely to develop hypoglycemia soon after delivery.

Chapter 11

1. Always consider pregnancy even if the woman denies the possibility. Whenever a woman presents with bleeding after intercourse, consider abuse a possible cause. Hormonal contraceptives can cause irregular bleeding.

Other causes of vaginal bleeding include

- Uterine fibroids
- Injury or disease of the vagina (caused by intercourse, trauma, infection, warts, ruptured polyp, or varicosity)
- Vaginal injury from insertion of foreign objects
- Malignancy
- Atrophic vaginitis (damage to thin, dry vaginal walls caused by a lack of estrogen after menopause)
- Hormonal imbalance
- Thyroid disorder

- Recent procedures on cervix, such as cone biopsy
- Ovarian cysts or polycystic ovarian syndrome
- Blood-clotting disorders
- Medication or herbal use
- Chronic liver disease
- Intrauterine devices
- Sexually transmitted infections
- Weight gain
- Stress
- Irregular menses

2. Signs and symptoms of TSS include
   - Acute onset of vomiting
   - Fever above 102°F (38.8°C)
   - Syncope
   - Diarrhea
   - Headache
   - Sore throat
   - Muscle aches
   - Signs of soft-tissue infection, such as swelling and erythema that can progress to necrotizing fasciitis
   - Sunburn-like rash
   - Bloodshot eyes
   - Desquamation of skin
   - Petechiae
   - Liver or kidney failure
   - DIC; adult respiratory distress syndrome; dysrhythmia; or persistent, prolonged hypovolemic or septic shock

3. Vaginal bleeding in a postmenopausal woman can indicate
   - Uterine or cervical cancer
   - Cervical polyps
   - Prolapse of the cervix or bladder
   - Atrophic vaginitis
   - Trauma

   Some women continue to take hormone replacement therapy for many years after menopause, and may experience bleeding from hormone withdrawal.

4. - Avoid disturbing the crime scene.
   - Use caution touching the patient or irrigating wounds.
   - If you must remove clothing, bag and label each item with minimal handling.
   - If clothing must be cut, avoid cutting through rips or tears.

- Discourage the victim from washing, urinating, defecating, douching, cleaning her fingernails, brushing her teeth or hair, or changing her clothing.
- Cover her with a sheet if her skin is exposed, then give the sheet to the hospital personnel as evidence.

5. Abuse victims frequently block trauma from memory, often for many years or even decades. Post-traumatic stress disorder is common after sexual abuse. Some symptoms of sexual abuse seen in survivors include
- Self injury and cutting
- Suicidal tendencies
- Recurrent nightmares
- Sexual dysfunction
- Inability to trust others
- Resistance to intimacy
- Depression
- Anxiety
- Substance abuse
- Eating disorders
- Dissociation

Chapter 12

1. Accurate records are essential:
- For obtaining third-party reimbursement
- To guide care given by other providers
- For use in legal action when crimes are involved
- To aid memory if it ever becomes necessary to re-create events
- For establishing professional credibility

2. Symptoms of toxoplasmosis are vague and resemble flu or mononucleosis; they may include malaise, muscle aches, fever, sore throat, and enlarged lymph nodes in the neck. Maternal toxoplasmosis can cause the unborn baby to have seizures and motor or cognitive defects, microcephaly, hydrocephalus, or anencephaly.

3. The pregnant EMS worker who has had chicken pox as a child is probably immune; those who have never had the disease or been vaccinated are at risk. Maternal varicella infection during the first half of pregnancy can cause serious injury to the developing child, including skin scarring, muscle atrophy, limb deformities, eye and brain damage, and mental retardation. After 20 weeks of pregnancy there is little risk of damage to the fetus, although when maternal disease develops around the time of delivery, the infant may develop neonatal varicella-zoster virus.

4. A pregnant woman should always discuss employment demands with her doctor or midwife and follow his or her recommendations. For general purposes, AMA recommendations for activity restrictions include
   - Light clerical and managerial work—safe throughout pregnancy
   - Prolonged standing—no more than 40 hours per week in early pregnancy. After 24 weeks, no more than 4 hours of standing at a time
   - Intermittent standing for 30-minute intervals—safe until the 32nd week
   - Repetitive lifting of up to 50 pounds—acceptable until the 24th week of pregnancy if the woman has been lifting such weights for at least a year before pregnancy and continues to use proper techniques. In weeks 24–40, her limit is 25 pounds.
   - Climbing ladders and poles—acceptable until the 28th week of gestation, but no more than 4 times per shift between weeks 20 and 28
   - Stair climbing—limit this to 4 times per shift after 28 weeks
   - Stooping below knee level—up to 10 times per hour to week 28, then a maximum of 2 times per hour for the rest of the pregnancy
5. The pregnant woman at risk for infection may be vaccinated against hepatitis B, influenza, and tetanus (if previously vaccinated), but a better strategy would be to get her vaccinations up to date before conceiving. She may also safely receive the purified protein derivative (PPD) tuberculosis skin test during pregnancy.

References

Chapter 1

Amesse, L., & Pfaff-Amesse, T. (2003). *Surgical management of Müllerian duct anomalies.* Retrieved December 3, 2004, from www.emedicine.com/med/topic3521.htm

Bachmann, G. (2004). *Menopause.* Retrieved December 3, 2004, from www.emedicine.com/med/topic3289.htm

Beischer, N., Mackay, E., & Colditz, P. (1997). *Obstetrics and the newborn: An illustrated textbook* (3rd ed.). London and Philadelphia: W. B. Saunders.

Berek, J., Adashi, E., & Hillard, P. (Eds.). (1996). *Novak's gynecology* (12th ed.). Baltimore: Williams and Wilkins.

Blackburn, S., & Loper, D. (1992). *Maternal, fetal and neonatal physiology.* Philadelphia: W. B. Saunders.

Braner, D., Denson, S., & Ibsen, L. (Eds.). (2000). *Textbook of neonatal resuscitation.* Dallas, TX: American Heart Association.

Carr, B. R. (2003, December). The sociology and physiology of menstruation. In Extended-cycle contraception: A shift in paradigm [Special issue]. *The Female Patient.*

Copeland, L., & Jarrell, J. (2000). *Textbook of gynecology.* Philadelphia: W. B. Saunders.

Cunningham, F., Grant, N., Leveno, K., Gilstrap, L., Hauth, J., & Wenstrom, K. (2001). *Williams obstetrics* (21st ed.). New York: McGraw-Hill.

Frye, A. (1998). *Holistic midwifery: A comprehensive textbook for midwives in home-birth practice.* Portland, OR: Labrys Press.

Gabbe, S., Niebyl, J., & Simpson, J. (2002). *Obstetrics, normal and problem pregnancies.* New York: Churchill Livingstone.

Hatcher, R., Trussel, J., Stewart, F., Cates, W., Stewart, G., Guest, F., et al. (Eds.). (1998). *Contraceptive technology* (17th ed.). New York: Ardent Media.

Ladewig, P., London, M., Moberly, S., & Olds, S. (2002). *Contemporary maternal–newborn nursing care.* Upper Saddle River, NJ: Prentice Hall.

Minino, A. M., & Smith, B. L. (2001). Deaths: Preliminary data for 2000 [Electronic version]. *National vital statistics reports, 49*(12).

Moore, K., & Persaud, T. (1998). *Before we are born: Essentials of embryology and birth defects* (5th ed.). Philadelphia: W. B. Saunders.

Pearlman, M., Tintinalli, J., & Dyne, P. (2004). *Obstetric and gynecologic emergencies: Diagnosis and management.* New York: McGraw-Hill.

Speroff, L., Glass, R., & Kase, N. (1999). *Clinical gynecologic endocrinology and infertility.* Philadelphia: Lippincott Williams & Wilkins.

Varney, H. (2004). *Varney's midwifery* (4th ed.). Sudbury, MA: Jones & Bartlett.

Chapter 2

Cunningham, F., Grant, N., Leveno, K., Gilstrap, L., Hauth, J., & Wenstrom, K. (2001). *Williams obstetrics* (21st ed.). New York: McGraw-Hill.

Frye, A. (1998). *Holistic midwifery: A comprehensive textbook for midwives in home-birth practice.* Portland, OR: Labrys Press.

Gabbe, S., Niebyl, J., & Simpson, J. (2002). *Obstetrics, normal and problem pregnancies.* New York: Churchill Livingstone.

Hatcher, R., Trussel, J., Stewart, F., Cates, W., Stewart, G., Guest, F., et al. (Eds.). (1998). *Contraceptive technology* (17th ed.). New York: Ardent Media.

Ladewig, P., London, M., Moberly, S., & Olds, S. (2002). *Contemporary maternal–newborn nursing care.* Upper Saddle River, NJ: Prentice Hall.

Moskosky, S. (1995). *Women's health care nurse practitioner certification review guide.* Potomac, MD: Health Leadership Associates.

Varney, H. (2004). *Varney's midwifery* (4th ed.). Sudbury, MA: Jones & Bartlett.

Varney, H., Kriebs, J., & Gregor, C. (1998). *Varney's pocket midwife.* Sudbury, MA: Jones & Bartlett.

Chapter 3

American College of Obstetricians and Gynecologists. (1995, April). *Septic shock* (ACOG Technical Bulletin 204). Washington, DC: Author.

American College of Obstetricians and Gynecologists. (1996, January). *Hypertension in pregnancy* (ACOG Technical Bulletin 219). Washington, DC: Author.

Blackburn, S., & Loper, D. (1992). *Maternal, fetal and neonatal physiology.* Philadelphia: W. B. Saunders.

Bledsoe, B., Porter, R., & Cherry, R. (2001). *Paramedic care: Principles and practice, Medical emergencies* (Vol. 3). Upper Saddle River, NJ: Prentice Hall Health.

Cunningham, F., Grant, N., Leveno, K., Gilstrap, L., Hauth, J., & Wenstrom, K. (2001). *Williams obstetrics* (21st ed.). New York: McGraw-Hill.

Frye, A. (1998). *Holistic midwifery: A comprehensive textbook for midwives in home-birth practice.* Portland, OR: Labrys Press.

Gabbe, S., Niebyl, J., & Simpson, J. (2002). *Obstetrics, normal and problem pregnancies.* New York: Churchill Livingstone.

Herndon, J., Strauss, L. T., Whitehead, S., Parker, W. Y., Bartlett, L., & Zane, S. (2002, June 7). Abortion surveillance—United States, 1998. *Morbidity and Mortality Weekly Report, 51*(SS-3), 3–34.

Hunt, C. M., & Sharara, A. I. (1999). Liver disease in pregnancy. *American Family Physician, 59*(4), 829–836. Retrieved December 3, 2004, from www.aafp.org/afp/990215ap/829.html

Ladewig, P., London, M., Moberly, S., & Olds, S. (2002). *Contemporary maternal–newborn nursing care.* Upper Saddle River, NJ: Prentice Hall.

Moore, L. E., & Ware, D. (2002). *Hydatidiform mole.* Retrieved March 22, 2003, from www.emedicine.com/med/topic1047.htm

Newberry, L. (Ed.). (2003). *Sheehy's emergency nursing: Principles and practice* (5th ed.). St. Louis: Mosby.

Olds, S., London, M., & Ladewig, P. (1996). *Maternal newborn nursing, a family centered approach.* Menlo Park, CA: Addison-Wesley Nursing.

Pearlman, M., Tintinalli, J., & Dyne, P. (2004). *Obstetric and gynecologic emergencies: Diagnosis and management.* New York: McGraw-Hill.

Roche, N. E. (2003). *Therapeutic abortion.* Retrieved March 22, 2003, from www.emedicine.com/med/topic3311.htm

Shah, A. K. (2002). *Preeclampsia and eclampsia.* Retrieved February 8, 2003, from www.emedicine.com/neuro/topic323.htm

Stewart, F., Wells, E., Flinn, S., & Weitz, T. (2001). *Early medical abortion: Issues for practice.* San Francisco, CA: UCSF Center for Reproductive Health Research and Policy.

Varney, H. (2004). *Varney's midwifery* (4th ed.). Sudbury, MA: Jones & Bartlett.

Varney, H., Kriebs, J., & Gregor, C. (1998). *Varney's pocket midwife.* Sudbury, MA: Jones & Bartlett.

Chapter 4

Beers, M. H., & Berkow, R. (Eds.). (2004). *The Merck manual of diagnosis and therapy* (17th ed.). Retrieved May 22, 2004, from www.merck.com/mrkshared/mmanual/section18/chapter251/251c.jsp

Bledsoe, B., Porter, R., & Cherry, R. (2003). *Essentials of paramedic care.* Upper Saddle River, NJ: Prentice Hall Health.

Cunningham, F., Grant, N., Leveno, K., Gilstrap, L., Hauth, J., & Wenstrom, K. (2001). *Williams obstetrics* (21st ed.). New York: McGraw-Hill.

Dobo, S. M., & Johnson, V. S. (2000). Evaluation and care of the pregnant patient with minor trauma. *Clinics in Family Practice, 2*(3).

Freda, M. C., Patterson, E. T., & Wieczorek, R. R. (2004). *Preterm labor: Prevention and nursing management: Continuing education for registered nurses and certified nurse-midwives* (3rd ed.). White Plains, NY: Education & Health Promotion, March of Dimes.

Heppard, M., & Garite, T. (2002). *Acute obstetrics: A practical guide* (3rd ed.). St. Louis: Mosby.

Ladewig, P., London, M., Moberly, S., & Olds, S. (2002). *Contemporary maternal–newborn nursing care.* Upper Saddle River, NJ: Prentice Hall.

Morris, S., & Stacey, M. (2003). Resuscitation in pregnancy. *British Medical Journal, 327*(7426), 1277–1279.

Neufeld, J. D. G. (2002). Trauma in pregnancy. In J. A. Marx et al. (Eds.), *Rosen's emergency medicine: Concepts and clinical practice* (5th ed.). St. Louis: Mosby.

Newberry, L. (Ed.). (2003). *Sheehy's emergency nursing: Principles and practice* (5th ed.). St. Louis: Mosby.

Pearlman, M., Tintinalli, J., & Dyne, P. (2004). *Obstetric and gynecologic emergencies: Diagnosis and management.* New York: McGraw-Hill.

Ratcliffe, S., Baxley, E., Byrd, J., & Sakornbut, E. (Eds.). (2001). *Family practice obstetrics* (2nd ed.). Philadelphia: Hanley & Belfus.

Sinclair, C. (2004). *A midwife's handbook.* St Louis,: Saunders.

Siu, S. C., & Colman, J. M. (2001). Heart disease and pregnancy. *Heart, 85*(6), 710.

Chapter 5

Beischer, N., Mackay, E., & Colditz, P. (1997). *Obstetrics and the newborn: An illustrated textbook* (3rd ed.). London and Philadelphia: W. B. Saunders.

Bledsoe, B., Porter, R., & Cherry, R. (2003). *Essentials of paramedic care.* Upper Saddle River, NJ: Prentice Hall Health.

Cunningham, F., Grant, N., Leveno, K., Gilstrap, L., Hauth, J., & Wenstrom, K. (2001). *Williams obstetrics* (21st ed.). New York: McGraw-Hill.

Gabbe, S., Niebyl, J., & Simpson, J. (2002). *Obstetrics, normal and problem pregnancies.* New York: Churchill Livingstone.

Gurewitsch, E. D., Diament, P., Fong, J., Huang, G. H., Popovtzer, A., Weinstein, D., et al. (2002). The labor curve of the grand multipara: Does progress of labor continue to improve with additional childbearing? *American Journal of Obstetrics and Gynecology, 186*(6), 1331–1338.

Ladewig, P., London, M., Moberly, S., & Olds, S. (2002). *Contemporary maternal–newborn nursing care.* Upper Saddle River, NJ: Prentice Hall.

Olds, S., London, M., & Ladewig, P. (1996). *Maternal newborn nursing, a family centered approach.* Menlo Park, CA: Addison-Wesley Nursing.

Oxorn, H. (1986). *Oxorn-Foote human labor and birth* (5th ed.). New York: McGraw-Hill.

Simkin, P., & Ancheta, R. (2000). *The labor progress handbook.* Oxford: Blackwell Science.

Varney, H. (2004). *Varney's midwifery* (4th ed.). Sudbury, MA: Jones & Bartlett.

Chapter 6

Blackburn, S., & Loper, D. (1992). *Maternal, fetal and neonatal physiology.* Philadelphia: W. B. Saunders.

Bledsoe, B., Porter, R., & Cherry, R. (2003). *Essentials of paramedic care.* Upper Saddle River, NJ: Prentice Hall Health.

Cunningham, F., Grant, N., Leveno, K., Gilstrap, L., Hauth, J., & Wenstrom, K. (2001). *Williams obstetrics* (21st ed.). New York: McGraw-Hill.

Goldberg, J., & Sultana, C. (2004). Preventing perineal lacerations during labor. *Contemporary OB/GYN, 49*(9), 50–58.

Klein, M. C. (2001). Reducing perineal trauma and pelvic floor relaxation: An evidence-based approach. *Clinics in Family Practice, 3*(2), 365–383.

Ladewig, P., London, M., Moberly, S., & Olds, S. (2002). *Contemporary maternal–newborn nursing care.* Upper Saddle River, NJ: Prentice Hall.

Larimore, W. L., & Cline, M. K. (2000). Keeping normal labor normal. *Primary Care, 27*(1), 221–236.

McCandlish, R. (2001). Perineal trauma: Prevention and treatment. *Journal of Midwifery and Women's Health, 46*(6), 427–431.

Mercer, J. (2001). Current best evidence: A review of the literature on umbilical cord clamping. *Journal of Midwifery and Women's Health, 46*(6), 402–414.

Olds, S., London, M., & Ladewig, P. (1996). *Maternal newborn nursing, a family centered approach.* Menlo Park, CA: Addison-Wesley Nursing.

Olds, S. B., London, M. L., Ladewig, P. A., & Davidson, M. R. (2004). *Maternal–newborn nursing and women's health care* (7th ed.). Upper Saddle River, NJ: Pearson Prentice Hall.

Roberts, J. (2002). The "push" for evidence: Management of the second stage. *Journal of Midwifery and Women's Health, 47*(1), 235–247.

Simkin, P., & Ancheta, R. (2000). *The labor progress handbook.* Oxford: Blackwell Science.

Varney, H. (2004). *Varney's midwifery* (4th ed.). Sudbury, MA: Jones & Bartlett.

Waltman, P. A., Brewer, J. M., Rogers, B. P., & May, W. L. (2004). Building evidence for practice: A pilot study of newborn bulb suctioning at birth. *Journal of Midwifery and Women's Health, 49*(1), 32–38.

World Health Organization, Division of Reproductive Health (Technical Support). (1998). Review of evidence on cord care practices. *Care of the umbilical cord: A review of the evidence.* Geneva: Author. Retrieved December 3, 2004, from www.who.int/reproductive-health/publications/MSM_98_4/MSM_98_4_chapter4.en.html

Chapter 7

Ailsworth, K., Anderson, J., Atwood, L. A., Bailey, R. E., & Canavan, T. (2000). *ALSO Advanced life support in obstetrics* (4th ed.). Leawood, KS: American Academy of Family Practice Physicians.

Beers, M. H., & Berkow, R. (Eds.). (2004). *The Merck manual of diagnosis and therapy* (17th ed.). Retrieved December 4, 2004, from www.merck.com/mrkshared/mmanual/section19/chapter260/260o.jsp

Bledsoe, B., Porter, R., & Cherry, R. (2003). *Essentials of paramedic care.* Upper Saddle River, NJ: Prentice Hall Health.

Brucker, M. C. (2001). Management of the third stage of labor: An evidence-based approach. *Journal of Midwifery and Women's Health, 46*(6), 381–392.

Cunningham, F., Grant, N., Leveno, K., Gilstrap, L., Hauth, J., & Wenstrom, K. (2001). *Williams obstetrics* (21st ed.). New York: McGraw-Hill.

Gabbe, S., Niebyl, J., & Simpson, J. (2002). *Obstetrics, normal and problem pregnancies.* New York: Churchill Livingstone.

Gomella, T. L., Cunningham, M. D., Eyal, F. G., & Zenk, K. E. (2004). *Neonatology: Management, procedures, on-call problems, diseases and drugs* (5th ed.). New York: Lange Medical Books/McGraw-Hill.

Heppard, M., & Garite, T. (2002). *Acute obstetrics: A practical guide* (3rd ed.). St. Louis: Mosby.

Kenner, C., & Lott, J. W. (2003). *Comprehensive neonatal nursing: A physiologic perspective* (3rd ed.). Philadelphia: W. B. Saunders.

Laufer-Cahana, A. (2002). *Ellis-van Creveld syndrome.* Retrieved December 3, 2004, from www.emedicine.com/ped/topic660.htm

Olds, S., London, M., & Ladewig, P. (1996). *Maternal newborn nursing, a family centered approach.* Menlo Park, CA: Addison-Wesley Nursing.

Oxorn, H. (1986). *Oxorn-Foote human labor and birth* (5th ed.). New York: McGraw-Hill.

Varney, H. (2004). *Varney's midwifery* (4th ed.). Sudbury, MA: Jones & Bartlett.

Chapter 8

Beischer, N., Mackay, E., & Colditz, P. (1997). *Obstetrics and the newborn: An illustrated textbook* (3rd ed.). London and Philadelphia: W. B. Saunders.

Cunningham, F., Grant, N., Leveno, K., Gilstrap, L., Hauth, J., & Wenstrom, K. (2001). *Williams obstetrics* (21st ed.). New York: McGraw-Hill.

Feied, C., & Handler, J. A. (2002). *Pulmonary embolism.* Retrieved April 6, 2004, from www.emedicine.com/EMERG/topic490.htm

Gabbe, S., Niebyl, J., & Simpson, J. (2002). *Obstetrics, normal and problem pregnancies.* New York: Churchill Livingstone.

Heppard, M., & Garite, T. (2002). *Acute obstetrics: A practical guide* (3rd ed.). St. Louis: Mosby.

Ladewig, P., London, M., Moberly, S., & Olds, S. (2002). *Contemporary maternal–newborn nursing care.* Upper Saddle River, NJ: Prentice Hall.

Newberry, L. (Ed.). (2003). *Sheehy's emergency nursing: Principles and practice* (5th ed.). St. Louis: Mosby.

Varney, H. (2004). *Varney's midwifery* (4th ed.). Sudbury, MA: Jones & Bartlett.

Chapter 9

Beischer, N., Mackay, E., & Colditz, P. (1997). *Obstetrics and the newborn: An illustrated textbook* (3rd ed.). London and Philadelphia: W. B. Saunders.

Bledsoe, B., Porter, R., & Cherry, R. (2003). *Essentials of paramedic care.* Upper Saddle River, NJ: Prentice Hall Health.

Bledsoe, B., Porter, R., & Cherry, R. (2001). *Paramedic care: Principles and practice, Special considerations/operations* (Vol. 5). Upper Saddle River, NJ: Prentice Hall Health.

Cloherty, J., Eichenwald, E., & Stark, A. (2004). *Manual of neonatal care* (5th ed.). Philadelphia: Lippincott Williams & Wilkins.

Gomella, T. L., Cunningham, M. D., Eyal, F. G., & Zenk, K. E. (2004). *Neonatology: Management, procedures, on-call problems, diseases and drugs* (5th ed.). New York: Lange Medical Books/McGraw-Hill

Haws, P. S. (Ed.). (2003). *Care of the sick neonate: A quick reference for health care providers.* Philadelphia: Lippincott Williams & Wilkins.

Kattwinkel, J., et al. (Eds.). (2000). *Textbook of neonatal resuscitation* (4th ed.). Dallas, TX: American Heart Association; Elk Grove Village, IL: American Academy of Pediatrics.

Kenner, C., & Lott, J. W. (2003). *Comprehensive neonatal nursing: A physiologic perspective* (3rd ed.). Philadelphia: W. B. Saunders.

Ladewig, P., London, M., Moberly, S., & Olds, S. (2002). *Contemporary maternal–newborn nursing care.* Upper Saddle River, NJ: Prentice Hall.

Thureen, P., Deacon, J., O'Neil, P., & Hernandez, J. (1999). *Assessment and care of the newborn.* London and Philadelphia: W. B. Saunders.

Varney, H. (2004). *Varney's midwifery* (4th ed.). Sudbury, MA: Jones & Bartlett.

Wong, D. L., Wilson, D., & Whaley, L. F. (1995). *Whaley & Wong's nursing care of infants and children* (5th ed.). St. Louis: Mosby.

Chapter 10

American College of Obstetricians and Gynecologists. (2003, January 31). *Obstetrician-gynecologists and pediatricians say most newborn brain injuries do not occur during childbirth.* Retrieved December 4, 2004, from www.acog.org/from_home/publications/press_releases/nr01-31-03-1.cfm

Beers, M. H., & Berkow, R. (Eds.). (2004). *The Merck manual of diagnosis and therapy* (17th ed.). Retrieved December 4, 2004, from www.merck.com/mrkshared/mmanual/section19/chapter260/260b.jsp

Beischer, N., Mackay, E., & Colditz, P. (1997). *Obstetrics and the newborn: An illustrated textbook* (3rd ed.). London and Philadelphia: W. B. Saunders.

Bledsoe, B., Porter, R., & Cherry, R. (2003). *Essentials of paramedic care.* Upper Saddle River, NJ: Prentice Hall Health.

Bledsoe, B., Porter, R., & Cherry, R. (2001). *Paramedic care: Principles and practice, Special considerations/operations* (Vol. 5). Upper Saddle River, NJ: Prentice Hall Health.

Chung, E., & Rooks, V. (2003). *Clubfoot.* Retrieved December 3, 2004, from www.emedicine.com/radio/topic177.htm

Cloherty, J., Eichenwald, E., & Stark, A. (2004). *Manual of neonatal care* (5th ed.). Philadelphia: Lippincott Williams & Wilkins.

Gomella, T. L., Cunningham, M. D., Eyal, F. G., & Zenk, K. E. (2004). *Neonatology: Management, procedures, on-call problems, diseases and drugs* (5th ed.). New York: Lange Medical Books/McGraw-Hill.

Haws, P. S. (Ed.). (2003). *Care of the sick neonate: A quick reference for health care providers.* Philadelphia: Lippincott Williams & Wilkins.

Kattwinkel, J., et al. (Eds.). (2000). *Textbook of neonatal resuscitation* (4th ed.). Dallas, TX: American Heart Association; Elk Grove Village, IL: American Academy of Pediatrics.

Kenner, C., & Lott, J. W. (2003). *Comprehensive neonatal nursing: A physiologic perspective* (3rd ed.). Philadelphia: W. B. Saunders.

Ladewig, P., London, M., Moberly, S., & Olds, S. (2002). *Contemporary maternal–newborn nursing care.* Upper Saddle River, NJ: Prentice Hall.

March of Dimes. (2004). *Cerebral palsy.* Retrieved December 4, 2004, from www.modimes.org/professionals/681_1206.asp

Sairam, V. K., & Travis, L. (2003). *Potter syndrome.* Retrieved December 3, 2004, from www.emedicine.com/ped/topic1878.htm

Thureen, P., Deacon, J., O'Neil, P., & Hernandez, J. (1999). *Assessment and care of the newborn.* London and Philadelphia: W. B. Saunders.

Varney, H. (2004). *Varney's midwifery* (4th ed.). Sudbury, MA: Jones & Bartlett.

Wong, D. L., Wilson, D., & Whaley, L. F. (1995). *Whaley & Wong's nursing care of infants and children* (5th ed.). St. Louis: Mosby.

Chapter 11

American College of Obstetricians and Gynecologists. (1999, December). *Domestic violence* (ACOG Educational Bulletin 257). Washington, DC: Author.

Berek, J., Adashi, E., & Hillard, P. (Eds.). (1996). *Novak's gynecology* (12th ed.). Baltimore: Williams and Wilkins.

Bledsoe, B., Porter, R., & Cherry, R. (2003). *Essentials of paramedic care.* Upper Saddle River, NJ: Prentice Hall Health.

Datner, E. M., & Ferroggiaro, A. A. (1999). Violence during pregnancy. *Emergency Medicine Clinics of North America, 17,* 645–656.

Dunphy, L. M. H., & Winland-Brown, J. E. (Eds.). (2001). *Primary care: The art and science of advanced practice nursing.* Philadelphia: F. A. Davis.

Furniss, K., Torchen, C., & Blakewell-Sachs, S. (1999, July–August). Learning to ask. *Journal of Obstetric, Gynecologic and Neonatal Nursing, 28,* 353.

Goroll, A. H., & Mulley, A. G. (Eds.). (2000). *Primary care medicine: Office evaluation and management of the adult patient* (4th ed.). Philadelphia: Lippincott Williams & Wilkins.

Hamberger, L. K., & Ambuel, B. (2001). Spousal abuse in pregnancy. *Clinics in Family Practice, 3,* 203–224.

Haywood, Y. C., & Haile-Mariam, T. (1999). Violence against women. *Emergency Medicine Clinics of North America, 17,* 603–615.

Mayer, L., & Liebschutz, J. (1998). Domestic violence in the pregnant patient: Obstetric and behavioral interventions. *Obstetrical and Gynecological Survey, 53,* 627–635.

Newberry, L. (Ed.). (2003). *Sheehy's emergency nursing: Principles and practice* (5th ed.). St. Louis: Mosby.

Norton, L. B., Peipert, J. F., Zierler, S., Lima, B., & Hume, L. (1995). Battering in pregnancy: An assessment of two screening methods. *Obstetrics & Gynecology, 85,* 321–325.

Pearlman, M., Tintinalli, J., & Dyne, P. (2004). *Obstetric and gynecologic emergencies: Diagnosis and management.* New York: McGraw-Hill.

Stewart, D. E., & Cecutti, A. (1993). Physical abuse in pregnancy. *Canadian Medical Association Journal, 149,* 1257–1263.

Chapter 12

Ladewig, P., London, M., Moberly, S., & Olds, S. (2002). *Contemporary maternal–newborn nursing care.* Upper Saddle River, NJ: Prentice Hall.

Larkin, G. L., & Fowler, R. L. (2002). Essential ethics for EMS: Cardinal virtues and core principles. *Emergency Medicine Clinics of North America, 10*(4), 887–911.

Mattera, C. J. (1995). Principles of EMS documentation for mobile intensive care nurses. *Journal of Emergency Nursing, 21*(3), 231–237.

Midwives Alliance of North America. (2003). *Direct-entry midwifery state-by-state legal status—last updated 12-6-2003.* Retrieved May 17, 2004, from www.mana.org/statechart.html

Moore, K., & Persaud, T. (1998). *Before we are born: Essentials of embryology and birth defects.* Philadelphia: W. B. Saunders.

Norton, L. B., Peipert, J. F., Zierler, S., Lima, B., & Hume, L. (1995). Battering in pregnancy: An assessment of two screening methods. *Obstetrics & Gynecology, 85,* 321–325.

Stewart, D. E., & Cecutti, A. (1993). Physical abuse in pregnancy. *Canadian Medical Association Journal, 149,* 1257–1263.

Varney, H. (2004). *Varney's midwifery* (4th ed.). Sudbury, MA: Jones & Bartlett.

Watson, J. (2000). *Theory of human caring.* Retrieved May 23, 2004, from www2.uchsc.edu/son/caring/content/wct.asp

Appendix A

Black, R. A., & Hill, D. A. (2003). Over-the-counter medications in pregnancy. *American Family Physician, 67,* 2517–2524. Retrieved June 8, 2004, from www.aafp.org/afp/20030615/2517.html

Bledsoe, B., Porter, R., & Cherry, R. (2003). *Essentials of paramedic care.* Upper Saddle River, NJ: Prentice Hall Health.

Meadows, M. (2001, May–June). Pregnancy and the drug dilemma. *FDA Consumer.* Retrieved June 8, 2004, from www.fda.gov/fdac/features/2001/301_preg.html

Sanders, M. J., & McKenna, K. (2001). *Mosby's paramedic textbook* (Rev. 2nd ed.). St. Louis: Mosby.

Appendix B

Bledsoe, B. E., Clayden, D. E., & Papa, F. J. (2001). *Prehospital emergency pharmacology* (5th ed.). Upper Saddle River, NJ: Brady.

Briggs, G., Freeman, R., & Yaffee, S. (1998). *Drugs in pregnancy and lactation* (5th ed.). Lippincott Williams & Wilkins.

Caroline, (1995). *Emergency care in the streets* (5th ed.). Boston: Little, Brown.

Fleming, H., et al. (Eds.). (2004). *Physicians' desk reference* (58th ed.). Montvale, NJ: Thompson PDR.

Gold Standard Multimedia. (2002). *Clinical pharmacology 2000*. Retrieved May 25–26, 2004, from www.gsm.com

Lawrence Township Firefighters Association. (2004). *EMS drug reference*. Retrieved May 22, 2004, from www.lawrencefire.com/drug_reference.asp

Nissen, D. (2004). *Mosby's drug consult* (14th ed.). St. Louis: Mosby.

RxList, LLC. (n.d.). *RxList: The Internet drug list*. Retrieved May 25–26, 2004, from www.rxlist.com

RxMed, Inc. (n.d.). *RxMed*. Retrieved May 27–June 1, 2004, from www.rxmed.com/b.main/b2.pharmaceutical/b2.prescribe.html

Sanders, M. J., & McKenna, K. (2001). *Mosby's paramedic textbook* (Rev. 2nd ed.). St. Louis: Mosby.

Shannon, M. T., Wilson, B. A., & Stang, C. L. (2003). *Health professional's drug guide 2003*. Upper Saddle River, NJ: Pearson Education.

U.S. National Library of Medicine and National Institutes of Health. (2004). *Medline plus: Drug information*. Retrieved May 25–29, 2004, from www.nlm.nih.gov/medlineplus/druginformation.html

Appendix C

U.S. Food and Drug Administration. (2003). *Birth control guide*. Retrieved June 30, 2004, from www.fda.gov/fdac/features/1997/babytabl.html

Glossary

The American Heritage dictionary (4th ed.). (2001). New York: Delta.

The American Heritage Stedman's medical dictionary (2nd ed.). (2004). Boston: Houghton Mifflin.

Beers, M. H., & Berkow, R. (Eds.). (2004). *The Merck manual of diagnosis and therapy* (17th ed.). Retrieved May 22–29, 2004, from www.merck.com/mrkshared/mmanual

Merriam-Webster's medical desk dictionary. (2002). Springfield, MA: Merriam-Webster.

Venes, D., & Thomas, C. L. (Eds.). (2001). *Taber's cyclopedic medical dictionary* (19th ed.). Philadelphia: F. A. Davis.

Glossary

abortifacient   A substance or device that causes abortion.

abortion   The spontaneous or induced termination of pregnancy before fetal viability.

acrocyanosis   Blue coloration of the extremities of a neonate that may persist for the first week.

active labor   First-stage labor, between about 3–4 and 10 cm dilation, characterized by frequent, strong contractions, 60–90 seconds in duration.

adhesion   Union of normally separate parts, as during healing of a wound or infection. Surgery, inflammation, or trauma may create adhesions—scar tissue that binds tissues together abnormally, causing pain and organ dysfunction.

afterpains   Uterine cramps during the first few days after childbirth.

amenorrhea   Absence or cessation of menstruation.

amniotomy   Deliberate rupture of the amniotic membranes.

antepartum   A noun or adjective referring to the period of pregnancy before labor or delivery; prenatal.

areola   The pigmented ring around the nipple.

asphyxia   Extreme hypoxia with increased carbon dioxide in the blood, leading to coma or death.

asynclitism   Tilting of the fetal head at an oblique angle.

atelectasis   Alveolar collapse resulting from insufficient ventilation. It can also represent incomplete expansion of the lungs in the neonate.

atony, uterine   Loss of uterine muscular tone, which may impede the progress of labor or cause postpartum hemorrhage.

atrophic vaginitis   Irritation of thin, dry vaginal walls caused by a lack of estrogen after menopause.

biophysical profile   An ultrasound exam to assess fetal well-being, which is interpreted alongside the nonstress test. During the biophysical profile, the sonographer evaluates fetal movement, fetal tone, breathing movements, and the amniotic fluid volume.

brachial plexus A network of nerves located in the neck and axilla supplying the chest, shoulder, and arm.

Candida albicans A fungus responsible for many vaginal yeast infections.

caput succedaneum A soft, spongy temporary swelling on the part of the baby's head that pushed open the cervix.

carboxyhemoglobin (COHb) A compound formed when carbon monoxide combines with hemoglobin in the blood.

catecholamine Any of a group of neurotransmitters and hormones produced in the medulla of the adrenal gland, including epinephrine, norepinephrine, and dopamine.

cephalopelvic disproportion A condition in which the size or position of the fetal head in relation to the maternal pelvis prevents progress in labor.

cerclage A suture that secures the cervix in an attempt to prevent premature delivery.

certified nurse-midwife A registered nurse with specialized graduate education from an accredited institution, certified and licensed to provide antepartum, intrapartum, and postpartum care; gynecological exams; newborn care; family planning; menopausal management; and counseling in health maintenance and disease prevention.

cervical incompetence Tendency of the cervix to open painlessly in the second or third trimester of pregnancy.

chorioamnionitis Infection of the fetal membranes.

closed-glottis pushing Pushing the infant down and out while holding the breath; Valsalva pushing.

colposcopy Examination of the vagina and cervix by means of a colposcope (a device that magnifies and photographs).

congenital Present at birth or during uterine development, as a result of either hereditary or environmental influences.

crowning Emergence of widest part of the fetal head from the vagina. In common usage this term can mean any fetal presenting part distending the vaginal opening.

cystitis Inflammation of the urinary bladder, often caused by infection.

deflexed Not flexed, partially or completely extended. In a deflexed fetus, the chin is not on the chest, potentially making birth more difficult by presenting a wider portion of the head to the pelvic inlet.

dehiscence   Splitting open or rupture of a surgical wound or sear.

dilation and curettage   A surgical procedure in which the cervix is dilated and the lining of the uterus is scraped with a curette, usually performed to obtain tissue samples, to stop abnormal bleeding, to remove placental fragments after childbirth, or as a method of abortion.

diverticulitis   Inflammation of small outpouchings of the colon.

dizygotic   Derived, like twins or other multiples, from two separately fertilized eggs; fraternal.

doula   A nonmedical person who provides physical, emotional, and logistical support to a woman in labor.

ductus arteriosus   A fetal blood vessel that connects the pulmonary artery to the ascending aorta, allowing the circulating blood largely to bypass the pulmonary circulation. It normally closes at birth.

dysmenorrhea   Pain just before or during a menstrual period.

effacement   Shortening and thinning of the cervix in preparation for birth, expressed in percentages. A cervix that is 100% effaced is paper thin.

endometritis   Inflammation of the endometrium (the mucous membrane lining the uterus), usually caused by infection.

endometrium   The mucous membrane lining the uterus.

engagement   Passage of the widest diameter of the fetal presenting part through the pelvis.

episiotomy   An incision through the vagina, perineum, and underlying muscles to facilitate delivery.

family-practice physician   A physician (M.D. or D.O.) who provides medical care for men, women, and children, but usually manages only low-risk pregnancies and deliveries.

fetal alcohol syndrome   A set of congenital anomalies (e.g., small head, slow growth, mental retardation, hyperactivity) caused by excessive consumption of alcohol during pregnancy.

fetal macrosomia   Excessively large fetus, with a birth weight of 4,000–4,500 g (8 lb, 13 oz to 9 lb, 15 oz) or greater than the 90th percentile for gestational age.

fetal phenytoin syndrome   A disorder caused by exposure of an embryo to the anticonvulsant drug phenytoin (Dilantin), characterized by mental retardation, microcephaly, abnormal facial features, and other anomalies.

follicular phase   The first part of the ovarian cycle, during which an ovum matures and is released.

fontanelles   Gaps between fetal and infant skull bones covered with thick connective tissue that allow the bones to overlap during birth; "soft spots."

foramen ovale   An opening between the atria of the fetal heart that ordinarily closes on its own shortly after birth.

fundus   The uppermost part of the uterus, between and above the openings of the fallopian tubes.

gastroschisis   A condition in which the abdominal wall is incompletely formed and the intestines protrude through the gap without a protective membrane.

gestation   The time from conception to birth, approximately 280 days from the last menstrual period.

grand multipara   A woman who has given birth many times, usually more than five.

hemolysis   Destruction of red blood cells.

Homan's sign   Pain in the calf upon dorsiflexion of the foot.

hyperbilirubinemia   Elevated levels of bilirubin (a by-product of the breakdown of red blood cells) in the newborn's blood, often evidenced by jaundice.

hypercoagulable state   A condition in which the blood has a higher tendency to clot, even in the absence of bleeding.

hyperemesis gravidarum   Severe, persistent nausea and vomiting; an extreme form of pregnancy-related "morning sickness" that can cause weight loss, ketosis, dehydration, and hypokalemia or other electrolyte imbalance and sometimes requires hospitalization.

hyperreflexia   Exaggerated patellar reflexes, sometimes a sign of preeclampsia.

intrapartum   A noun or adjective pertaining to the period of pregnancy from the onset of labor through the expulsion of the placenta.

intrauterine growth restriction (or retardation; IUGR)   Fetal weight below the 10th percentile with poor growth due to insufficient nutrition and oxygenation *in utero*.

introitus   The entrance to the vagina, between the labia minora.

kernicterus   Irreversible brain damage caused by hyperbilirubinemia.

lanugo   Fine, downy hair that covers the fetus until shortly before or after birth; especially abundant on a premature infant.

leiomyoma (fibroid)   A benign tumor of the uterine smooth muscle.

lithotomy position   Lying on the back with the legs apart or elevated.

lochia   Liquid discharged from the vagina after childbirth, containing primarily blood, cellular debris, mucus, and fetal substances such as meconium, lanugo, and vernix.

lordosis   Exaggerated forward curvature of the lumbar spine (considered normal in pregnancy); "swayback."

luteal phase   The phase of the ovarian cycle from ovulation to the onset of menses.

malpresentation   Abnormal position of the fetus that may make vaginal delivery difficult or impossible.

mastitis   Inflammation of the connective tissue in the breast, usually caused by bacterial infection.

meconium   The tarry blackish-green substance excreted in a baby's first bowel movement, which ideally occurs shortly after birth, but may occur *in utero*.

meconium aspiration syndrome (MAS)   Hypoxia and other problems that occur when meconium is inhaled into the tracheo-bronchial airways.

menarche   The beginning of menstruation.

menorrhagia (hypermenorrhea)   Excessive or prolonged menstrual bleeding that occurs at normal intervals.

microcephaly   Abnormally small head.

milia   Pinhead-sized lesions across the nose, forehead, and cheeks of an infant caused by sebaceous glands blocked with vernix.

mittelschmerz   An abdominal pain caused by ovulation.

monozygotic   Derived, like twins or other multiples, from a single fertilized egg; identical.

Müllerian ducts   A pair of embryonic structures that gives rise to the reproductive organs in the female, but disappears in the male.

multigravida   A woman who is or has been pregnant for at least the second time.

multipara   A woman who has had two or more deliveries beyond 20 weeks' gestation. This term is often used in actual practice to indicate a woman who is giving birth for at least the second time.

necrotizing fasciitis   Severe infection with toxin-producing bacteria that leads to necrosis of subcutaneous tissue and adjacent fascia.

neonate   An infant less than 4 weeks old.

neural tube defect   Any of various congenital anomalies resulting from incomplete closing of the neural tube in an embryo, such as spina bifida or anencephaly.

nitrazine® paper   Paper impregnated with phenaphthazine, an indicator dye, used to determine the pH of solutions by its change in color.

nonstress test (NST)   A test that assesses fetal well-being by graphing the fetal heart rate while monitoring for uterine contractions. Reassuring features of a fetal heart rate include accelerations when the baby moves, variability or fluctuations above and below the normal baseline rate, and lack of pathological decelerations.

nuchal cord   An umbilical cord wrapped around the fetal neck.

nulligravida   A woman who has never been pregnant.

nullipara   A woman who has never delivered beyond 20 weeks' gestation.

occiput posterior (OP)   A fetal position in which the occiput of the fetal skull is directed toward the mother's sacrum.

perimenopause   The time surrounding menopause, the permanent cessation of menstrual periods that marks the transition from reproductive to postreproductive life.

perimortem cesarean delivery   Surgical delivery performed when the mother is in cardiac arrest.

perinatologist (maternal–fetal medicine specialist)   An obstetrician who has done a fellowship of 2–3 years after residency to specialize in high-risk pregnancies and has become board certified in maternal–fetal medicine.

perineum   The area between the vaginal opening and the anus.

periodic breathing   Intervals of rapid respiration interspersed with very slow breathing and pauses.

polyhydramnios   Excessive amounts of amniotic fluid.

postmaturity syndrome   A condition occurring in infants of prolonged gestation (usually beyond 42 weeks) who exhibit signs of perinatal compromise related to diminished intrauterine oxygenation and nutrition resulting from placental insufficiency.

primary amenorrhea   Failure of menstruation to begin by age 16.

primigravida   A woman who is pregnant for the first time.

primipara   A woman who has had one delivery beyond 20 weeks' gestation. This term is also used informally to indicate a woman giving birth for the first time.

products of conception (conceptus)   The results of conception—not only the embryo or fetus, but also the placenta, membranes, amniotic fluid, and other substances and structures.

prostaglandin   A hormonelike substance that may affect metabolism, blood pressure, smooth-muscle activity, or nerve transmission.

proteinuria   Abnormal amounts of protein in the urine.

puerperium   The time interval lasting from childbirth to the return of normal uterine size, about 6 weeks.

pulmonary hypoplasia   Underdeveloped lungs.

pyelonephritis   Inflammation of the kidney and renal pelvis, usually from infection.

retraction   Pulling in of the flesh above and below the sternum, between the ribs, and around the neck when a newborn breathes, a sign of respiratory distress.

RhoGam   A blood product (anti-D immunoglobulin) given to Rh-negative women in pregnancy and postpartum to prevent harm to subsequent Rh-positive babies (Rh isoimmunization).

salpingitis   Inflammation of the fallopian tube.

secondary amenorrhea   Cessation of menstruation after menses established.

shoulder dystocia   A bone-on-bone obstruction in which the fetal shoulder is caught behind the maternal pubic bone, preventing delivery.

somatization disorder   A condition characterized by physical symptoms that have no apparent physiological cause and are attributable to psychological factors.

subinvolution   Failure of the uterus to return to its prepregnant size after delivery, often because of retained placental fragments or infection.

supine hypotension syndrome   A drop in blood pressure that occurs when a pregnant woman lies on her back, allowing her uterus and its contents to compress her vena cava against her spine.

surfactant   A substance secreted by the alveolar cells of the lung that reduces surface tension of fluids that coat the lung, allowing the lung to remain expanded.

teratogen   Anything (such as ionizing radiation or a toxic substance) that interferes with normal embryonic or fetal development.

toxoplasmosis   Infection by a parasite (*Toxoplasma gondii,* found in raw and rare meat, garden soil, and cat feces) not usually harmful to nonpregnant adults, but potentially damaging and sometimes deadly to the fetus.

uteroplacental insufficiency   Insufficient oxygen and nutrient exchange between the uterus and the placenta.

vernix caseosa   A white, greasy, tenacious substance secreted by fetal sebaceous glands that adheres to the body hair and protects delicate fetal skin *in utero.*

vertex presentation   A fetal presentation in which the top of the head enters the pelvis first.

viable   Able to live outside the womb. The threshold of fetal viability is usually considered 500 g or 20 weeks of gestation, though 24 weeks is generally the practical limit. Legal and popular definitions are numerous.

virilization   Development of male secondary sex characteristics.

Index